NDH

POCKET GUIDE TO DRUG DOSAGES

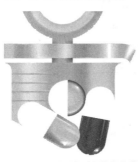

S0-ARM-536

Springhouse Corporation
Springhouse, Pennsylvania

Staff

Senior Vice President, Editorial
Patricia Dwyer Schull, RN, MSN

Art Director
John Hubbard

Editorial Manager
Andrew T. McPhee, RN, BSN

Clinical Manager
Ann M. Barrow, RN, MSN, CCRN

Senior Editor
Naina Chohan

Editors
Kathy Goldberg, Laini Berlin

Clinical Editors
Ann Marie Angelucci, RN, MSN; Joanne M. Bartelmo, RN, MSN, CCRN; Collette Bishop Hendler, RN, CCRN; Nancy Laplante, RN, BSN; Elizabeth D. McNeeley, RN, BSN; Michelle Robinson-Jackson, MSN, CRNP, CS; Beverly Tscheschlog, RN; Kimberly A. Zalewski, RN, MSN, CEN

Associate Acquisitions Editor
Betsy K. Snyder

Copy Editors
Cynthia C. Breuninger (manager), Karen C. Comerford, Leslie Dwarkin, Stacey A. Follin, Brenna H. Mayer, Beth Pitcher, Pamela Wingro

Designers
Arlene Putterman (associate art director), Joseph John Clark, Elaine Kasmer Ezrow, Jacalyn B. Facciolo, Lorraine Lostracco, Donna Morris

Typographers
Diane Paluba (manager), Joyce Rossi Biletz, Valerie Rosenberger

Manufacturing
Deborah Meiris (director), Pat Dorshaw, (manager), Otto Mezei

Editorial Assistants
Carol A. Caputo, Carrie R. Krout

Indexer
Barbara Hodgson

Contents

Clinical consultants

Thomas E. Ary, BPharm, PhD
Director of Compliance
PRACS Institute, Ltd.
Fargo, N. Dak.

Deborah Becker, RN, MSN, CCRN
Clinical Site Coordinator
Adult Critical Care Nurse Practitioner Program
University of Pennsylvania Medical Center
Philadelphia

David J. Blanchard, RPh, BS
Pharmacist
St. Luke's Memorial Hospital
New Hartford, N.Y.

Karen T. Bruchak, RN, MSN, MBA
Assistant Administrator, Cancer Clinical Programs
University of Pennsylvania Medical Center
Philadelphia

James Camamo, PharmD
Clinical Pharmacist, Medication Information
and Policy Development
University Medical Center
Tucson, Ariz.

Lawrence Carey, PharmD
Clinical Pharmacist Coordinator
Jefferson Home Infusion Service
Thomas Jefferson University Hospital
Philadelphia

Sandra L. Chase, PharmD, BS
Clinical Pharmacist, Drug Use Policy and
Medical Information Service
Thomas Jefferson University Hospital
Philadelphia

Nancy R. Cirone, RN,C, MSN, CDE
Clinical Development Specialist
Allegheny University Hospitals, Bucks
Warminster, Pa.

Rachael Clark-Vetri, RPh, PharmD
Clinical Assistant Professor
Temple University School of Pharmacy
Philadelphia

Patricia Drobins, RN, BSN, OCN
Clinical Research Nurse Specialist
University of Pennsylvania Cancer Center
Philadelphia

Teresa S. Dunsworth, PharmD, BCPS
Assistant Professor of Clinical Pharmacy
West Virginia University School of
Pharmacy
Morgantown

Bruce M. Frey, RPh, PharmD
Clinical Pharmacist in Pediatrics and Neonatology
Thomas Jefferson University Hospital
Philadelphia

Douglas R. Geraets, RPh, PharmD, FCCP
Clinical Pharmacy Specialist, Ambulatory Care
VA Medical Center, Pharmacy Service
Iowa City

Mary Jo Gerlach, RN, MSNEd
Assistant Professor Adult Nursing
Medical College of Georgia
Athens

Martin R. Giannamore, RPh, PharmD
Assistant Professor of Clinical Pharmacy
Practice
Ohio State University, College of Pharmacy
Columbus

John D. Grabenstein, MS Pharm, EdM, FASHP
Medical Service Corps, United States Army

Mary Beth Gross, PharmD, FASCP
Manager, Pharmacy
Mercy Hospital Medical Center;
Associate Professor of Pharmacy
Drake University, College of Pharmacy
Des Moines, Iowa

David W. Hawkins, PharmD
Professor and Assistant Dean of Pharmacy
University of Georgia
Athens

James R. Hildebrand, III, PharmD
Drug Information Product Manager
SmithKline Beecham Pharmaceuticals
Philadelphia

Jeffrey W. Hui, RPh, PharmD
Drug Information Resident
Department of Pharmacy
Temple University Hospital
Philadelphia

Lori Ann Hytrek, PharmD
Specialty Resident in Pharmacy
Administration
University of California
San Francisco

Cary E. Johnson, PharmD
Associate Professor of Pharmacy;
Clinical Pharmacist, Pediatrics
University of Michigan, College of
Pharmacy
Ann Arbor

William A. Kehoe, PharmD, MA, BCPS
Professor of Clinical Pharmacy
University of the Pacific, School of
Pharmacy
Stockton, Calif.

James Allen Koestner, PharmD
Clinical Pharmacist, Trauma
Vanderbilt University Medical Center
Nashville, Tenn.

W. Greg Leader, PharmD
Assistant Professor
West Virginia University School of
Pharmacy
Morgantown

Marie Maloney, PharmD
Clinical Pharmacist
University Medical Center
Tucson, Ariz.

Michael A. Mancano, RPh, PharmD, BS Pharm
Director of Drug Information
Temple University Hospital
Assistant Professor of Clinical Pharmacy
Temple University School of Pharmacy
Philadelphia

Jan E. Markind, RPh, PharmD, BS
Drug Information Specialist and Clinical Assistant Professor
University of Illinois
Chicago

Dawna Martich, RN, MSN
Clinical Manager
University of Pittsburgh Medical Center, USO
Moon Township, Pa.

Michael K. McGuire, PharmD
Clinical Coordinator
Germantown Hospital and Medical Center
Philadelphia

Joan A.W. Mege, PharmD, RPh
Freelance Medical Writer;
Formerly Pharmacy Practice Resident,
Milton S. Hershey Medical Center
Hershey, Pa.

Steven Meisel, PharmD
Assistant Director, Pharmacy
Fairview Southdale Hospital
Edina, Minn.

William O'Hara, RPh, PharmD, BS
Clinical Pharmacist
Thomas Jefferson University Hospital
Philadelphia

Theresa R. Prosser, PharmD, BCPS
Associate Professor
St. Louis (Mo.) College of Pharmacy

Leslie N. Schechter, PharmD
Clinical Coordinator
Department of Pharmacy
Thomas Jefferson University Hospital
Philadelphia

Michelle Swartz, BS
Teacher, Upper Dublin School District
Fort Washington, Pa.

Lynda Thomson, RPh, PharmD, BS
Clinical Pharmacist, Infectious Diseases
Thomas Jefferson University Hospital
Philadelphia

Candy Tsourounis, RPh, PharmD
Assistant Clinical Professor
Drug Information Analysis Service
University of California
San Francisco

Kenneth K. Wieland, PharmD
Director of Pharmacy
Chestnut Hill Hospital
Philadelphia

Stacy A. Wiegman, RPh, PharmD, MS
Fellow
Institute for Safe Medication Practices
Warminster, Pa.

How to use this book

NDH Pocket Guide to Drug Dosages offers comprehensive dosage information in a unique, quick-scan format. The book opens with a list of abbreviations used in the entries. Then, organized alphabetically by generic name, each drug entry covers generic and common trade names, pharmacologic and therapeutic class, pregnancy risk category, controlled substance schedule (where appropriate), common indications and dosages, and key nursing considerations. Information is divided into columns for quick reference.

The first column shows the generic name in boldface, followed by trade names. Canadian and Australian brand-name drugs are denoted by a dagger (†) and double-dagger (‡), respectively. Below the list of trade names are the drug's pharmacologic class and then its therapeutic class. Pregnancy risk category and, where applicable, controlled substance schedule are listed next.

Pregnancy risk categories parallel those assigned by the FDA to reflect a drug's potential to cause birth defects:

- A: Adequate studies in pregnant women have failed to show a risk to the fetus.
- B: Animal studies have not shown a risk to the fetus, but controlled studies have not been conducted in pregnant women; or animal studies have shown an adverse effect on the fetus, but adequate studies in pregnant women have not shown a fetal risk.
- C: Animal studies have shown an adverse effect on the fetus, but adequate studies have not been conducted in humans. The benefits may be acceptable despite potential risks.

- D: The drug may pose risks to the human fetus, but potential benefits may be acceptable despite the risks.
- X: Studies in animals or humans show fetal abnormalities, or reports of adverse reactions indicate evidence of fetal risk. The risks involved clearly outweigh the potential benefits.
- NR: Not rated.

Drugs regulated under the Controlled Substances Act of 1970 are divided into the following schedules:

- I: high abuse potential, no accepted medical use
- II: high abuse potential, severe dependence liability
- III: less abuse potential than schedule II drugs, moderate dependence liability
- IV: less abuse potential than schedule III drugs, limited dependence liability
- V: limited abuse potential.

The second column covers major indications and the most common dosages ordered for a particular drug. The third column lists the more important nursing considerations applicable for the drug. This list might include considerations related to monitoring, drug administration, patient teaching, and numerous other topics.

Appendices include a table of equivalents, common pharmacologic abbreviations, pharmacologic abbreviations to avoid, estimating surface area in children, estimating surface area in adults, and dangerous drug interactions. The index is organized by generic name, trade name, and disease.

Abbreviations

ABG	arterial blood gas	LDL	low-density lipoprotein
ACE	angiotensin-converting enzyme	MAO	monoamine oxidase
		MI	myocardial infarction
ADH	antidiuretic hormone	mo	month
ALT	alanine aminotransferase	NG	nasogastric
AST	aspartate aminotransferase	NSAID	nonsteroidal anti-inflammatory drug
buff	buffered	O_2 sat, SaO_2	oxygen saturation
CAD	coronary artery disease	PABA	para-aminobenzoic acid
CDC	Centers for Disease Control and Prevention	PCWP	pulmonary capillary wedge pressure
chew	chewable	ped	pediatric
CK	creatinine kinase	periop	perioperative
CMV	cytomegalovirus	pharm	pharmacologic
conc	concentration, concentrated	pkg	package
		pkt	packet
contr-release	controlled-release	PSVT	paroxysmal supraventricular tachycardia
CSF	cerebrospinal fluid		
CV	central venous	PT	prothrombin time
CVP	central venous pressure	PTT	partial thromboplastin time
ECG	electrocardiogram		
EEG	electroencephalogram	PVD	peripheral vascular disease
equiv	equivalent		
ET	endotracheal	RDA	recommended daily allowance
ext-release	extended-release		
G	gauge	REM	rapid eye movement
gram-neg	gram-negative	SA	sinoatrial
gram-pos	gram-positive	SIADH	syndrome of inappropriate antidiuretic hormone
gyn	gynecologic		
Hct	hematocrit	sust-release	sustained-release
HDL	high-density lipoprotein	T_3	triiodothyronine
Hgb	hemoglobin	T_4	thyroxine
HR	heart rate	TB	tuberculosis
H_1, H_2	histamine-1, histamine-2	temp	temperature
I&O	intake and output	TIA	transient ischemic attack
ICP	intracranial pressure	UCE	urea cycle enzymopathy
IND	investigational new drug	USP	United States Pharmacopeia
IPPB	intermittent positive-pressure breathing		
		UTI	urinary tract infection
INR	international normalized ratio	vag	vaginal, vaginally

DRUG/CLASS/ CATEGORY	INDICATIONS/ DOSAGES	KEY NURSING CONSIDERATIONS
abciximab ReoPro Antiplatelet aggregate Platelet aggregation inhibitor Preg. Risk Category: C	*Adjunct to PTCA or atherectomy to prevent acute cardiac ischemic complications in patients at high risk for abrupt closure of treated coronary vessel —* **Adults:** 0.25 mg/kg IV bolus 10 to 60 min before start of PTCA or atherectomy, then continuous IV infusion of 10 mcg/min for 12 hr.	▪ Keep epinephrine, dopamine, theophylline, antihistamines, and corticosteroids available in case of anaphylaxis. ▪ Give in separate IV line; don't add other medication to solution. ▪ Institute bleeding precautions. Keep on bed rest for 6 to 8 hr after sheath removal or infusion stoppage, whichever later. Minimize or avoid, if possible, arterial and venous punctures, IM injections, urinary catheters, NG tubes, automatic BP cuffs, and nasotracheal intubation. ▪ Intended for use with aspirin and heparin.
acarbose Precose Alpha-glucosidase inhibitor Antidiabetic agent Preg. Risk Category: B	*Adjunct to diet to lower blood glucose in non-insulin-dependent diabetes mellitus when hyperglycemia can't be managed by diet alone or by diet and sulfonylureas —* **Adults:** Individualized. Initially, 25 mg PO tid at start of main meals; then adjust q 4 to 8 wk. Maintenance: 50 to 100 mg PO tid; don't exceed 50 mg tid in patients < 60 kg.	▪ May increase hypoglycemic potential of sulfonylureas. Closely monitor patient. ▪ Give oral glucose for hypoglycemia, as ordered. Give IV glucose or glucagon for severe hypoglycemia. ▪ Patient may need insulin during increased stress. Monitor for hyperglycemia. ▪ Monitor 1-hr postprandial plasma glucose.

acebutolol, acebutolol hydrochloride

Monitant, Sectral

Beta-adrenergic blocker

Antihypertensive/antiarrhythmic

Preg. Risk Category: B

Hypertension — **Adults:** 400 mg PO as 1 daily dose or in divided doses bid to max 1,200 mg qd.

Ventricular arrhythmias — **Adults:** 400 mg PO daily divided bid; increase prn for adequate response. Usual dosage 600 to 1,200 mg.

- Check apical pulse before giving; if < 60, withhold drug and call doctor. Monitor BP.
- Before surgery, tell anesthesiologist that patient is taking drug.
- May mask hyperthyroidism signs.

---

acetaminophen (APAP, paracetamol)

Actamin, Anacin-3, Datril Extra-Strength, Dolanex, Panadol, Tempra, Tylenol, Valorin

Para-aminophenol derivative

Nonnarcotic analgesic/antipyretic

Preg. Risk Category: B

Mild pain or fever — **Adults and children >11 yr:** 325 to 650 mg PO q 4 to 6 hr; or 1 g PO tid or qid. Alternatively, 2 ext-release cap PO q 8 hr. For long-term use, don't exceed 2.6 g daily. **Children 11 yr:** 480 mg PO or PR q 4 to 6 hr. **Children 9 to 10 yr:** 400 mg PO or PR q 4 to 6 hr. **Children 6 to 8 yr:** 320 mg PO or PR q 4 to 6 hr. **Children 4 to 5 yr:** 240 mg PO or PR q 4 to 6 hr. **Children 2 to 3 yr:** 160 mg PO or PR q 4 to 6 hr. **Children 12 to 23 mo:** 120 mg PO q 4 to 6 hr. **Children < 3 mo:** 80 mg PO q 4 to 6 hr. **Children < 3 mo:** 40 mg PO q 4 to 6 hr.

- Warn that high doses or unsupervised long-term use can cause liver damage.
- Caution that excessive alcohol use may increase risk of liver toxicity.
- Warn not to take for marked fever (> 103.1° F [39.5° C]), fever lasting > 3 days, or recurrent fever, unless directed by doctor.
- May cause false-positive blood glucose decrease in home monitoring systems.
- Don't give to children < 2 yr without consulting doctor.

---

acetazolamide

Acetazolam†, AK-Zol, Dazamide, Diamox

acetazolamide sodium

Diamox Parenteral

Secondary glaucoma and preop treatment of acute angle-closure glaucoma — **Adults:** 250 mg PO q 4 hr; or 250 mg PO bid for short-term therapy. To rapidly lower IOP, initially, 500 mg IV, then 125 to 250 mg IV q 4 hr.

- Monitor I & O, glucose, and electrolytes (especially potassium, bicarbonate, and chloride). When used as diuretic, consult doctor and dietitian about high-potassium diet.
- Elderly patients especially susceptible to excessive diuresis; monitor closely.

(continued)

ACETAZOLAMIDE 3

†Canadian, †Australian

DRUG/CLASS/ CATEGORY	INDICATIONS/ DOSAGES	KEY NURSING CONSIDERATIONS
acetazolamide *(continued)* Carbonic anhydrase inhibitor Antiglaucoma agent/diuretic Preg. Risk Category: C	*Edema in heart failure* — **Adults:** 250 to 375 mg PO or IV qd in morning. *Chronic open-angle glaucoma* — **Adults:** 250 mg to 1 g PO daily in divided doses qid, or 500 mg (ext-release) PO bid.	▪ Weigh patient daily; rapid fluid loss may cause weight loss and hypotension. ▪ **IV use:** Inject 100 to 500 mg/min into large vein using 21G or 23G needle. Intermittent or continuous infusion not recommended.
acetic acid Domeboro Otic, VoSol Otic *Acid* Antibacterial/antifungal Preg. Risk Category: NR	*External ear canal infection* — **Adults and children:** 4 to 6 drops into ear canal q 2 to 3 hr; or insert saturated wick for 1st 24 hr, then continue with instillations.	▪ Reculture persistent drainage. ▪ Has anti-infective, anti-inflammatory, and antipruritic effects. *P. aeruginosa* particularly sensitive. ▪ Avoid contact with eyes and other mucus membranes. ▪ To give to child, pull earlobe down and back. For adults, pull earlobe up and back.
acetohexamide Dimelor†, Dymelor *Sulfonylurea* Antidiabetic agent Preg. Risk Category: NR	*Adjunct to diet to lower blood glucose in type 2 diabetes* — **Adults:** initially, 250 mg PO daily before breakfast; increase 250 to 500 mg q 5 to 7 days as needed, to max 1.5 g daily in divided doses bid or tid before meals. *To replace insulin therapy in type 2 diabetes* — **Adults:** If insulin dosage < 20 units daily, stop insulin and start oral acetohexamide with 250 mg PO daily before break-	▪ Use cautiously in history of porphyria or impaired hepatic or renal function or in debilitated, malnourished, or elderly patients. ▪ In times of increased stress, patient may also need insulin therapy. Monitor closely. ▪ Most patients switching from other oral antidiabetics don't need transition period.

- Patients switching from insulin need blood glucose monitoring tid before meals; may require hospitalization during transition.

fast, increased as above if needed. If insulin dosage ≥ 20 units daily, start with 250 mg PO daily before breakfast, as insulin dosage falls by 25% to 30% qd or qod, depending on response to oral therapy.

---

acetylcholine chloride
Miochol
Cholinergic agonist
Miotic
Preg. Risk Category: NR

Anterior segment surgery — Adults and children: during surgery, 0.5 to 2 ml instilled gently into anterior chamber.

- Reconstitute immediately before using, shaking vial gently until solution clear. Discard unused solution.
- Don't gas-sterilize vial. Ethylene oxide may produce formic acid.

---

acetylcysteine
Airbront, Mucomyst, Mucomyst-10, Mucosil-10, Mucosil-20, Parvolex‡
Amino acid (L-cysteine) derivative
Mucolytic agent/antidote for acetaminophen overdose
Preg. Risk Category: B

Adjuvant therapy for abnormal viscid or inspissated mucus secretions in pneumonia, bronchitis, TB, cystic fibrosis, emphysema, atelectasis (adjunct), pulmonary complications of thoracic and CV surgery — **Adults and children:** 1 to 2 ml 10% or 20% solution by direct instillation into trachea up to q hr; or 1 to 10 ml of 20% solution or 2 to 20 ml of 10% solution by nebulization q 2 to 6 hr, prn.

Acetaminophen toxicity — **Adults and children:** initially, 140 mg/kg PO, then 70 mg/kg PO q 4 hr for 17 doses. Alternatively by IV: loading dose 150 mg/kg IV in 200 ml D₅W over 15 min followed by 50 mg/kg IV in 500 ml D₅W over 4 hr, then 100 mg/kg IV in 100 ml D₅W over 16 hr.

- Start treatment immediately after acetaminophen ingestion; don't wait for blood drug levels.
- To use orally for acetaminophen overdose, dilute with cola, fruit juice, or water. Add 3 ml diluent to each ml acetylcysteine.
- Repeat dose if patient vomits within 1 hr of loading or maintenance dose.
- Use plastic, glass, stainless steel, or other nonreactive metal when giving by nebulization. Hand-bulb nebulizer not recommended.
- Physically or chemically incompatible with tetracyclines, erythromycin lactobionate, amphotericin B, and ampicillin sodium.
- Physically incompatible with iodized oil, trypsin, and hydrogen peroxide; don't add those drugs to nebulizer.

ACETYLCYSTEINE

5

DRUG/CLASS/ CATEGORY	INDICATIONS/ DOSAGES	KEY NURSING CONSIDERATIONS
activated charcoal Actidose, Actidose-Aqua, Charcoaid, Charcocaps, Liqui-Char *Adsorbent* *Antidote/antidiarrheal/anti-flatulent* Preg. Risk Category: C	*Flatulence or dyspepsia* — **Adults:** 600 mg to 5 g PO as single dose or 0.975 g to 3.9 g PO tid after meals. *Poisoning* — **Adults and children:** initially, 1 to 2 g/kg (30 to 100 g) PO or 10 times amount of poison ingested, given as susp in 120 to 240 ml of water. Check with poison control center for specific uses in poisonings or overdoses.	• Inactivates ipecac syrup; give only after emesis complete. • Mix powder form with water to form thick consistency. May add small amount of fruit juice. • Give by large-bore NG tube after lavage, if necessary. • If patient vomits shortly after receiving, be prepared to repeat dose. • Space doses at least 1 hr apart from other drugs when giving for indications other than poisoning.
acyclovir sodium Avirax, Zovirax *Synthetic purine nucleoside* *Antiviral agent* Preg. Risk Category: C	*Mucocutaneous herpes simplex virus (HSV-1 and HSV-2) infections in immunocompromised patients, genital herpes in immunocompetent patients* — **Adults and children ≥ 12 yr:** 5 mg/kg IV q 8 hr for 7 to 14 days (5 to 7 days for severe initial episode of genital herpes). **Children < 12 yr:** 250 mg/m² IV q 8 hr for 7 days. *Initial genital herpes* — **Adults:** 200 mg PO q 4 hr while awake (total 5 caps daily); or 400 mg PO q 8 hr. Continue 7 to 10 days.	• **IV use:** Give infusion over at least 1 hr. • Don't give by bolus injection or by IM or SC injection. • As ordered, start therapy as soon as possible after symptom onset. • Encourage adequate fluid intake. • Encephalopathic changes more likely in neurologic disorders and in patients with neurologic reactions to cytotoxic drugs. • Dosage for obese patients based on ideal weight.

Varicella (chickenpox) infections in immunocompromised patients — **Adults and children ≥ 12 yr:** 10 mg/kg IV q 8 hr for 7 days. **Children < 12 yr:** 500 mg/m² IV q 8 hr for 7 to 10 days.

- As ordered, start therapy as soon as possible after symptom onset.
- Apply with finger cot or rubber glove.
- For cutaneous use only; don't apply to eye.

acyclovir
Zovirax
Synthetic purine nucleoside
Antiviral agent
Preg. Risk Category: C

Initial herpes genitalis; limited, non-life-threatening mucocutaneous herpes simplex virus infections in immunocompromised patients — **Adults and children:** cover all lesions q 3 hr, 6 times daily for 7 days.

- Use cautiously in asthma.
- *IV use:* Rapid injection required. Administer directly into vein if possible; use port closest to patient and flush immediately and rapidly with 0.9% NaCl.
- Monitor ECG for arrhythmias.

adenosine
Adenocard
Nucleoside
Antiarrhythmic
Preg. Risk Category: C

Conversion of PSVT to sinus rhythm —
Adults: 6 mg IV rapid bolus injection over 1 to 2 sec. If PSVT persists after 1 to 2 min, give 12 mg by rapid IV push and repeat if necessary. Single doses > 12 mg not recommended.

---

albumin 5%
Albuminar 5%, Albutein 5%
albumin 25%
Albuminar 25%, Albutein 25%
Blood derivative
Plasma protein
Preg. Risk Category: C

Hypovolemic shock — **Adults:** initially, 500 to 750 ml 5% sol by IV infusion, repeat q 30 min, prn. Alternatively, 100 to 200 ml IV of 25% sol, repeat in 10 to 30 min, if needed.
Children: 12 to 20 ml 5% sol/kg by IV infusion, repeat in 15 to 30 min if response inadequate. Alternatively, 2.5 to 5 ml IV of 25% sol/kg, repeat in 10 to 30 min if needed.

- Ensure proper hydration before infusion.
- *IV use:* Avoid rapid IV infusion. Specific dosage and rate varies with age, condition, diagnosis, and response. 5% albumin infused undiluted; 25% albumin may be infused undiluted or diluted with sterile water for injection, 0.9% NaCl solution, or D₅W injection. Don't give > 250 ml in 48 hr.
- Watch for hemorrhage or shock after surgery or injury. Rapid BP rise may cause bleeding from sites not apparent at lower pressures.

(continued)
ALBUMIN 7

---

†Canadian, ‡Australian

DRUG / CLASS / CATEGORY	INDICATIONS / DOSAGES	KEY NURSING CONSIDERATIONS
albumin 25% *(continued)*	*Hypoproteinemia* — **Adults:** 200 to 300 ml of 25% solution. *Hyperbilirubinemia* — **Infants:** 1 g albumin (4 ml 25%)/kg during or 1 to 2 hr before exchange transfusion.	▪ Watch for signs of vascular overload. ▪ Monitor I&O, Hgb, Hct, serum protein, and electrolytes.
albuterol (salbutamol) Asmol‡, Proventil, Ventolin **albuterol sulfate (salbutamol sulphate)** Proventil, Proventil Repetabs, Respolin Inhaler‡, Respolin Respirator Solution‡, Ventolin *Bronchodilator* *Adrenergic* Preg. Risk Category: C	*To prevent or treat bronchospasm in reversible obstructive airway disease or to prevent exercise-induced bronchospasm* — **Adults and children ≥ 12 yr:** dosage and frequency vary with dosage form. *Aerosol inhalation:* 1 to 2 inhalations q 4 to 6 hr. *Solution for inhalation:* 2.5 mg tid or qid by nebulizer. *Cap for inhalation:* 200 mcg inhaled q 4 to 6 hr using Rotahaler. Some patients may need 400 mcg q 4 to 6 hr. *Oral tab:* 2 to 4 mg PO tid or qid; max 8 mg qid. *Ext-release tab:* 4 to 8 mg PO q 12 hr; max 16 mg bid. **Children 6 to 13 yr:** 2 mg (1 tsp) PO tid or qid. **Children 2 to 5 yr:** 0.1 mg/kg PO tid, not to exceed 2 mg (1 tsp) tid. **Adults > 65 yr:** 2 mg PO tid or qid.	▪ Use ext-release tabs cautiously in preexisting GI narrowing. ▪ Pleasant-tasting syrup may be taken by children as young as 2 yr. Contains no alcohol or sugar. ▪ Aerosol form may be used 15 min before exercise. ▪ May use tablets and aerosol concomitantly. Monitor closely for toxicity. ▪ If doctor orders >1 inhalation, instruct to wait at least 2 min between inhalations. ▪ If patient also uses steroid inhaler, advise to use steroid 5 min after taking albuterol.

aldesleukin (interleukin-2, IL-2)

Proleukin

Lymphokine

Immunoregulatory agent

Preg. Risk Category: C

Metastatic renal cell carcinoma — **Adults:** 600,000 IU/kg (0.037 mg/kg) IV q 8 hr for 5 days (total of 14 doses). After 9-day rest, repeat sequence for another 14 doses. May give repeat courses after rest period of ≥ 7 wk.

- Monitor hematologic tests, serum electrolytes, and renal and liver function tests and obtain chest X-ray before therapy, as ordered. Repeat daily.
- Monitor vital signs and patient condition closely.
- Withhold dose and notify doctor if moderate to severe lethargy or somnolence occurs.
- Reconstitute with sterile water for injection.
- Add ordered dose of reconstituted drug to 50 ml D₅W and infuse over 15 min. Don't use in-line filter.

---

alendronate sodium

Fosamax

Osteoclast-mediated bone resorption inhibitor

Anti-osteoporotic agent

Preg. Risk Category: C

Osteoporosis in postmenopausal women — **Adults:** 10 mg PO daily, taken with plain water only, ≥ 30 min before 1st food, beverage, or medication of day.

Paget's disease of bone — **Adults:** 40 mg PO daily for 6 mo, taken with plain water only, ≥ 30 min before 1st food, beverage, or medication of day.

- Correct hypocalcemia and other disturbances of mineral metabolism before therapy begins.
- When used for Paget's disease, indicated for patients with alkaline phosphatase at least 2 times upper limit of normal, in symptomatic patients, and in those at risk for disease complications.
- Monitor serum calcium and phosphate, as ordered.
- When used to treat osteoporosis in postmenopausal women, osteoporosis may be confirmed by diagnostic findings of low bone mass or by history of osteoporotic fracture.

ALENDRONATE SODIUM 9

DRUG / CLASS / CATEGORY	INDICATIONS / DOSAGES	KEY NURSING CONSIDERATIONS
alfentanil hydrochloride Alfenta *Opioid* *Analgesic/adjunct to anesthesia/anesthetic* Preg. Risk Category: C Controlled Sub. Sched.: II	*Adjunct to general anesthetic* — **Adults:** initially, 8 to 50 mcg/kg IV; then increments of 3 to 15 mcg/kg IV q 5 to 20 min. *As primary anesthetic* — **Adults:** initially, 130 to 245 mcg/kg IV; then 0.5 to 1.5 mcg/kg/min IV.	▪ Should be administered only by persons specifically trained in IV anesthetic use. ▪ Use tuberculin syringe to give small volumes accurately. ▪ Monitor SaO_2. ▪ Keep narcotic antagonist and resuscitation equipment available when giving IV.
allopurinol Alloremed‡, Lopurin, Purinol†, Zyloprim *Xanthine oxidase inhibitor* *Antigout* Preg. Risk Category: C	*Gout, primary or secondary to hyperuricemia; secondary to certain diseases* — Dosage varies with disease severity; doses > 300 mg should be divided. **Adults:** mild gout, 200 to 300 mg PO daily; severe gout with large tophi, 400 to 600 mg PO daily. Same dosage for maintenance in secondary hyperuricemia. Max 800 mg/day. *Hyperuricemia secondary to malignancies* — **Children < 6 yr:** 50 mg PO tid. **Children 6 to 10 yr:** 300 mg PO daily or divided tid. *Prevention of acute gouty attacks* — **Adults:** 100 mg PO daily; increase at weekly intervals by 100 mg without exceeding max dose (800 mg) until serum uric acid falls to 6 mg/dl or less.	▪ Monitor serum uric acid. ▪ Monitor I & O; daily output of ≥ 2 L and maintenance of neutral or slightly alkaline urine desirable. ▪ Periodically monitor CBC and hepatic and renal function. ▪ If renal insufficiency occurs, be prepared to reduce dosage. ▪ Optimal benefits may require 2 to 6 wk of therapy. Concurrent colchicine may be prescribed prophylactically for acute gouty attacks.

alprazolam

Apo-Alpraz†, Novo-Alpra-zol†, Nu-Alpraz†, Xanax

Benzodiazepine

Antianxiety agent

Preg. Risk Category: D

Controlled Sub. Sched.: IV

Anxiety — Adults: usual initial dose 0.25 to 0.5 mg PO tid, to max 4 mg daily in divided doses. For elderly or debilitated patients or those with advanced liver disease, usual initial dose 0.25 mg PO bid or tid, to max 4 mg daily in divided doses.

Panic disorders — Adults: 0.5 mg PO tid, increased q 3 to 4 days in increments of no more than 1 mg. Max 10 mg qd in divided doses.

- Not to be used for everyday stress or for more than 4 mo.
- Warn not to withdraw abruptly after long-term use; withdrawal symptoms may occur. Abuse or addiction possible.
- In repeated or prolonged therapy, monitor liver, renal, and hematopoietic studies periodically as ordered.

alprostadil

Caverject

Prostaglandin

Corrective agent for impotence

Preg. Risk Category: NR

Erectile dysfunction due to vasculogenic, psychogenic, or mixed etiology — Adults: dosages highly individualized, with initial dose of 2.5 mcg intracavernously. If partial response occurs, give 2nd dose of 2.5 mcg, then increase in increments of 5 to 10 mcg until suitable erection. If no response to initial dose, may increase 2nd dose to 7.5 mcg within 1 hr, then increase in increments of 5 to 10 mcg until suitable erection.

Erectile dysfunction of neurologic etiology (spinal cord injury) — Adults: dosages highly individualized, with initial dose of 1.25 mcg intracavernously. If partial response occurs, give 2nd dose of 2.5 mcg, followed by increment of 2.5 mcg, to dose of 5 mcg, and then in increments of 5 mcg until suitable erection. If no response to initial dose, may give next higher dose within 1 hr.

- Regular follow-up care with thorough exam of penis strongly recommended to detect penile fibrosis.
- Erection should occur 5 to 20 min after administration and should last preferably ≤ 1 hr. Erection lasting > 6 hr requires immediate medical intervention. With initial dosing, patient must stay in doctor's office until complete detumescence.
- Should not be used > 3 times/wk. Interval of at least 24 hr required between uses.
- Monitor for adverse reactions, such as penile redness, swelling, tenderness, curvature, unusual pain, nodules, or priapism.
- Bleeding at injection site may increase risk of transmitting bloodborne disease to sexual partner.

DRUG / CLASS / CATEGORY

alprostadil
Prostin VR Pediatric
Prostaglandin
Ductus arteriosus patency adjunct
Preg. Risk Category: NR

alteplase (tissue plasminogen activator, recombinant; tPA)
Activase‡, Activase
Enzyme
Thrombolytic enzyme
Preg. Risk Category: C

INDICATIONS / DOSAGES

Palliative therapy for temporary maintenance of patency of ductus arteriosus until surgery — **Infants:** 0.05 to 0.1 mcg/kg/min IV infusion. When therapeutic response achieved, reduce infusion rate to lowest dosage that will maintain response; max 0.4 mcg/kg/min. Alternatively, give through umbilical artery catheter placed at ductal opening.

Lysis of thrombi obstructing coronary arteries in acute MI — **Adults:** 100 mg IV infusion over 3 hr as follows: 60 mg in 1st hr, of which 6 to 10 mg given as bolus over 1st 1 to 2 min. Then 20 mg/hr infusion for 2 hr. Smaller adults (< 65 kg) should receive 1.25 mg/kg in single fashion (60% in 1st hr, 10% as bolus; then 20% of total dose per hr for 2 hr).
Management of acute massive pulmonary embolism — **Adults:** 100 mg IV infusion over 2 hr. Begin heparin at end of infusion when PTT or thrombin time returns to twice normal or less. Don't exceed 100-mg dose.

KEY NURSING CONSIDERATIONS

- Not for use in neonatal respiratory distress syndrome.
- Don't use diluents with benzyl alcohol.
- If apnea and bradycardia occur, stop infusion immediately.
- Keep emergency equipment available.
- In restricted pulmonary blood flow, monitor blood oxygenation. In restricted systemic blood flow, monitor systemic BP and blood pH.

- Must be initiated as soon as possible after symptom onset when used to recanalize occluded coronary arteries.
- *IV use:* Check manufacturer's labeling for specific reconstitution information.
- Monitor vital signs and neurologic status carefully. Keep patient on strict bed rest.
- Have antiarrhythmics readily available, and carefully monitor ECG.
- Avoid invasive procedures. Carefully monitor for signs of internal bleeding, and frequently check all puncture sites.

- If uncontrollable bleeding occurs, stop infusion (and concomitant heparin), apply pressure to site if possible, and notify doctor.

Acute ischemic stroke — **Adults:** 0.9 mg/kg IV infusion over 1 hr with 10% of total dose given as initial IV bolus over 1 min. Max 90 mg total. *Note:* Give within 3 hr after symptoms occur and only when intracranial bleed has been ruled out.

---

altretamine (hexamethylmelamine; HMM)

Hexalen, Hexastat†
Alkylating agent
Antineoplastic
Preg. Risk Category: D

Palliative treatment of persistent or recurrent ovarian cancer after 1st-line therapy with cisplatin or alkylating agent–based combination therapy — **Adults:** 260 mg/m² PO daily in 4 divided doses with meals and hs for 14 or 21 consecutive days in 28-day cycle.

- Obtain baseline CBC and platelet count before each course of therapy and monthly.
- Perform careful neurologic assessment before each course.
- May be given with pyridoxine to reduce neurotoxicity.
- Be prepared to discontinue for at least 14 days if platelet count < 75,000/mm³, WBC count < 2,000/mm³, or granulocyte count < 1,000/mm³. Discontinue temporarily for severe GI distress unresponsive to treatment or signs of progressive neuropathy. Discontinue if neurologic symptoms fail to stabilize.
- Reduce dosage or discontinue temporarily for severe nausea and vomiting.

---

aluminum carbonate

Basaljel
Inorganic aluminum salt
Antacid/hypophosphatemic
Preg. Risk Category: B

Antacid — **Adults:** 5 to 10 ml of oral susp PO q 2 hr, prn; or 1 to 2 tabs or caps PO q 2 hr, prn. Max 24 caps, tabs, tsp/24 hr.
To prevent urinary phosphate stones (in conjunction with low-phosphate diet) — **Adults:** 15 to 30 ml oral susp in water or

- When giving through NG tube, ensure correct tube placement and patency; after instilling, flush tube with water.
- Monitor long-term, high-dose use in patients on restricted sodium intake.

(continued)

ALUMINUM CARBONATE   13

†Canadian, ‡Australian

DRUG/CLASS/CATEGORY	INDICATIONS/DOSAGES	KEY NURSING CONSIDERATIONS
aluminum carbonate *(continued)*	juice PO 1 hr after meals and hs; or 2 to 6 tabs or caps 1 hr after meals and hs.	• Watch for hypophosphatemia symptoms with prolonged use.
aluminum hydroxide AlternaGEL, Alu-Cap, Amphojel, Dialume, Nephrox *Aluminum salt* *Antacid/hypophosphatemic agent/adsorbent* Preg. Risk Category: C	*Antacid* — **Adults:** 500 to 1,500 mg PO (5 to 30 ml of most susp products) 1 hr after meals and hs; alternatively, 300-mg tab or 600-mg tab (chewed before swallowing) taken with milk or water 5 to 6 times daily after meals and hs.	• When giving through NG tube, ensure correct tube placement and patency; after instilling, flush tube with water. • Monitor long-term, high-dose use in patients on restricted sodium intake. • Watch for hypophosphatemia symptoms with prolonged use.
amantadine hydrochloride Antadine†, Symadine, Symmetrel *Synthetic cyclic primary amine* *Antiviral/antiparkinsonism agent* Preg. Risk Category: C	*Prophylaxis or symptomatic treatment of influenza type A virus, respiratory tract illnesses* — **Adults ≤ 65 yr with normal renal function and children > 9 yr weighing > 45 kg:** 200 mg PO daily in single dose. **Children 1 to 9 yr or < 45 kg:** 4.4 to 8.8 mg/kg PO daily, as single dose or divided bid. Max 150 mg daily. **Adults > 65 yr with normal renal function:** 100 mg PO qd. Start treatment within 24 to 48 hr after symptoms appear and continue for 24 to 48 hr after they	• Elderly patients are more susceptible to adverse neurologic effects. • If insomnia occurs, advise taking drug several hours before bedtime. • Use cautiously in elderly patients and those with seizure disorders, heart failure, peripheral edema, hepatic disease, mental illness, eczematoid rash, renal impairment, orthostatic hypotension, or cardiovascular disease. • If patient also taking anticholinergic, dosage of anticholinergic may be reduced prior to start of amantadine therapy.

- If orthostatic hypotension occurs, instruct to stand or change position slowly.
- Observe for adverse reactions, especially dizziness, depression, anxiety, nausea, and urine retention.

disappear. Start as soon as possible after initial exposure.

amifostine
Ethyol
Organic thiophosphate
Cytoprotective agent
Preg. Risk Category: C

Reduction of cumulative renal toxicity associated with repeated cisplatin administration in patients with advanced ovarian cancer or non-small-cell lung cancer — **Adults:** 910 mg/m² daily as 15-min IV infusion, starting 30 min before chemotherapy. If hypotension occurs and BP doesn't return to normal within 5 min after treatment stops, use dose of 740 mg/m² for subsequent cycles.

- Should stop antihypertensive therapy 24 hr before amifostine administration.
- Patient should be adequately hydrated before administration. Keep supine during infusion. Monitor I & O.
- Monitor BP q 5 min during infusion. If hypotension occurs and necessitates interrupting therapy, notify doctor and keep patient supine with legs elevated. Then give infusion of 0.9% NaCl, as ordered, using separate IV line.
- Don't infuse drug for > 15 minutes. A longer infusion has been associated with a higher incidence of adverse reactions.

amikacin sulfate
Amikin
Aminoglycoside
Antibiotic
Preg. Risk Category: D

Serious infections caused by sensitive strains of susceptible organisms — **Adults and children:** 15 mg/kg/day divided q 8 to 12 hr by IM or IV infusion (in 100 to 200 ml D₅W or 0.9% NaCl solution run in over 30 to 60 min). **Neonates:** Initially, loading dose of 10 mg/kg IV, then 7.5 mg/kg q 12 hr. *Uncomplicated UTI* — **Adults:** 250 mg IM or IV bid.

- Obtain specimen for culture and sensitivity tests for 1st dose.
- Evaluate weight, hearing, and renal function before and during therapy.
- Peak levels > 35 mcg/ml and trough levels > 10 mcg/ml may indicate toxicity.

AMIKACIN SULFATE 15

DRUG/CLASS/ CATEGORY	INDICATIONS/ DOSAGES	KEY NURSING CONSIDERATIONS
amiloride hydrochloride Kalurit‡, Midamor *Potassium-sparing diuretic Diuretic/antihypertensive* Preg. Risk Category: B	*Hypertension; edema associated with heart failure, usually in patients also taking thiazide or other potassium-wasting diuretics* — **Adults:** usual dosage 5 mg PO daily. Increase to 10 mg daily, if necessary. Max 20 mg daily.	• To prevent nausea, administer with meals. • If not given concurrently with potassium-wasting drug, monitor serum potassium. Alert doctor immediately if level > 5.5 mEq/L, and expect to discontinue.
amino acid infusions Aminosyn, FreAmine III, Aminosyn II with dextrose, Travasol with electrolytes, Aminosyn II with electrolytes in dextrose, Hepat-Amine, Aminosyn-HBC, Aminosyn-RF *Protein substrates Parenteral nutritional therapy and caloric agent* Preg. Risk Category: C	*Total parenteral nutrition in patients who can't or won't eat* — **Adults:** 1 to 1.5 g/kg IV daily. **Children < 10 kg:** 2 to 4 g/kg IV daily. **Children > 10 kg:** 20 to 25 g/kg IV daily for 1st 10 kg, then 1 to 1.25 g/kg IV daily for each kg over 10 kg. *Nutritional support in cirrhosis, hepatitis, and hepatic encephalopathy* — **Adults:** 80 to 120 g of amino acids (12 to 18 g of nitrogen) IV daily of form for hepatic failure. *Nutritional support in high metabolic stress* — **Adults:** 1.5 g/kg IV daily of form for high metabolic stress. *Nutritional support in renal failure* — **Adults:** 0.3 to 0.5 g/kg IV daily (max 26 g daily). Dialysis patients may require 1 to 1.2 g/kg daily.	• Obtain baseline serum electrolytes, glucose, BUN, calcium, and phosphorus levels before therapy, as ordered. Monitor periodically throughout therapy. • Limit peripheral infusions to 2.5% amino acids and dextrose 10%. Check infusion site frequently for erythema, inflammation, irritation, tissue sloughing, necrosis, and phlebitis. Change peripheral sites routinely. If subclavian catheter used, administer solution into midsuperior vena cava. • Assess body temp q 4 hr. If chills, fever, or other signs of sepsis, replace IV tubing and bottle and send to lab to be cultured. • Administer cautiously to diabetics and in patients with cardiac insufficiency.

aminocaproic acid Amicar *Carboxylic acid derivative* *Fibrinolysis inhibitor* Preg. Risk Category: C	*Excessive bleeding resulting from hyperfib-rinolysis* — **Adults:** initially, 5 g PO or slow IV infusion, then 1 to 1.25 g hourly until bleeding controlled. Max 30 g daily.	▪ **IV use:** Dilute solution with sterile water for injection, 0.9% NaCl for injection, D_5W, or Ringer's injection. Infuse slowly. Don't give by direct or intermittent injection. ▪ Monitor coagulation studies, as ordered, and HR and BP. Notify doctor immediately of any change.
aminoglutethimide Cytadren *Antiadrenal hormone* *Antineoplastic* Preg. Risk Category: D	*Suppression of adrenal function in Cush-ing's syndrome and adrenal cancer* — **Adults:** 250 mg q 6 hr. May increase dosage in increments of 250 mg daily q 1 to 2 wk, to max 2 g daily.	▪ Perform baseline hematologic studies, as ordered. ▪ Monitor BP frequently; monitor CBC peri-odically, as ordered. ▪ May cause adrenal hypofunction, especial-ly in stressful circumstances. Patients may need mineralocorticoid supplements to treat hyponatremia and orthostatic hy-potension. Glucocorticoid replacement may also be necessary, especially in pa-tients with breast cancer. Monitor such patients carefully. ▪ May decrease thyroid hormone produc-tion. Monitor thyroid function studies.
aminophylline (theophylline eth-ylenediamine) Aminophyllin, Cardophyl-lin†, Corophyllin†, Phyllo-contin, Somophyllin, Tru-phylline	*Symptomatic relief of bronchospasm* — **Pa-tients not taking theophylline who need rapid relief:** loading dose 6 mg/kg (equiv to 4.7 mg/kg anhydrous theophylline) IV, then maintenance infusion. **Adults (nonsmokers):** 0.7 mg/kg/hr IV for 12 hr; then 0.5 mg/kg/hr.	▪ Before loading dose, ensure that patient hasn't had recent theophylline therapy. ▪ Relieve GI symptoms by giving oral drug with full glass of water at meals (although food in stomach delays absorption)

18

†Canadian, ‡Australian

DRUG / CLASS / CATEGORY	INDICATIONS / DOSAGES	KEY NURSING CONSIDERATIONS
aminophylline *(continued)* *Xanthine derivative* *Bronchodilator* Preg. Risk Category: C	**Otherwise healthy adult smokers:** 1 mg/kg/ hr IV for 12 hr; then 0.8 mg/kg/hr. **Children 9 to 16 yr:** 1 mg/kg/hr IV for 12 hr; then 0.8 mg/kg/hr. **Children 6 mo to 9 yr:** 1.2 mg/kg/ hr for 12 hr; then 1 mg/kg/hr. **Patients taking theophylline:** Determine time, amount, route, and dosage form of last dose. Infusions of 0.63 mg/kg (0.5 mg/kg anhydrous theophylline) increase plasma drug level by 1 mcg/ml. If no obvious signs of toxicity, dose of 3.1 mg/kg (2.5 mg/kg anhydrous theophylline). *Chronic bronchial asthma* — **Adults and children:** initial dose 16 mg/kg or 400 mg (whichever is less) PO qd in divided doses q 6 to 8 hr using rapidly absorbed forms. May increase in increments of 25% q 2 to 3 days. Alternatively, 12 mg/kg or 400 mg (whichever is less) PO qd in divided doses q 8 to 12 hr if using ext-release forms. May increase by 2 to 3 mg/kg daily q 3 days.	• *IV use:* IV administration can cause burning; dilute with compatible IV solution and inject no faster than 25 mg/min. • Monitor serum theophylline. Desirable level 10 to 20 mcg/ml; toxicity reported > 20 mcg/ml. • Inform elderly patient that dizziness is common adverse effect. • Caution to avoid switching brands. • Instruct patient to check with doctor or pharmacist before taking with other drugs. • Rectal dosage same as recommended oral dosage.
amiodarone hydrochloride Aratac‡, Cordarone, Cordarone X‡	*Recurrent ventricular fibrillation and recurrent hemodynamically unstable ventricular tachycardia refractory to other antiarrhythmics* — **Adults:** loading dose 800 to 1,600	• Continuously monitor cardiac status of patient receiving drug IV. • High incidence of adverse reactions limits use.

Benzofuran derivative
Ventricular and supraventricular antiarrhythmic
Preg. Risk Category: D

mg PO daily for 1 to 3 wk until initial therapeutic response, then 600 to 800 mg/day PO for 1 mo and maintenance of 200 to 600 mg PO daily. Or, loading dose 150 mg IV over 10 min (15 mg/min); then 360 mg IV over next 6 hr (1 mg/min); then 540 mg IV over next 18 hr (0.5 mg/min). After 1st 24 hr, continue maintenance infusion of 720 mg/24 hr (0.5 mg/min).

- Monitor carefully for pulmonary toxicity, which can be fatal. Incidence increases with doses > 400 mg/day.
- Monitor for symptoms of pneumonitis. Monitor pulmonary function tests and chest X-ray.
- Methylcellulose ophthalmic solution recommended during therapy to minimize corneal microdeposits.

---

amitriptyline hydrochloride
Apo-Amitriptyline†, Elavil
amitriptyline pamoate
Elavil
Tricyclic antidepressant
Antidepressant
Preg. Risk Category: NR

Depression — **Adults:** initially, 50 to 100 mg PO hs, increased to 150 mg daily; max 300 mg daily, if needed. Maintenance: 50 to 100 mg/day PO or 20 to 30 mg IM qid. **Elderly patients and adolescents:** 10 mg PO tid and 20 mg hs daily.

- Parenteral form for IM use only.
- Has strong anticholinergic effects and is one of most sedating TCAs.
- If signs of psychosis occur or worsen, expect to reduce dosage. Record mood changes. Monitor for suicidal tendency and allow only minimal drug supply.
- Don't withdraw abruptly.

---

amlodipine besylate
Norvasc
Dihydropyridine calcium channel blocker
Antianginal/antihypertensive
Preg. Risk Category: C

Chronic stable angina; vasospastic angina (Prinzmetal's [variant] angina) — **Adults:** initially, 5 to 10 mg PO daily. *Hypertension* — **Adults:** initially, 2.5 to 5 mg PO daily. With small, frail, or elderly patients, those receiving other antihypertensives, or those with hepatic insufficiency, begin at 2.5 mg daily. Adjust according to patient response and tolerance. Max 10 mg/day.

- Monitor carefully for increased frequency, duration, or severity of angina or acute MI.
- Monitor BP frequently when therapy begins.
- Notify doctor if patient has signs of heart failure (shortness of breath, swelling of hands and feet).

AMLODIPINE BESYLATE 19

DRUG/CLASS/ CATEGORY	INDICATIONS/ DOSAGES	KEY NURSING CONSIDERATIONS
ammonium chloride Asendin *Acid-forming salt* *Acidifying agent/expectorant* Preg. Risk Category: C	*Metabolic alkalosis; chloride replacement —* **Adults and children:** IV dose (in mEq/L) equal to serum chloride deficit (in mEq/L) multiplied by extracellular fluid volume (estimated as 20% of body weight in kg). Give half of calculated volume, then reassess patient. *Acidifier —* **Adults:** 4 to 12 g PO daily in divided doses q 4 to 6 hr. **Children:** 75 mg/kg PO daily in 4 divided doses.	▪ Don't administer with milk or other alkaline solutions; incompatible. ▪ Observe for signs of ammonia toxicity: pallor, sweating, irregular breathing, and twitching. Notify doctor at once. ▪ Determine CO_2 combining power and serum electrolytes before and during therapy to prevent acidosis. Each g of ammonium chloride reduces CO_2 combining power by 1.1 volume percent. ▪ *IV use:* Dilute per manufacturer's labeling. Administer via infusion pump, ≤ 5 ml/min in adults.
amoxapine Asendin *Dibenzoxazepine* *Tricyclic antidepressant* Preg. Risk Category: C	*Depression —* **Adults:** initially, 50 mg PO bid or tid, increased to 100 mg bid or tid by end of first wk if tolerated. Make increases > 300 mg daily only if this dose ineffective during trial of at least 2 wk. Max recommended for outpatients 400 mg daily. When effective dosage established, entire dosage may be given hs. **Elderly patients:** initially, 25 mg bid or tid. If tolerated by end of 1st wk, increase to 50 mg bid or tid. Carefully increase up to 300 mg daily.	▪ Use with extreme caution in history of seizure disorders. ▪ Full effect may take 4 wk or more. ▪ If signs of psychosis occur or worsen, expect to reduce dosage. Record mood changes. Monitor for suicidal tendency and allow only minimal drug supply. ▪ Monitor for tardive dyskinesia, especially in elderly women. ▪ Has been linked to neuroleptic malignant syndrome.

**amoxicillin/clavu-
lanate potassium
(amoxicillin/clavu-
lanate potassium)**
Augmentin, Clavulin†
*Aminopenicillin and beta-
lactamase inhibitor*
Antibiotic
Preg. Risk Category: B

*Lower respiratory infections, otitis media,
sinusitis, skin and skin-structure infections,
and UTIs caused by susceptible strains of
gram-pos and gram-neg organisms —*
Adults and children ≥ 40 kg: 250 mg
(based on amoxicillin component) PO q 8
hr. For more severe infections, 500 mg q 8
hr. **Children < 40 kg:** 20 to 40 mg/kg (based
on amoxicillin component) PO daily in divided doses q 8 hr.

- Assess history of drug allergies.
- Obtain specimen for culture and sensitivity
  tests before first dose.
- Know that two 250-mg tablets not equiva-
  lent to one 500-mg tablet.
- Give at least 1 hr before bacteriostatic an-
  tibiotics.
- Advise to take with food.
- Instruct to call doctor if rash occurs.
- Observe for superinfection.

**amoxicillin
trihydrate
(amoxicillin
trihydrate)**
Amoxil, Cilamox‡, Larotid,
Polymox, Trimox, Wymox
Aminopenicillin
Antibiotic
Preg. Risk Category: NR

*Systemic infections, acute and chronic UTIs
caused by susceptible strains of gram-pos
and gram-neg organisms —* **Adults and
children ≥ 20 kg:** 250 to 500 mg PO q 8 hr.
Children < 20 kg: 20 mg/kg PO daily in divided doses q 8 hr; in severe infection, 40
mg/kg PO daily in divided doses q 8 hr or
500 mg to 1 g/m² PO in divided doses q 8
hr.
Uncomplicated gonorrhea — **Adults and
children > 45 kg:** 3 g PO with 1 g probenecid given as single dose. Don't give to children < age 2.
*Endocarditis prophylaxis for dental proce-
dures —* **Adults:** initially, 3 g PO 1 hr before
procedure; then 1.5 g 6 hr later. **Children:**
initially, 50 mg/kg PO 1 hr before procedure; then half of initial dose 6 hr later.

- Assess history of allergic reactions to
  penicillin. (However, negative history
  doesn't preclude future reactions.)
- Obtain specimen for culture and sensitivity
  tests before 1st dose.
- With prolonged therapy, observe for fungal or bacterial superinfection, especially
  in elderly, debilitated, or immunosup-
  pressed patients.
- Give at least 1 hr before bacteriostatic antibiotics.
- Advise patient taking oral form that drug
  can be stored at room temp for up to 2
  wk.

AMOXICILLIN TRIHYDRATE   21

†Canadian, ‡Australian

DRUG/CLASS/ CATEGORY	INDICATIONS/ DOSAGES	KEY NURSING CONSIDERATIONS
amphotericin B Amphocin, Amphotericin B for Injection, Fungilin Oral†, Fungizone Intravenous *Polyene macrolide* *Antifungal* Preg. Risk Category: B	*Systemic fungal infections, meningitis* — **Adults:** initially, test dose of 1 mg in 20 ml D₅W infused IV over 20 to 30 min may be recommended. If tolerated, initiate daily dosage as 0.25 to 0.3 mg/kg by slow IV infusion (0.1 mg/ml) over 2 to 6 hr. Increase dosage gradually to max 1 mg/kg daily. If discontinued for 1 wk or more, resume drug with initial dose and increase gradually. *GI tract infections caused by Candida albicans* — **Adults:** 100 mg PO qid for 2 wk. *Oral and perioral candidal infections* — **Adults:** 1 lozenge qid for 7 to 14 days. Lozenge should dissolve slowly.	• For severe reactions, discontinue and notify doctor. • *IV use:* Monitor pulse, respiratory rate, temp, and BP for at least 4 hr with initial test dose. • Monitor vital signs q 30 min; fever, shaking chills, and hypotension may appear 1 to 2 hr after IV infusion starts and should subside within 4 hr of stopping drug. • Report change in urine appearance or volume. Monitor BUN and serum creatinine (or creatinine clearance) weekly. • Use infusion pump and in-line filter with mean pore diameter > 1 micron.
ampicillin sodium/sulbactam sodium Unasyn *Aminopenicillin/beta-lactamase inhibitor combination* *Antibiotic* Preg. Risk Category: B	*Intra-abdominal, gyn, and skin-structure infections caused by susceptible strains* — **Adults:** dosage expressed as total drug (each 1.5-g vial contains 1 g ampicillin sodium and 0.5 g sulbactam) — 1.5 to 3 g IM or IV q 6 hr. Max daily dosage 4 g sulbactam and 8 g ampicillin (12 g of combined drugs).	• Assess history of allergic reactions to penicillin. (However, negative history doesn't preclude future reactions.) • Obtain specimen for culture and sensitivity tests before first dose. • *IV use:* Give IV over 10 to 15 min, or dilute in 50 to 100 ml of compatible diluent and infuse over 15 to 30 min. If permitted, give intermittently. Change site every 48 hr. • For IM injection, reconstitute with sterile water for injection or 0.5% or 2% lidocaine.

amrinone lactate
Inocor
Bipyridine derivative
Inotropic/vasodilator
Preg. Risk Category: C

Short-term management of heart failure —
Adults: initially, 0.75 mg/kg IV bolus over 2 to 3 min. Then start maintenance infusion of 5 to 10 mcg/kg/min. May give additional bolus of 0.75 mg/kg 30 min after therapy starts. Don't exceed 10 mg/kg total daily dosage. Dosage depends on clinical response.

- Primarily given to patients unresponsive to cardiac glycosides, diuretics, and vasodilators.
- Don't give through same IV line as furosemide.
- Don't dilute with solution containing dextrose. Can be injected into free-flowing dextrose infusions through Y-connector or directly into tubing.
- Monitor BP and HR throughout infusion. If BP falls, slow or stop infusion and notify doctor.

anastrozole
Arimidex
Nonsteroidal aromatase inhibitor
Antineoplastic agent
Preg. Risk Category: D

Treatment of advanced breast cancer in postmenopausal women with disease progression after tamoxifen therapy — **Adults:** 1 mg PO daily.

- Use cautiously in breast-feeding women.
- Should be given under supervision of qualified doctor experienced in use of anticancer drugs.

antihemophilic factor (AHF)
Hemofil M, Humate-P, Hyate:C, Koate-HP, Koate-HS
Blood derivative
Antihemophilic
Preg. Risk Category: C

Spontaneous hemorrhage in patients with hemophilia A (factor VIII deficiency) —
Adults and children: calculate dosage using this formula: AHF required (IU) = body weight (kg) × desired factor VIII increase (% of normal) × 0.5. To prevent spontaneous hemorrhage, desired level of factor VIII is 5% of normal; for mild hemorrhage, 30% of

- Monitor coagulation studies and vital signs before and regularly during therapy. Monitor for hemolysis if patient has blood type A, B, or AB.
- Change in urine color to orange or red hue may signify hemolytic reaction.

(continued)

ANTIHEMOPHILIC FACTOR   23

†Canadian, ‡Australian

DRUG / CLASS / CATEGORY	INDICATIONS / DOSAGES	KEY NURSING CONSIDERATIONS
antihemophilic factor *(continued)*	normal; for moderate hemorrhage and minor surgery, 30% to 50% of normal; for severe hemorrhage, 80% to 100% of normal. *Treatment of bleeding in patients with hemophilia A* — **Adults and children:** for minor hemorrhage into muscle and joints, 8 to 10 IU/kg IV (or calculated dose to raise plasma factor VIII levels to 20% to 40% of normal) q 8 to 12 hr for 1 to 3 days, prn. For overt bleeding, initial dose of 15 to 25 IU/kg IV, followed by 8 to 15 IU/kg q 8 to 12 hr for 3 to 4 days. To treat massive bleeding or hemorrhage involving major organs, initial dose of 40 to 50 IU/kg IV, followed by 20 to 25 IU/kg IV q 8 to 12 hr. *Prevention of bleeding in hemophilic patients requiring surgery* — **Adults:** 25 to 30 IU/kg IV 1 hr before surgery, followed by half of initial dosage 5 hr later. Dosage adjusted to achieve level of AHF 80% to 100% of normal during surgery and maintained at 30% to 60% of normal for ≥ 10 to 14 days postop.	• Refrigerate concentrate until ready to use. Warm concentrate and diluent bottle to room temp before reconstituting. To mix drug, gently roll vial between hands. • *IV use:* Use plastic syringe; may interact with glass syringe and bind to surface. • Use reconstituted solution within 3 hr. Store away from heat and don't refrigerate. Don't shake or mix with other IV solutions. Filter solution before administration. • Don't give SC or IM. • Some patients develop inhibitors to factor VIII, resulting in decreased drug response. • Monitor for allergic reactions. • Risk of hepatitis must be weighed against risks involved if patient doesn't receive drug. • Because of manufacturing process, risk of HIV transmission is extremely low.

antithrombin III, human (AT-III, heparin cofactor I)

ATnativ, Thrombate III
Glycoprotein
Anticoagulant/antithrombotic
Preg. Risk Category: C

Thromboembolism associated with hereditary AT-III deficiency — **Adults and children:** initial dose individualized to quantify required to increase AT-III activity to 120% of normal activity as determined 30 min after administration. Usual dose 50 to 100 IU/min, not to exceed 100 IU/min. Dose calculated based on anticipated 1% increase in plasma AT-III activity produced by 1 IU/kg of body weight using the formula:

Dose required (IU) = (desired activity [%] – baseline activity [%]) × weight (kg) ÷ 1.4

Maintenance dosage individualized to quantity required to increase AT-III activity to 80% of normal activity, and given at 24-hr intervals. To calculate subsequent dosages, multiply desired AT-III activity (as percentage of normal) minus baseline AT-III activity (as percentage of normal) by body weight (in kg). Divide by actual increase in AT-III activity (as percentage) produced by 1 IU/kg as determined 30 min after initial dose given. Treatment usually continues for 2 to 8 days but may be prolonged in pregnancy or when used with surgery or immobilization.

- **IV use:** Reconstitute using 10 ml of sterile water (provided), 0.9% NaCl sol, or D₅W. Dilute further in same diluent solution if desired. Don't shake vial. Dilute further in same diluent solution if desired.
- Obtain AT-III activity levels bid until dosage requirement stabilizes, then qd immediately before dose. Functional assays preferred.
- Monitor for dyspnea and increased BP, which may occur with too-rapid administration rate.
- Heparin binds to AT-III lysine binding sites, resulting in increased heparin efficacy.
- 1 IU equiv to quantity of endogenous AT-III present in 1 ml normal human plasma.
- Prepared from pooled plasma from human donors; carries minimal risk of transmission of viruses, including hepatitis and HIV.
- Risk of neonatal thromboembolism (sometimes fatal) in children of parents with hereditary AT-III deficiency. Obtain AT-III levels immediately after birth.

ANTITHROMBIN III, HUMAN

25

DRUG/CLASS/ CATEGORY	INDICATIONS/ DOSAGES	KEY NURSING CONSIDERATIONS
apraclonidine hydrochloride Iopidine *Alpha-adrenergic agonist Ocular hypotensive agent* Preg. Risk Category: C	*Prevention or control of elevated IOP before and after ocular laser surgery* — **Adults:** 1 drop of 1% sol instilled 1 hr before initiation of laser surgery on anterior segment, followed by 1 drop immediately after surgery. *Short-term adjunct therapy in patients who require additional IOP reduction* — **Adults:** 1 or 2 drops of 0.5% sol instilled into affected eye tid.	• Closely monitor patients who tend to develop exaggerated IOP decreases after drug therapy. • Observe closely for vasovagal attack during laser surgery. • Closely monitor patients with severe systemic disease, including hypertension.
aprotinin Trasylol *Naturally occurring protease inhibitor Systemic hemostatic agent* Preg. Risk Category: B	*To reduce blood loss or need for transfusion in patients undergoing CABG* — **Adults:** start with 10,000 units (1 ml) test dose ≥ 10 min before loading dose. If no allergic reaction, anesthesia may be induced while loading dose of 2 million units given slowly over 20 to 30 min. When loading dose complete, sternotomy may be performed. Before bypass initiated, cardiopulmonary bypass circuit primed with 2 million units of drug by replacing aliquot of priming fluid with drug. Continuous infusion at 500,000 units/hr given until patient leaves OR. This is known as *regimen A*. Alternatively, *regimen B* may be used: give half dosage of *regimen A* (except for test dose).	• Be prepared to administer test dose. Test dose particularly important in patients with history of allergies or who have previously received drug. In such patients, pretreat with antihistamine, as ordered. • Use cautiously and monitor closely for hypersensitivity reaction. Patient may experience anaphylaxis even if no symptoms occurred with test dose. If hypersensitivity symptoms occur, discontinue infusion immediately, notify doctor, and provide supportive treatment. • Administer through central line. Don't mix with other drugs. • Monitor for increased serum creatinine and other signs of nephrotoxicity.

asparaginase (L-asparaginase)

Elspar, Kidrolase†

Antineoplastic

Enzyme

Preg. Risk Category: C

Acute lymphocytic leukemia (in combination with other drugs) — **Adults and children:** 1,000 IU/kg IV daily for 10 days, injected over 30 min; or 6,000 IU/m² IM at intervals specified in protocol.

Sole induction agent for acute lymphocytic leukemia — **Adults:** 200 IU/kg IV daily for 28 days.

- Risk of hypersensitivity increases with repeated doses. Intradermal skin test should be done before initial dose and when drug given after interval of ≥ 1 wk between doses. Desensitization may be required. Be prepared to treat anaphylaxis.
- Monitor patient closely. Watch for signs of hyperglycemia. Monitor bone marrow function tests, bleeding studies, and serum amylase levels.
- If drug contacts skin, flush with copious amounts of water for ≥ 15 min.
- Administer fluids as ordered to help prevent tumor lysis and combat dehydration secondary to vomiting.

---

aspirin (acetylsalicylic acid)

A.S.A., Ascriptin, Bayer Timed-Release, Bufferin, Ecotrin

Salicylate

Nonnarcotic analgesic/ antipyretic/anti-inflammatory/antiplatelet

Preg. Risk Category: C (D in 3rd trimester)

Rheumatoid arthritis, other inflammatory conditions — **Adults:** initially, 2.4 to 3.6 g PO qd in divided doses. Maintenance: 3.2 to 6 g PO qd in divided doses.

Mild pain or fever — **Adults and children > 11 yr:** 325 to 650 mg PO or PR q 4 hr, prn. **Children 2 to 11 yr:** 1.5 g/m² or 65 mg/kg PO or PR daily in 4 to 6 divided doses.

Reduction of MI risk in patients with previous MI or unstable angina — **Adults:** 160 to 325 mg PO daily.

- Don't give to children or teenagers with chickenpox or flu-like illness; use cautiously at all times.
- Give on scheduled basis for inflammatory conditions, rheumatic fever, and thrombosis.
- Monitor blood drug levels. Tinnitus may occur at 30 mg/100 ml and above.
- During prolonged therapy, periodically assess Hct, Hgb, PT, and renal function.
- Instruct to discontinue aspirin 5 to 7 days before elective surgery.

---

†Canadian, ‡Australian

ASPIRIN   27

DRUG / CLASS / CATEGORY	INDICATIONS / DOSAGES	KEY NURSING CONSIDERATIONS
astemizole Hismanal *Histamine₁-receptor antagonist* *Antiallergy agent* Preg. Risk Category: C	*Relief of symptoms associated with chronic idiopathic urticaria and seasonal allergic rhinitis* — **Adults and children > 12 yr:** 10 mg PO daily.	▪ Contraindicated in hepatic failure or hypersensitivity to drug and in patients taking itraconazole, ketoconazole, or macrolide antibiotics. ▪ Teach to take only once daily. High doses may increase risk of arrhythmias.
atenolol Apo-Atenolol‡, Noten‡, Nu-Atenol†, Tenormin *Beta-adrenergic blocker* *Antihypertensive/antianginal* Preg. Risk Category: D	*Hypertension* — **Adults:** initially, 50 mg PO daily as single dose, increased to 100 mg once daily after 7 to 14 days. Dosages > 100 mg unlikely to bring further benefit. *Angina pectoris* — **Adults:** 50 mg PO once daily, increased to 100 mg daily after 7 days for optimal effect. Max 200 mg daily. *To reduce CV mortality and risk of reinfarction in acute MI* — **Adults:** 5 mg IV, repeat 10 min later. After additional 10 min, 50 mg PO, then 50 mg PO in 12 hr. Thereafter, 100 mg PO qd (or 50 mg bid) for ≥ 7 days.	▪ If apical pulse < 60, withhold drug and call doctor. ▪ *IV use:* Give by slow IV injection, not exceeding 1 mg/min. ▪ Monitor BP. ▪ Caution not to increase dosage without consulting doctor. High dosages may lead to arrhythmias. ▪ Instruct to take on empty stomach at least 2 hr after meal and avoid eating for at least 1 hr after taking. ▪ Withdraw gradually over 2 wk.
atorvastatin calcium Lipitor *Hydroxymethylglutaryl-coenzyme A (HMG-CoA) reductase inhibitor*	*Adjunct to diet in primary hypercholesterolemia and mixed dyslipidemia* — **Adults:** 10 mg PO qd; increase as needed to max 80 mg qd. Dosage based on blood lipid levels drawn 2 to 4 wk after therapy starts.	▪ Should be initiated only after diet and other nonpharmacologic treatments prove ineffective. ▪ Periodic liver function tests and lipid levels should be done before initiation, and 6 and 12 wk after initiation, or after dosage increase, and periodically thereafter.

Antilipemic agent Preg. Risk Category: X	*Alone or as adjunct to lipid-lowering treatments in homozygous familial hypercholesterolemia* — **Adults:** 10 to 80 mg PO qd.	• Watch for signs of myositis.
atovaquone Mepron *Ubiquinone analogue* *Antiprotozoal* Preg. Risk Category: C	*Acute, mild to moderate P. carinii pneumonia in patients who can't tolerate co-trimoxazole* — **Adults:** 750 mg PO bid with food for 21 days.	• Risk of other concurrent pulmonary infections; monitor patient closely during therapy. • Instruct to take with meals.
atropine sulfate *Anticholinergic/belladonna alkaloid* *Antiarrhythmic/vagolytic* Preg. Risk Category: C	*Symptomatic bradycardia, bradyarrhythmia (junctional or escape rhythm)* — **Adults:** usually 0.5 to 1 mg IV push; repeat q 3 to 5 min to max 2 mg as needed. **Children:** 0.01 mg/kg IV; may repeat q 4 to 6 hr; max 0.4 mg or 0.3 mg/m². *Preop to diminish secretions and block cardiac vagal reflexes* — **Adults and children ≥ 20 kg:** 0.4 to 0.6 mg IM or SC 30 to 60 min before anesthesia. **Children < 20 kg:** 0.01 mg/kg IM or SC up to max 0.4 mg 30 to 60 min before anesthesia.	• **IV use:** Administer by direct IV into large vein or IV tubing over at least 1 min. • Watch for tachycardia in cardiac patients. • Monitor for paradoxical initial bradycardia (usually disappears within 2 min). • Monitor I&O. Watch for urine retention and urinary hesitancy. • Promptly report serious or persistent adverse reactions. • Doses < 0.5 mg can cause bradycardia.
atropine sulfate Atropisol, Atropta, BufOpto Atropine, Isopto Atropine *Anticholinergic/belladonna alkaloid*	*Acute iritis; uveitis* — **Adults:** 1 to 2 drops instilled into eyes up to qid, or small strip of oint applied to conjunctival sac up to tid. **Children:** 1 to 2 drops of 0.5% sol instilled into eyes up to tid, or small strip of oint applied to conjunctival sac up to tid.	• Not for internal use; signs of poisoning are disorientation and confusion. Antidote is physostigmine salicylate. • Watch for signs of glaucoma: increased IOP (ocular pain, headache, progressive blurring of vision). If present, notify doctor.

(continued)

ATROPINE SULFATE   29

†Canadian, ‡Australian

DRUG/CLASS/ CATEGORY	INDICATIONS/ DOSAGES	KEY NURSING CONSIDERATIONS
atropine sulfate *(continued)* *Cycloplegic/mydriatic* Preg. Risk Category: C	*Cycloplegic refraction* — **Adults:** 1 to 2 drops of 1% sol instilled 1 hr before refraction. **Children:** 1 to 2 drops of 0.5% sol instilled in each eye bid for 1 to 3 days before eye exam and 1 hr before refraction.	• Apply light finger pressure on lacrimal sac for 1 min after instillation. • Excessive use in children and in certain susceptible patients may produce symptoms of atropine poisoning.
attapulgite Children's Kaopectate, Diasorb, Donnagel, Fowler's†, Rheaban Maximum Strength *Hydrated magnesium aluminum silicate* *Antidiarrheal agent* Preg. Risk Category: NR	*Acute, nonspecific diarrhea* — **Adults and adolescents:** 1.2 to 1.5 g (up to 3 g of Diasorb) PO after each loose bowel movement, not to exceed 9 g in 24 hr. **Children 6 to 12 yr:** 600 mg (susp) or 750 mg (tab) PO after each loose bowel movement, not to exceed 4.2 g (susp) or 4.5 g (tab) in 24 hr. **Children 3 to 6 yr:** 300 mg PO after each loose bowel movement, not to exceed 2.1 g in 24 hr.	• Don't give if diarrhea accompanied by fever or by blood or mucus in stool. • Instruct to take after each loose bowel movement until diarrhea controlled. • Advise to notify doctor if diarrhea not controlled within 48 hr or if fever develops. • Instruct to chew tablets well before swallowing or to shake liquid well before measuring dose.
auranofin Ridaura *Gold salt* *Antiarthritic* Preg. Risk Category: C	*Rheumatoid arthritis* — **Adults:** 6 mg PO daily, either as 3 mg bid or 6 mg qd. After 6 mo, may increase to 9 mg daily.	• Stop drug if monthly platelet count < 100,000/mm³, if Hgb drops suddenly, or if granulocytes < 1,500/mm³ or if leukopenia or eosinophilia present. • Monitor urinalysis. If proteinuria or hematuria detected, stop drug and notify doctor.

aurothioglucose
Gold-50‡, Solganal
gold sodium thiomalate
Myochrysine
Gold salt
Antiarthritic
Preg. Risk Category: C

Rheumatoid arthritis
aurothioglucose — Adults: initially, 10 mg IM, followed by 25 mg for 2nd and 3rd doses at weekly intervals. Then, 50 mg q wk until 800 mg to 1 g given. If improvement occurs without toxicity, 25 to 50 mg continued at 3- to 4-wk intervals indefinitely. **Children 6 to 12 yr:** one-fourth of usual adult dosage. Don't exceed 25 mg per dose.
gold sodium thiomalate — Adults: initially, 10 mg IM, followed by 25 mg in 1 wk. Then, 25 to 50 mg q wk to total dose of 1 g. If improvement occurs without toxicity, 25 to 50 mg q 2 wk for 2 to 20 wk; then, 25 to 50 mg q 3 to 4 wk as maintenance therapy. If relapse occurs, resume injections at weekly intervals. **Children:** initially, 10 mg IM, followed by 1 mg/kg IM weekly. Follow adult spacing of doses.

- Watch for anaphylactoid reaction for 30 min after administration.
- Keep dimercaprol on hand to treat acute toxicity.
- Give IM, as ordered, preferably intragluteally. Drug is pale yellow; don't use if it darkens.
- Immerse aurothioglucose vial in warm water; shake vigorously before injecting.
- When injecting gold sodium thiomalate, have patient lie down for 10 to 20 min to minimize hypotension.
- Analyze urine for protein and sediment changes before each injection. Monitor CBC, platelet count, and liver function tests.

azatadine maleate
Optimine, Zadine‡
Piperidine antihistamine
Antihistamine
Preg. Risk Category: B

Rhinitis, allergy symptoms, chronic urticaria — **Adults and children ≥ 12 yr:** 1 to 2 mg PO bid; max 4 mg daily.

- Monitor blood counts (including platelets) during long-term therapy, as ordered; watch for blood dyscrasias.

azathioprine
Imuran, Thioprine‡
Purine antagonist

Immunosuppression in kidney transplantation — **Adults and children:** initially, 3 to 5 mg/kg PO or IV daily, usually starting on

- Administer after meals to minimize adverse GI effects.

(continued)

†Canadian, ‡Australian

DRUG / CLASS / CATEGORY	INDICATIONS / DOSAGES	KEY NURSING CONSIDERATIONS
azathioprine (continued) Immunosuppressive Preg. Risk Category: D	day of transplantation. Maintain at 1 to 3 mg/kg daily (dosage varies considerably according to patient response). *Severe, refractory rheumatoid arthritis* — **Adults:** initially, 1 mg/kg PO as single dose or divided into 2 doses. If response not satisfactory after 6 to 8 wk, may increase by 0.5 mg/kg daily (to max 2.5 mg/kg daily) at 4-wk intervals.	▪ Monitor Hgb and WBC and platelet counts at least once monthly, as ordered, more often at beginning of treatment. Notify doctor if counts drop suddenly or become dangerously low. May need to be temporarily withheld. ▪ Watch for early signs of hepatotoxicity (clay-colored stools, dark urine, pruritus, and yellow skin and sclera) and for increased alkaline phosphatase, bilirubin, AST, and ALT. ▪ *IV use:* Reconstitute 100-mg vial with 10 ml sterile water for injection. May give by direct IV injection or further dilute in 0.9% NaCl for injection or D$_5$W, and infuse over 30 to 60 min. Use only for patients unable to tolerate oral medications.
azithromycin Zithromax *Azalide macrolide Macrolide anti-infective* Preg. Risk Category: B	*Acute bacterial exacerbations of COPD, mild community-acquired pneumonia, second-line therapy of pharyngitis or tonsillitis caused by susceptible organisms* — **Adults and adolescents ≥ 16 yr:** 500 mg PO as single dose on day 1, then 250 mg daily on days 2 through 5. Total dose 1.5 g. *Nongonococcal urethritis or cervicitis*	▪ Obtain specimen for culture and sensitivity tests before first dose. ▪ Give capsules 1 hr before or 2 hr after meals; don't give with antacids. Oral suspension can be taken with or without food. Reduce GI distress by taking with food or milk. ▪ Caution to avoid alcohol and activities requiring alertness until CNS effects known.

- Monitor blood counts (including platelets) during long-term therapy. Watch for signs of blood dyscrasias.
- Monitor for superinfection.

---

aztreonam
Azactam
Monobactam
Antibiotic
Preg. Risk Category: B

caused by C. trachomatis — **Adults and adolescents ≥ 16 yr:** 1 g PO as single dose. *Prevention of disseminated M. avium complex disease in advanced HIV infection* — **Adults:** 1,200 mg PO q wk, as indicated.

UTIs, lower respiratory tract infections, septicemia, skin and skin-structure infections, intra-abdominal infections, surgical infections, and gyn infections caused by susceptible strains of gram-neg aerobic organisms; also respiratory infections caused by H. influenzae — **Adults:** 500 mg to 2 g IV or IM q 8 to 12 hr. For severe systemic or life-threatening infections, may give 2 g q 6 to 8 hr. Max 8 g daily.

- Obtain culture and sensitivity tests before first dose.
- *IV use:* Inject bolus dose slowly (over 3 to 5 min) directly into vein or IV tubing. Give infusions over 20 min to 1 hr.
- Administer IM deep into large muscle mass. Give doses > 1 g IV.

---

b

bacitracin
AK-Tracin
Polypeptide antibiotic
Ophthalmic antibiotic
Preg. Risk Category: NR

Surface bacterial infections involving conjunctiva and cornea — **Adults and children:** small amount of oint applied into conjunctival sac ≥ qd or prn until favorable response seen.

- Clean eye area of excessive exudate before application.
- Ophth oint may be stored at room temp.

---

bacitracin
Baciguent, Bacitin†
Polypeptide antibiotic
Topical antibiotic
Preg. Risk Category: C

†Canadian, ‡Australian

Topical infections, abrasions, cuts, and minor burns or wounds — **Adults and children:** apply thin film qd to tid, depending on severity of condition. Don't use for > 1 wk.

- Clean area before applying.
- Anticipate alternative treatment for burns covering > 20% of body surface.
- Prolonged use may result in overgrowth of nonsusceptible organisms.

DRUG / CLASS / CATEGORY	INDICATIONS / DOSAGES	KEY NURSING CONSIDERATIONS
bacitracin Baciguent, Baci-IM, Bacitin† *Polypeptide antibiotic* *Systemic antibiotic* Preg. Risk Category: C	*Pneumonia or empyema caused by suscep-tible staphylococci* — **Infants > 2.5 kg:** 1,000 units/kg IM daily, divided q 8 to 12 hr. **Infants < 2.5 kg:** 900 units/kg IM daily, divided q 8 to 12 hr.	• Obtain culture and sensitivity tests before first dose. • Assess baseline renal function studies before and during therapy; monitor urine output. • Keep urine pH > 6.0.
baclofen Clofen†, Lioresal, Lioresal Intrathecal *Chlorphenyl derivative* *Skeletal muscle relaxant* Preg. Risk Category: C	*Spasticity in multiple sclerosis, spinal cord injury* — **Adults:** 5 mg PO tid for 3 days, then 10 mg tid for 3 days, 15 mg tid for 3 days, 20 mg tid for 3 days. Increase prn to max 80 mg daily. *Management of severe spasticity in patients who can't tolerate or don't respond to oral therapy* — **Adults:** *Test dose:* 1 ml of 50-mcg/ml dilution into intrathecal space by bar-botage over ≥ 1 min. If poor response, give 2nd test dose (75 mcg/1.5 ml) 24 hr after 1st. If poor response, give test dose (100 mcg/2 ml) 24 hr later. Patients unresponsive to final test dose shouldn't have implantable pump. Initial maintenance dose titrated based on screening-dose response. Effective dose doubled and given over 24 hr. If screening-dose efficacy maintained for ≥ 12 hr, don't double dose. After 1st 24 hr, increase dose slowly, prn and as tolerated, by 10% to 30% daily.	• With test doses, markedly decreased sever-ity or reduced frequency of spasms or reduced mus-cle tone should appear within 4 to 8 hr. • After test dose, give maintenance dose by implantable infusion pump. Most patients need 300 to 800 mcg daily. • Don't give orally to treat muscle spasm caused by rheumatic disorders, cerebral palsy, Parkinson's disease, or CVA; effica-cy not established. • Watch for sensitivity reactions, such as fever, skin eruptions, and respiratory dis-tress. • Observe for increased risk of seizures in patients with seizure disorder. • Amount of relief determines whether dosage can be reduced. • Don't withdraw abruptly after long-term use unless required by severe adverse re-actions; doing so may trigger hallucina-tions or rebound spasticity.

beclomethasone dipropionate

Becloforte Inhaler‡, Beclovent, Vanceril

Glucocorticoid
Anti-inflammatory/anti-asthmatic
Preg. Risk Category: C

Steroid-dependent asthma — **Adults and children ≥ 12 yr:** 2 inhalations tid or qid or 4 inhalations bid; max 20 inhalations daily (840 mcg). **Children 6 to 12 yr:** 1 to 2 inhalations tid or qid or 2 to 4 inhalations bid. Max 10 inhalations daily (420 mcg).

- Taper oral therapy slowly. Acute adrenal insufficiency and death have occurred in asthmatics who changed abruptly from oral corticosteroids to beclomethasone.
- Spacer device may ensure proper dose and decrease local (oral) adverse effects.
- Check mucous membranes frequently for signs of fungal infection.

beclomethasone dipropionate

Beconase AQ Nasal Spray, Beconase Nasal Inhaler, Vancenase AQ Nasal Spray, Vancenase Nasal Inhaler

Glucocorticoid
Anti-inflammatory
Preg. Risk Category: C

Relief of symptoms of seasonal or perennial rhinitis; prevention of recurrence of nasal polyps after surgical removal — **Adults and children > 12 yr:** usual dosage 1 or 2 sprays in each nostril bid, tid, or qid.

- Observe for fungal infections.
- Not effective for acute rhinitis exacerbations. Decongestants or antihistamines may be needed.

benazepril hydrochloride

Lotensin

ACE inhibitor
Antihypertensive
Preg. Risk Category: C (D in 2nd and 3rd trimesters)

Hypertension — **Adults:** in patients not receiving diuretics, 10 mg PO daily initially. Most patients receive 20 to 40 mg daily in 1 or 2 doses; patient receiving diuretic, 5 mg PO daily.

- Monitor for hypotension.
- Measure BP 2 to 6 hr after administration and just before next dose.
- Assess renal and hepatic function before and during therapy. Monitor serum potassium levels.

BENAZEPRIL HYDROCHLORIDE 35

DRUG/CLASS/ CATEGORY	INDICATIONS/ DOSAGES	KEY NURSING CONSIDERATIONS
benzonatate Tessalon *Local anesthetic (esther)* *Nonnarcotic antitussive agent* Preg. Risk Category: C	*Symptomatic relief of cough* — **Adults and children > 10 yr:** 100 mg PO tid; up to 600 mg daily may be needed.	• Don't give when cough is valuable diagnostic sign or is beneficial (as after thoracic surgery). • Monitor cough type and frequency. • Use with percussion and chest vibration.
benztropine mesylate Apo-Benztropine†, Bensylate†, Cogentin‡, PMS Benztropine† *Anticholinergic* *Antiparkinsonian agent* Preg. Risk Category: NR	*Drug-induced extrapyramidal disorders (except tardive dyskinesia)* — **Adults:** 1 to 4 mg PO or IM qd or bid. *Acute dystonic reaction* — **Adults:** 1 to 2 mg IV or IM, then 1 to 2 mg PO bid. *Parkinsonism* — **Adults:** 0.5 to 6 mg PO or IM daily. Initial dose 0.5 mg to 1 mg, increased by 0.5 mg q 5 to 6 days. Adjust dosage to meet individual requirements.	• Never discontinue abruptly. Reduce dosage gradually. • Monitor vital signs carefully. Watch for adverse reactions, especially in elderly or debilitated patients. • May aggravate tardive dyskinesia. • Watch for intermittent constipation and abdominal distention and pain; may indicate onset of paralytic ileus.
benzyl benzoate lotion Ascabiol‡ *Synthetic benzoic acid with benzyl alcohol* *Scabicide/pediculicide* Preg. Risk Category: C	*Parasitic infestation (scabies, P. pubis, P. humanus capitis)* — **Adults and children:** scrub entire body with soap and water. Remove scales or crusts. Apply lotion undiluted over affected area (include whole body for scabies), except face and scalp, while still damp. Be sure to apply around nails. Let dry. Apply 2nd coat on most involved areas. Instruct to bathe after 24 hr. May repeat treatment in 7 to 10 days if mites appear or new lesions develop.	• Place hospitalized patient in isolation, with linen-handling precautions, until treatment completed. • Don't apply to face, eyes, mucous membranes, or urethral meatus. If accidental contact with eyes occurs, flush with water and notify doctor. • Don't apply to infants' or small children's hands.

bepridil hydrochloride
Bepadin†, Vascor
Calcium channel blocker
Antianginal
Preg. Risk Category: C

Chronic stable angina in patients who can't tolerate or don't respond to other agents — **Adults:** initially, 200 mg PO daily. After 10 days, increase dosage based on response. Maintenance dosage in most patients 300 mg/day. Max 400 mg daily.

- Use cautiously in left bundle-branch block, sinus bradycardia, impaired renal or hepatic function, or heart failure.
- Monitor for adverse reactions. Can cause severe ventricular arrhythmias.
- Don't adjust dosage more often than every 10 to 14 days.

beractant (natural lung surfactant)
Survanta
Bovine lung extract
Lung surfactant
Preg. Risk Category: NR

Prevention of respiratory distress syndrome (RDS) in premature neonates weighing 1,250 g or less at birth or having symptoms of surfactant deficiency — **Neonates:** 4 ml/kg intratracheally; give each dose in 4 quarter-doses; in between, use hand-held resuscitation bag at rate of 60 breaths/min and sufficient O_2 to prevent cyanosis. Give within 15 min of birth, if possible. Repeat in 6 hr if respiratory distress continues. Give no more than 4 doses in 48 hr.

Rescue treatment of RDS in premature infants — **Neonates:** 4 ml/kg intratracheally; before giving, increase ventilator rate to 60 with inspiratory time of 0.5 sec and FiO_2 of 1. Give each dose in 4 quarter-doses; in between, continue ventilation for at least 30 sec or until stable. Give dose as soon as RDS confirmed. Repeat in 6 hr if distress continues. Give max 4 doses in 48 hr.

- Continuous monitoring of ECG and O_2 sat essential; frequent arterial BP monitoring and frequent ABG sampling highly desirable.
- Accurate weight determination essential to proper dosage measurements.
- Can rapidly affect oxygenation and lung compliance. May need to adjust peak ventilator inspiratory pressures if chest expansion improves markedly after administration. Notify doctor and adjust immediately as directed.
- Homogeneous drug distribution important.

DRUG/CLASS/ CATEGORY	INDICATIONS/ DOSAGES	KEY NURSING CONSIDERATIONS
betamethasone Betnesol‡, Celestone **betamethasone acetate and betamethasone sodium phosphate** Celestone Soluspan **betamethasone sodium phosphate** Celestone Phosphate *Glucocorticoid* *Anti-inflammatory* Preg. Risk Category: C	*Conditions with severe inflammation; conditions requiring immunosuppression* — **Adults:** 0.6 to 7.2 mg PO daily; or 0.5 to 9 mg IM, IV, or into joint or soft tissue daily. Betamethasone sodium phosphate-acetate susp 6 to 12 mg injected into large joints or 1.5 to 6 mg injected into smaller joints. May give both injections q 1 to 2 weeks, prn. *Note:* Betamethasone sodium phosphate and betamethasone acetate susp combination product should *not* be given IV.	▪ Don't use for alternate-day therapy. ▪ Obtain baseline weight before starting therapy and weigh daily; report sudden gain. ▪ For better results and less toxicity, give once-daily dose in morning. ▪ To reduce GI irritation, give with milk or food. ▪ Monitor blood glucose and serum potassium regularly, as ordered. Diabetics may require insulin dosage adjustments.
betamethasone dipropionate Alphatrex, Diprolene, Diprolene AF, Diprosone, Maxivate **betamethasone valerate** Betatrex, Beta-Val, Betnovate†‡, Valisone *Topical glucocorticoid* *Anti-inflammatory* Preg. Risk Category: C	*Inflammation associated with corticosteroid-responsive dermatoses* — **Adults and children:** clean area; apply cream, oint, lotion, or aerosol spray sparingly. Give dipropionate qd or bid; valerate qd to qid. Max dosage 45 g/wk for Diprolene cream, 50 ml/wk for Diprolene lotion.	▪ Gently wash skin before applying. Rub in gently, leaving thin coat. When treating hairy sites, part hair and apply directly to lesions. For patients with eczematous dermatitis, hold dressing in place with gauze, elastic bandage, stocking, or stockinette. ▪ Don't apply near eyes or mucous membranes or in ear canal. ▪ Notify doctor and remove occlusive dressing if fever, infection, striae, or atrophy occurs.

betaxolol hydrochloride
Kerlone
Beta-adrenergic blocker
Antihypertensive
Preg. Risk Category: C

Hypertension (used alone or with other antihypertensives) — **Adults:** initially, 10 mg PO qd; if necessary, 20 mg PO qd if desired response not achieved in 7 to 14 days.

- May mask tachycardia associated with hyperthyroidism. In suspected thyrotoxicosis, withdraw gradually, as ordered.
- Abrupt discontinuation may trigger angina pectoris in unrecognized CAD.
- Monitor BP closely.

betaxolol hydrochloride
Betoptic, Betoptic S, Kerlone
Beta-adrenergic blocker
Antiglaucoma agent
Preg. Risk Category: C

Chronic open-angle glaucoma and ocular hypertension — **Adults:** 1 or 2 drops of 0.5% sol or 0.25% susp bid.

- Wash hands before and after instilling. Apply light finger pressure on lacrimal sac for 1 min after instillation. Don't touch dropper tip to eye or surrounding tissue. Shake suspension well before instilling.
- Some patients may need several weeks of treatment to stabilize IOP-lowering response. Determine IOP after 4 wk.

bethanechol chloride
Duvoid, Myotonachol, Urabeth, Urecholine, Urocarb Tablets‡
Cholinergic agonist
Urinary tract and GI tract stimulant
Preg. Risk Category: C

Acute postop and postpartum nonobstructive (functional) urine retention, neurogenic atony of urinary bladder with urine retention — **Adults:** 10 to 50 mg PO tid to qid. Or 2.5 to 5 mg SC. Never give IM or IV. When used for urine retention, some patients may require 50 to 100 mg PO per dose. Use such doses with extreme caution. Test dose: 2.5 mg SC, repeated at 15- to 30-min intervals to total of 4 doses to determine minimal effective dose; then use minimal effective dose q 6 to 8 hr. All doses adjusted individually.

- Never give IM or IV.
- Give on empty stomach; otherwise, may cause nausea and vomiting.
- Monitor vital signs frequently, especially respirations. Always have atropine injection available. Provide respiratory support if needed.
- Watch for toxicity. Edrophonium ineffective against muscle relaxation caused by bethanechol.
- Inform that drug usually effective within 30 to 90 min after oral dose and 5 to 15 min after SC dose.

BETHANECHOL CHLORIDE   39

†Canadian ‡Australian

DRUG / CLASS / CATEGORY	INDICATIONS / DOSAGES	KEY NURSING CONSIDERATIONS
biperiden hydrochloride Akineton **biperiden lactate** Akineton Lactate *Anticholinergic Antiparkinsonian agent* Preg. Risk Category: C	*Drug-induced extrapyramidal disorders* — **Adults:** 2 mg PO qd, bid, or tid, depending on severity. Usual dosage 2 mg daily, or 2 mg IM or IV q ½ hr, not to exceed 4 doses or 8 mg daily. *Parkinsonism* — **Adults:** 2 mg PO tid or qid. Dosage individualized and titrated to max 16 mg/24 hr.	▪ *IV use:* Administer very slowly. Keep patient supine. ▪ Monitor vital signs carefully. ▪ Instruct to take oral form with or after meals. ▪ Warn to avoid activities that require alertness until CNS effects known. ▪ Advise to report signs of urinary hesitancy or urine retention.
bisacodyl Bisac-Evac, Carter's Little Pills, Dacodyl, Deficol, Dulcagen, Dulcolax‡, Durolax, Fleet Bisacodyl, Fleet Bisacodyl Prep, Fleet Laxative, Theralax *Diphenylmethane derivative Stimulant laxative* Preg. Risk Category: B	*Chronic constipation; preparation for delivery, surgery, or rectal or bowel examination* — **Adults and children > 12 yr:** 10 to 15 mg PO in evening or before breakfast. May give up to 30 mg PO or 10 mg PR for evacuation before examination or surgery. **Children 6 to 12 yr:** 5 mg PO or PR hs or before breakfast. Oral form not recommended if unable to swallow tablet whole.	▪ Soft, formed stools usually produced 15 to 60 min after PR administration. ▪ For constipation, determine if patient has adequate fluid intake, exercise, and diet. ▪ Avoid embedding supp in fecal material; may delay drug onset. ▪ Store tab and supp below 86° F (30° C). ▪ Don't give within 1 hr of milk or antacid intake. ▪ Discourage excessive use.
bismuth subsalicylate Bismatrol, Pepto-Bismol, Pink Bismuth *Adsorbent Antidiarrheal* Preg. Risk Category: NR	*Mild, nonspecific diarrhea* — **Adults:** 30 ml or 2 tabs PO q ½ to 1 hr, to max of 8 doses and for no longer than 2 days. **Children 3 to 6 yr:** 5 ml or ⅓ tab PO. **Children 6 to 9 yr:** 10 ml or ⅔ tab PO. **Children 9 to 12 yr:** 15 ml or 1 tab PO.	▪ Use cautiously in patients taking aspirin. ▪ Discontinue if tinnitus occurs. ▪ Avoid use before GI radiologic procedures (may interfere with X-rays).

bisoprolol fumarate
Zebeta
Beta-adrenergic blocker
Antihypertensive
Preg. Risk Category: C

Hypertension (used alone or in combination with other antihypertensives) — **Adults:** initially, 5 mg PO qd. If response inadequate, increase to 10 mg qd or to 20 mg PO daily if needed. Max recommended dosage 20 mg daily.

- Use cautiously in bronchospastic disease, diabetes, peripheral vascular disease, or thyroid disease and in history of heart failure.
- Monitor BP frequently.
- May mask hypoglycemia signs.

bitolterol mesylate
Tornalate
Adrenergic
Beta₂ agonist
Preg. Risk Category: C

To prevent or treat bronchial asthma and reversible bronchospasm — **Adults and children > 12 yr:** for bronchospasm, 2 inhalations given at interval of at least 1 to 3 min, then give third inhalation if needed. To prevent bronchospasm, usual dosage 2 inhalations q 8 hr. In either case, never exceed 3 inhalations q 6 hr or 2 inhalations q 4 hr.

- Use cautiously in ischemic heart disease or hypertension, hyperthyroidism, diabetes mellitus, arrhythmias, seizure disorders, and history of unusual responsiveness to beta-adrenergic agonists.
- Monitor BP regularly.
- Beneficial effects last up to 8 hr.
- Assist to perform oral inhalation correctly.

bleomycin sulfate
Blenoxane
Antibiotic/antineoplastic (cell cycle–phase specific, G2 and M phase)
Antineoplastic
Preg. Risk Category: D

Dosage and indications may vary.
Squamous cell carcinoma, lymphosarcoma, reticulum cell carcinoma, testicular carcinoma — **Adults:** 10 to 20 units/m² IV, IM, or SC once or twice weekly to total of 300 to 400 units.
Hodgkin's disease — **Adults:** 10 to 20 units/m² IV, IM, or SC once or twice/wk. After 50% response, maintenance dosage 1 unit IM or IV daily or 5 units IM or IV/wk.
Treatment of malignant pleural effusion; prevention of recurrent pleural effusions — **Adults:** 60 units given as single-dose bolus intrapleural injection.

- Obtain pulmonary function tests as ordered. Pulmonary toxic effects may increase in patients receiving radiation therapy.
- Watch for hypersensitivity reactions. May need to give test dose. Monitor for fever, which may be treated with antipyretics.
- Reconstitute per manufacturer's labeling. Administer IV infusion over 10 min.

BLEOMYCIN SULFATE   41

DRUG / CLASS / CATEGORY	INDICATIONS / DOSAGES	KEY NURSING CONSIDERATIONS
bretylium tosylate Bretylate†‡, Bretylol, Critifib‡ *Adrenergic blocker Ventricular antiarrhythmic* Preg. Risk Category: C	*Ventricular fibrillation or hemodynamically unstable ventricular tachycardia unresponsive to other antiarrhythmics* — **Adults:** 5 mg/kg IV push over 1 min. If necessary, increase dose to 10 mg/kg and repeat q 15 to 30 min until 30 to 35 mg/kg given. For continuous suppression, diluted solution given at 1 to 2 mg/min continuously or 5 to 10 mg/kg diluted over more than 8 min q 6 hr.	• To prevent nausea and vomiting, follow dosage directions carefully. • Keep patient supine until tolerance to hypotension develops. • Monitor patient closely for transient hypertension and arrhythmias. • Monitor BP and HR continuously. • Observe susceptible patients for increased anginal pain.
bromocriptine mesylate Parlodel *Dopamine receptor agonist Semisynthetic ergot alkaloid/dopaminergic agonist/antiparkinsonian agent/inhibitor of prolactin release/inhibitor of growth hormone release* Preg. Risk Category: NR	*Amenorrhea and galactorrhea associated with hyperprolactinemia; female infertility* — **Adults:** 1.25 to 2.5 mg PO daily, increased by 2.5 mg daily at 3- to 7-day intervals until desired effect achieved. Therapeutic dosage range 2.5 to 15 mg/day. Safety and efficacy of doses > 100 mg daily not established. *Parkinson's disease* — **Adults:** 1.25 mg PO bid with meals. Increase dosage q 14 to 28 days, up to 100 mg daily, prn. *Acromegaly* — **Adults:** 1.25 to 2.5 mg PO with snack hs for 3 days. Additional 1.25 to 2.5 mg may be added q 3 to 7 days until benefit obtained. Max 100 mg/day.	• Monitor for adverse reactions. Incidence of such reactions high, especially at start of therapy; however, most are mild to moderate, with nausea being most common. • For Parkinson's disease, usually given in conjunction with levodopa or carbidopa-levodopa. • Give with meals. • May lead to early postpartum conception. Test for pregnancy every 4 wk or whenever period missed after menses resume.

brompheniramine maleate	*Rhinitis, allergy symptoms* — **Adults:** 4 to 8 mg PO tid or qid; or 8 to 12 mg ext-release PO bid or tid. Max oral dosage 24 mg daily. Or, 5 to 20 mg q 6 to 12 hr IM, IV, or SC. Max parenteral dosage 40 mg daily. **Children 6 to 12 yr:** 2 to 4 mg PO tid or qid; or 8 to 12 mg ext-release PO q 12 hr; or 0.5 mg/kg IM, IV, or SC daily in divided doses tid or qid. **Children < 6 yr:** 0.5 mg/kg PO, IM, IV, or SC daily in divided doses tid or qid.	• *IV use:* Can give injectable form containing 10 mg/ml diluted or undiluted very slowly IV. • Don't give 100 mg/ml injection IV. • Monitor blood count during long-term therapy, as ordered; observe for blood dyscrasias. • Children < 12 yr should use only as directed by doctor.
Bromphen, Chlorphed, Codimal-A, Dimetane, Veltane *Alkylamine antihistamine* *Antihistamine (H₁-receptor antagonist)* Preg. Risk Category: C		
budesonide	*Symptoms of seasonal or perennial allergic rhinitis* — **Adults and children ≥ 6 yr:** 2 sprays in each nostril in morning and evening, or 4 sprays in each nostril in morning. Maintenance dosage should be fewest number of sprays needed to control symptoms.	• Instruct to avoid exposure to chickenpox or measles. • Don't break or incinerate canister or store in extreme heat.
Rhinocort *Glucocorticoid* *Anti-inflammatory* Preg. Risk Category: C		
bumetanide	*Edema in heart failure or hepatic or renal disease* — **Adults:** 0.5 to 2 mg PO qd. If diuretic response inadequate, may give 2nd or 3rd dose at 4- to 5-hr intervals. Max 10 mg/day. May be given IV or IM if PO not feasible. Usual initial dose 0.5 to 1 mg, given IV or IM. If response inadequate, may give 2nd or 3rd dose at 2- to 3-hr intervals. Max 10 mg/day.	*IV use:* Give direct IV doses over 1 to 2 min. For intermittent infusion, give diluted at ordered rate. • Intermittent dosage is safest and most effective way to control edema. • Monitor I&O, weight, BP, pulse, O₂, and serum electrolyte, BUN, creatinine, glucose, and uric acid levels. • Watch for signs of hypokalemia.
Bumex, Burinex‡ *Loop diuretic* *Diuretic* Preg. Risk Category: C		

DRUG / CLASS / CATEGORY	INDICATIONS / DOSAGES	KEY NURSING CONSIDERATIONS
bupropion hydrochloride Wellbutrin *Aminoketone* *Antidepressant* Preg. Risk Category: B	*Depression* — **Adults:** initially, 100 mg PO bid, increased after 3 days to 100 mg PO tid if needed. If no response after several weeks of therapy, increase to 150 mg tid. No single dose should exceed 150 mg.	▪ May cause agitation, insomnia, or anxiety. ▪ To minimize risk of seizure, don't exceed 450 mg/day, and give daily dosage in 3 to 4 equally divided doses. ▪ Closely monitor patients with history of bipolar disorders.
buspirone hydrochloride BuSpar *Azaspirodecanedione derivative* *Antianxiety agent* Preg. Risk Category: B	*Anxiety disorders; short-term relief of anxiety* — **Adults:** initially, 5 mg PO tid, increased at 3-day intervals in 5-mg increments. Usual maintenance dosage 20 to 30 mg daily in divided doses. Don't exceed 60 mg daily.	▪ Monitor closely for adverse CNS reactions. ▪ Less sedating than other antianxiety agents. ▪ Has shown no potential for abuse. ▪ Before initiating in patient also receiving benzodiazepines, warn against stopping benzodiazepines abruptly; withdrawal reaction may occur.
busulfan Myleran *Alkylating agent (cell cycle–phase nonspecific)* *Antineoplastic* Preg. Risk Category: D	*Chronic myelocytic (granulocytic) leukemia* — **Adults:** 4 to 8 mg PO daily, up to 12 mg PO daily, until WBC count falls to 15,000/mm³; drug stopped until WBC count rises to 50,000/mm³, and then resumed as before; or 4 to 8 mg PO daily until WBC count falls to 10,000 to 20,000/mm³; then daily dosage reduced as needed to maintain WBC count at this level (usually 1 to 3 mg daily). **Children:** 0.06 to 0.12 mg/kg/day or 1.8 to 4.6 mg/m²/day PO; dosage adjusted	▪ To prevent bleeding, avoid all IM injections when platelet count < 100,000/mm³. ▪ Monitor patient response (increased appetite and sense of well-being, decreased total WBC count, reduced spleen size), which usually begins within 1 to 2 wk. ▪ Monitor serum uric acid. To prevent hyperuricemia with resulting uric acid nephropathy, allopurinol may be ordered. Keep patient adequately hydrated. ▪ Anticipate possible blood transfusion.

- to maintain WBC count at 20,000/mm^3, but never less than 10,000/mm^3.

- Pulmonary fibrosis may occur as late as 8 mo to 10 yr after treatment.
- Toxicity can accompany therapeutic effects.

---

butoconazole nitrate
Femstat
Synthetic imidazole derivative
Topical fungistat
Preg. Risk Category: C

Vulvovaginal mycotic infections caused by Candida species — **Adults:** for nonpregnant patient, 1 applicatorful intravaginally hs for 3 days. If needed, treat for another 3 days. For pregnant patient during 2nd or 3rd trimester, 1 applicatorful intravaginally hs for 6 days.

- Confirm diagnosis by smears or cultures, as ordered.
- May be used with oral contraceptives and antibiotic therapy.

---

butorphanol tartrate
Stadol, Stadol NS
Narcotic agonist-antagonist, opioid partial agonist
Analgesic/adjunct to anesthesia
Preg. Risk Category: C

Moderate to severe pain — **Adults:** 1 to 4 mg IM q 3 to 4 hr, prn or around the clock; or 0.5 to 2 mg IV q 3 to 4 hr, prn or around the clock. Not to exceed 4 mg per dose. Alternatively, 1 mg by nasal spray q 3 to 4 hr (1 spray in one nostril); repeated in 60 to 90 min if pain relief inadequate.
Preoperative anesthesia or preanesthesia — **Adults:** 2 mg IM 60 to 90 min before surgery.

- Periodically monitor postop vital signs and bladder function.
- Respiratory depression apparently doesn't increase with larger dosage.
- Psychological and physical addiction may occur.

C

calcifediol
Calderol
Vitamin D analogue/Anti-hypocalcemic
hypocalcemic
Preg. Risk Category: C

Metabolic bone disease and hypocalcemia associated with chronic renal failure — **Adults:** initially, 300 to 350 mcg PO weekly. Dosage may be increased at 4-wk intervals.

- Monitor serum calcium level; during titration, at least weekly.
- If hypercalcemia occurs, discontinue calcifediol and notify doctor.

DRUG / CLASS / CATEGORY	INDICATIONS / DOSAGES	KEY NURSING CONSIDERATIONS
calcipotriene Dovonex *Synthetic vitamin D₃ analogue* *Topical antipsoriatic* Preg. Risk Category: C	*Moderate plaque psoriasis* — **Adults:** apply thin layer to affected area bid. Rub in gently and completely.	• Use cautiously in elderly patients; they may have more severe adverse skin reactions. • Advise to apply thin layer of ointment to avoid transient elevations of serum calcium. • Advise not to use drug on face, in eyes, orally, or vaginally.
calcitonin (human) Cibacalcin **calcitonin (salmon)** Calcimar, Miacalcin, Miacalcin Nasal Spray, Salmonine, Osteocalcin *Thyroid hormone* *Hypocalcemic* Preg. Risk Category: C	*Paget's disease of bone (osteitis deformans)* — **Adults:** 100 IU of calcitonin (salmon) qd SC or IM; maintenance dosage is 50 to 100 IU qd or qod. Or, calcitonin (human) 0.5 mg 2 or 3 times weekly or 0.25 mg qd, up to 0.5 mg bid. *Hypercalcemia* — **Adults:** 4 IU/kg of calcitonin (salmon) q 12 hr IM. If poor response after 1 or 2 days, increase to 8 IU/kg IM q 12 hr. If response remains poor after 2 more days, increase to max 8 IU/kg IM q 6 hr. *Postmenopausal osteoporosis* — **Adults:** 100 IU of calcitonin (salmon) qd IM or SC. Or, 200 IU (1 activation) of calcitonin (salmon) qd intranasally, alternating nostrils qd.	• Skin test usually done before therapy. • Systemic allergic reactions possible. Keep epinephrine handy. • Administer at bedtime. • Use reconstituted sol within 2 hr. • Observe for signs of hypocalcemic tetany. • Monitor serum calcium, alkaline phosphatase, and 24-hr urine hydroxyproline closely. • Store calcitonin (human) at room temperature; refrigerate calcitonin (salmon). • Facial flushing and warmth may occur within min of injection and usually last about 1 hr.
calcitriol (1,25-dihydroxy-cholecalciferol)	*Hypocalcemia in patients undergoing chronic dialysis* — **Adults:** 0.25 mcg PO qd. Increased by 0.25 mcg qd q 4 to 8 wk.	• Monitor serum calcium level; during titration, twice weekly. Discontinue if hypercalcemia occurs and notify doctor. • Protect from heat and light.

Maintenance is 0.25 mcg qod, up to 1.25 mcg qd.

Hypoparathyroidism and pseudohypoparathyroidism — **Adults and children > 6 yr:** 0.25 mcg PO daily. May be increased at 2- to 4-wk intervals. Maintenance, 0.25 to 2 mcg daily.

Hypoparathyroidism — **Children 1 to 6 yr:** 0.25 to 0.75 mcg PO daily.

- Tell the patient to immediately report weakness, nausea, vomiting, dry mouth, constipation, muscle or bone pain, or metallic taste.
- Drug not to be taken by anyone without a prescription for it.

Calcijex, Delta D, Rocaltrol
Vitamin D analogue
Antihypocalcemic
Preg. Risk Category: C

calcium acetate
Phos-Ex, PhosLo
calcium carbonate
Calcarb 600, CalCarb-HD, Calci-Chew, Os-Cal 500, Rolaids Calcium Rich, Tums
calcium chloride
calcium citrate
Citrical
calcium glubionate
Neo-Calglucon
calcium gluceptate
calcium gluconate
Kalcinate
calcium lactate
calcium phosphate, dibasic
calcium phosphate, tribasic

Hypocalcemic emergency — **Adults:** 7 to 14 mEq calcium IV (as 10% gluconate sol, 2% to 10% chloride sol, or 22% gluceptate sol). **Children:** 1 to 7 mEq calcium IV. **Infants:** up to 1 mEq calcium IV.

Hypocalcemic tetany — **Adults:** 4.5 to 16 mEq calcium IV. Repeat until controlled. **Children:** 0.5 to 0.7 mEq/kg calcium IV 3 to 4 times/day until controlled. **Neonates:** 2.4 mEq/kg IV qid in divided doses.

Adjunctive treatment of cardiac arrest — **Adults:** 0.027 to 0.054 mEq/kg calcium chloride IV, 4.5 to 6.3 mEq calcium gluceptate IV, or 2.3 to 3.7 mEq calcium gluconate IV. **Children:** 0.27 mEq/kg calcium chloride IV. May repeat in 10 min; check serum calcium before administering further doses.

Adjunctive treatment of magnesium intoxication — **Adults:** initially, 7 mEq IV. Subsequent doses based on response.

- Use all calcium products with extreme caution in patients with sarcoidosis and renal or cardiac disease, and in digitalized patients.
- Warm solutions to body temperature before administration.
- *IV use (direct injection):* Give slowly through small needle into large vein or IV line with free-flowing, compatible sol at max 1 ml/min (1.5 mEq/min) for chloride, 1.5 to 5 ml/min for gluconate, and 2 ml/min for gluceptate. Don't use scalp veins. *(intermittent infusion):* Infuse diluted sol through IV line with compatible sol at max rate of 200 mg/min for gluceptate and gluconate.
- Give chloride and gluconate IV only. Use in-line filter.

(continued)

CALCIUM ACETATE   47

DRUG/CLASS/ CATEGORY	INDICATIONS/ DOSAGES	KEY NURSING CONSIDERATIONS
calcium *(continued)* Posture *Calcium supplement* *Therapeutic agent for electrolyte balance/cardiotonic* Preg. Risk Category: C	*During exchange transfusions* — **Adults:** 1.35 mEq IV concurrently with each 100 ml citrated blood. **Neonates:** 0.45 mEq IV after each 100 ml citrated blood. *Hyperphosphatemia* — **Adults:** 1,334 to 2,000 mg PO acetate tid with meals. Dialysis patients need 3 to 4 tabs with meals. *Dietary supplement* — **Adults:** 500 mg to 2 g PO daily	▪ Drug will precipitate if given IV with alkaline drugs. ▪ Monitor ECG when giving calcium IV. Stop for complaints of discomfort, and notify doctor. Following IV injection, patient should remain recumbent for 15 min. ▪ Ensure that doctor specifies form of calcium to be used. ▪ Monitor blood calcium levels frequently. ▪ Severe necrosis and tissue sloughing can occur after extravasation.
calcium carbonate Alka-Mints, Rolaids Calcium Rich, Tums *Calcium supplement* *Therapeutic agent for electrolyte balance* Preg. Risk Category: NR	*Antacid, calcium supplement* — **Adults:** 350 mg to 1.5 g PO or 2 pieces of chewing gum 1 hr after meals and hs, prn.	▪ Watch for nausea, vomiting, headache, mental confusion, and anorexia. ▪ Monitor serum calcium. ▪ Record amt and consistency of stools. ▪ Tell patient to shake suspension and take with small amount of water.
calcium polycarbophil Equalactin, Fiberall, FiberCon, FiberLax, FiberNorm *Hydrophilic agent* *Bulk laxative/antidiarrheal* Preg. Risk Category: NR	*Constipation; diarrhea associated with irritable bowel syndrome, as well as acute nonspecific diarrhea* — **Adults:** 1 g PO qid prn. Max 6 g in 24-hr period. **2 to 6 yr:** as directed by doctor. 500 mg PO bid prn. Max 1.5 g in 24-hr period. **6 to 12 yr:** 500 mg PO qd to tid prn. Max 3 g in 24-hr period.	▪ Before giving for constipation, determine if patient has adequate fluid intake, exercise, and diet. ▪ Rectal bleeding or failure to respond to therapy may indicate need for surgery.

capsaicin

Axsain, Zostrix, Zostrix-HP 0.075%

Naturally occurring non-enamide

Topical analgesic

Preg. Risk Category: NR

Temporary relief of pain after herpes zoster infections, neuralgias, pain associated with osteoarthritis or rheumatoid arthritis —

Adults and children > 2 years: apply to affected areas not more than qid.

- For external use only.
- Warn to avoid getting drug in eyes or on broken skin.
- Advise not to bandage area tightly after application.

captopril

Apo-Capto†, Capoten, Novo-Captopril†, Syn-Captopril†

ACE inhibitor

Antihypertensive/adjunctive treatment of heart failure

Preg. Risk Category: C (D in 2nd and 3rd trimesters)

Hypertension — **Adults:** 25 mg PO bid or tid initially. If BP not controlled in 1 to 2 wk, increase to 50 mg bid or tid. If BP not controlled after another 1 to 2 wk, expect to add diuretic. If further BP reduction needed, may increase dosage to 150 mg tid while continuing diuretic. Max 450 mg daily.

Heart failure; to reduce risk of death and to slow development of heart failure after MI — **Adults:** 6.25 to 12.5 mg PO tid initially. Gradually increase to 50 mg tid prn. Max 450 mg daily.

- Monitor BP and HR frequently.
- Elderly patients may be more sensitive to hypotensive effects.
- In impaired renal function or collagen vascular disease, monitor WBC and differential before treatment starts and every 2 wk for first 3 mo of therapy.
- Take cap 1 hr before meals because food in GI tract may reduce absorption.
- Inform that dizziness may occur during first few days of therapy.

carbachol (intraocular)

Miostat

carbachol (topical)

Isopto Carbachol

Cholinergic agonist

Miotic

Preg. Risk Category: C

To produce pupillary miosis during ocular surgery — **Adults:** before or after securing sutures, doctor gently instills 0.5 ml (intraocular form) into anterior chamber.

Open-angle glaucoma — **Adults:** 1 to 2 drops instilled (topical form) q 4 to 8 hr.

- In case of toxicity, give atropine parenterally.
- Patients with dark eyes may require stronger solutions or more frequent instillation.
- Warn to avoid hazardous activities until temporary blurring subsides.

DRUG/CLASS/ CATEGORY	INDICATIONS/ DOSAGES	KEY NURSING CONSIDERATIONS
carbamazepine Apo-Carbamazepine†, Epitol, Mazepine†, Novocarbamaz†, Tegretol *Iminostilbene derivative; chemically related to TCAs* *Anticonvulsant/analgesic* Preg. Risk Category: C	*Generalized tonic-clonic and complex partial seizures, mixed seizure patterns* — **Adults and children > 12 yr:** 200 mg PO bid for tab or 1 tsp susp PO qid. Increase at weekly intervals by 200 mg PO qd, in divided doses at 6- to 8-hr intervals. Adjust to min. effective level. Max 1 g/day in ages 12 to 15 or 1.2 g/day in patients > age 15. **Children 6 to 12 yr:** 100 mg PO bid or ½ tsp of susp PO qid. Increase weekly by 100 mg PO qd. Max 1 g/day.	▪ Therapeutic blood level 4 to 12 mcg/ml. ▪ Observe for appetite changes. ▪ Monitor UA, BUN, LFTs, CBC, platelet and reticulocyte counts, and serum iron level. ▪ Institute seizure precautions. ▪ When giving by NG tube, mix with equal volume water, 0.9% NaCl solution, or D₅W. Then flush with 100 ml diluent. ▪ Warn not to discontinue suddenly. Tell to notify doctor immediately if adverse reactions occur.
carbamide peroxide Debrox *Urea hydrogen peroxide* *Ceruminolytic/topical antiseptic* Preg. Risk Category: NR	*Impacted cerumen* — **Adults and children:** 5 to 10 drops into ear canal bid for up to 4 days. Allow to remain in ear canal for 15 to 30 min; remove with warm water.	▪ Use in children < 12 years only under a doctor's direction. ▪ Tell patient to flush ear gently with warm water, using a rubber bulb syringe. ▪ Tell patient to call doctor if redness, pain, or swelling persists.
carbenicillin indanyl sodium Geocillin, Geopen Oral‡ *Ext.-spectrum penicillin* *Antibiotic* Preg. Risk Category: B	*UTI caused by susceptible strains of gram-neg organisms* — **Adults:** 382 to 764 mg PO qid for 10 days or longer. *Prostatitis caused by susceptible strains of gram-neg organisms* — **Adults:** 764 mg PO qid for 2 to 4 wk or longer.	▪ Before giving, ask about previous allergic reactions to penicillin. ▪ Obtain specimen for culture and sensitivity tests before first dose. ▪ Used only in patients with creatinine clearance ≥ 10 ml/min.

carbidopa-levodopa
Sinemet, Sinemet CR
Decarboxylase inhibitor-dopamine precursor
Antiparkinsonian agent
Preg. Risk Category: NR

Idiopathic Parkinson's disease, postencephalitic parkinsonism, and symptomatic parkinsonism resulting from carbon monoxide or manganese intoxication — **Adults:** 1 tab 25 mg carbidopa/100 mg levodopa PO tid, then increase by 1 tab qd or qod prn to max 8 tab daily. 25 mg carbidopa/250 mg levodopa or 10 mg carbidopa/100 mg levodopa tab substituted as required to obtain max response. Optimum dosage determined by individual titration. Patients treated with conventional tab may receive ext-release tab; dosage calculated on current levodopa intake. Initially, ext-release tab dosage should amount to 10% more levodopa per day, increased as needed and tolerated to 30% more levodopa per day. Give in divided doses at intervals of 4 to 8 hr.

- Muscle twitching and blepharospasm may be early signs of overdose.
- Levodopa should be discontinued at least 8 hr before starting carbidopa-levodopa.
- Therapeutic and adverse reactions more rapid with carbidopa-levodopa than levodopa alone. Monitor vital signs, especially while adjusting dosage.
- With long-term therapy, patient should be tested regularly for diabetes and acromegaly and have periodic tests of liver, renal, and hematopoietic function.

carboplatin
Paraplatin, Paraplatin-AQ†
Alkylating agent
Antineoplastic
Preg. Risk Category: D

Palliative treatment of ovarian cancer — **Adults:** 360 mg/m² IV on day 1 q 4 weeks; doses not repeated until platelet count > 100,000/mm³ and neutrophil count > 2,000/mm³. Subsequent dosages based on blood counts. Adjust dosage in renal failure and for creatinine clearance < 60 ml/min.

- Check serum electrolyte, creatinine, BUN, CBC, and creatinine clearance before first infusion and each course of treatment.
- IV form associated with mutagenic, teratogenic, and carcinogenic risks for personnel. Have emergency drugs available when administering drug.
- Do not use needles or IV administration sets containing aluminum to administer drug.
- Monitor vital signs during infusion.

CARBOPLATIN

51

DRUG / CLASS / CATEGORY	INDICATIONS / DOSAGES	KEY NURSING CONSIDERATIONS
carisoprodol Rela, Sodol, Soma, Soprodol, Soridol *Carbamate derivative Skeletal muscle relaxant* Preg. Risk Category: NR	*As adjunct in acute, painful musculoskeletal conditions* — **Adults:** 350 mg PO tid and hs.	• Watch for idiosyncratic reactions after first to fourth dose (weakness, ataxia, visual and speech difficulties, fever, skin eruptions, and mental changes) and for severe reactions (including bronchospasm, hypotension, and anaphylactic shock). • Record amount of relief to help determine whether dosage can be reduced. • Don't stop drug abruptly.
carmustine (BCNU) BiCNU *Alkylating agent Antineoplastic* Preg. Risk Category: D	*Brain tumors, Hodgkin's disease, malignant lymphoma, and multiple myeloma* — **Adults:** 75 to 100 mg/m² IV by slow infusion daily for 2 days; repeated q 6 wk if platelet count is > 100,000/mm³ and WBC count is > 4,000/mm³. Dosage reduced by 30% when WBC count is 2,000 to 3,000/mm³ and platelet count falls. Or, 150 to 200 mg/m² IV by slow infusion as a single dose, repeated q 6 weeks.	• Parenteral form associated with carcinogenic, mutagenic, and teratogenic risks for personnel. • Dilute solution with 27 ml of sterile water for injection. Resultant solution contains 3.3 mg of carmustine/ml in 10% alcohol. Dilute in 0.9% NaCl solution or D₅W for IV infusion. Give at least 250 ml over 1 to 2 hr. • Monitor CBC, uric acid and liver, renal, and pulmonary function tests periodically.
carteolol Cartrol *Beta-adrenergic blocker Antihypertensive* Preg. Risk Category: C	*Hypertension* — **Adults:** initially, 2.5 mg PO as single daily dose; increase gradually to 5 or 10 mg as single daily dose as needed. Dosages > 10 mg daily don't produce greater response (may actually decrease response).	• Monitor BP frequently. • May inhibit glycogenolysis and hypoglycemia signs and symptoms. • May mask tachycardia associated with hyperthyroidism. • Patients with unrecognized CAD may experience angina pectoris on withdrawal

carteolol hydrochloride
Ocupress Ophthalmic Solution, 1%
Beta adrenergic blocker
Antihypertensive
Preg. Risk Category: C

Chronic open-angle glaucoma, intraocular hypertension — **Adults:** 1 drop bid in conjunctival sac of affected eye.

- Discontinue drug at first sign of cardiac failure and notify doctor.
- If signs of serious adverse reactions or hypersensitivity occur, tell patient to discontinue drug and notify doctor immediately.

---

cascara sagrada
cascara sagrada aromatic fluidextract
cascara sagrada fluidextract
Anthraquinone glycoside mixture
Laxative
Preg. Risk Category: C

Acute constipation; preparation for bowel or rectal exam — **Adults and children ≥ 12 yr:** one 325-mg tablet of cascara sagrada PO qd; 200 to 400 mg of cascara sagrada extract PO qd; 0.5 to 1.5 ml of cascara sagrada fluidextract PO qd or 5 ml of aromatic cascara fluidextract PO qd. **Children < 2 yr:** one-quarter adult dosage. **Children 2 to 12 yr:** one-half adult dosage.

- Before giving for constipation, determine if fluid intake, exercise, and diet are adequate.
- Monitor serum electrolytes.
- Aromatic fluidextract less active and less bitter than nonaromatic fluidextract.

---

cefaclor
Ceclor
Second-generation cephalosporin
Antibiotic
Preg. Risk Category: B

Respiratory, urinary tract, skin, or soft-tissue infections and otitis media caused by susceptible organisms — **Adults:** 250 to 500 mg PO q 8 hr. For pharyngitis or otitis media, may give daily dosage in 2 equally divided doses q 12 hr. **Children:** 20 mg/kg daily PO in divided doses q 8 hr. For pharyngitis or otitis media, may give daily dosage in 2 equally divided doses q 12 hr. In more serious infections, 40 mg/kg daily recommended, not to exceed 1 g daily.

- Obtain specimens for culture and sensitivity test before first dose.
- With large doses or prolonged therapy, monitor for superinfection, especially in high-risk patients.
- Store reconstituted suspension in refrigerator for up to 14 days. Shake well before using.
- Tell doctor to call if rash occurs.

CEFACLOR   53

DRUG / CLASS / CATEGORY	INDICATIONS / DOSAGES	KEY NURSING CONSIDERATIONS
cefadroxil monohydrate Duricef, Ultracef *First-generation cephalosporin Antibiotic* Preg. Risk Category: B	*UTI, skin and soft-tissue infections, and pharyngitis or tonsillitis caused by susceptible organisms —* **Adults:** 1 to 2 g PO daily, depending on infection type. Usually given qd or bid. **Children:** 30 mg/kg PO daily in 2 divided doses q 12 hr.	• Obtain specimen for culture and sensitivity tests before first dose. • With large doses or prolonged therapy, monitor for superinfection, especially in high-risk patients. • Instruct to take with food or milk. • Advise to call doctor if rash occurs.
cefazolin sodium Ancef, Kefzol, Zolicef *First-generation cephalosporin Antibiotic* Preg. Risk Category: B	*Prophylaxis in contaminated surgery —* **Adults:** 1 g IM or IV 30 to 60 min before surgery; then 0.5 to 1 g IM or IV q 6 to 8 hr for 24 hr. In operations > 2 hr, may give another 0.5 to 1 g IM intraoperatively. Where infection would be devastating, prophylaxis may continue 3 to 5 days. *Respiratory, biliary, GU, skin, soft-tissue, bone and joint infections; septicemia; endocarditis caused by susceptible organisms —* **Adults:** 250 mg IM or IV q 8 hr to 1.5 g PO q 6 hr. Max 12 g/day in life-threatening situations. **Children >1 mo:** 25 to 50 mg/kg or 1.25 g/m² daily IM or IV in 3 or 4 divided doses. May increase to 100 mg/kg/day.	• Obtain specimen for culture and sensitivity tests before first dose. • **IV use:** Reconstitute with diluent: 2 ml to 500-mg vial; 2.5 ml to 1-g vial. Shake until dissolved. Resultant concentration: 225 mg/ml or 330 mg/ml, respectively. For direct injection, dilute Ancef with 5 ml or Kefzol with 10 ml of sterile water for injection. Inject into large vein or tubing of free-flowing IV solution over 3 to 5 min. For intermittent infusion, add reconstituted drug to 50 to 100 ml of compatible solution or use premixed solution. • With large doses or prolonged therapy, monitor for superinfection.

cefepime hydrochloride
Maxipime
Semisynthetic cephalosporin
Antibiotic
Preg. Risk Category: B

Mild to moderate UTI caused by susceptible organisms. — **Adults and children ≥ 12 yr:** 0.5 to 1 g IM (IM used only for infections caused by *E. coli*) or I.V infused over 30 min q 12 hr for 7 to 10 days.
Severe UTI — **Adults and children ≥ 12 yr:** 2 g IV infused over 30 min q 12 hr for 10 days.
Moderate to severe pneumonia — **Adults and children ≥ 12 yr:** 1 to 2 g IV infused over 30 min q 12 hr for 10 days.

- Obtain specimens for culture and sensitivity tests before first dose, if appropriate.
- **IV use**: Give resulting solution over about 30 min.
- Monitor PT as ordered. Give exogenous vitamin K as ordered.
- Monitor for superinfection.
- Instruct to report adverse reactions promptly.

cefmetazole sodium (cefmetazone)
Zefazone
Second-generation cephalosporin
Antibiotic
Preg. Risk Category: B

Lower respiratory tract, intra-abdominal, skin, and skin-structure infections caused by susceptible organisms — **Adults:** 2 g IV q 6 to 12 hr for 5 to 14 days.
UTIs caused by E. coli — **Adults:** 2 g IV q 12 hr.

- Obtain specimen for culture and sensitivity tests before first dose.
- Monitor for superinfection.
- Monitor PT in patients at risk from renal or hepatic impairment, malnutrition, or prolonged therapy.
- Advise to report adverse reactions promptly.

cefonicid sodium
Monocid
Second-generation cephalosporin
Antibiotic
Preg. Risk Category: B

Periop prophylaxis in contaminated surgery — **Adults:** 1 g IM or IV 30 to 60 min before surgery; then 1 g IM or IV daily for 2 days after surgery. If used for prophylaxis in cesarean section, 1 g IM or IV after umbilical cord is clamped.
Serious infections of lower respiratory and urinary tracts, skin and skin-structure infections, septicemia, bone and joint infections, and preoperative prophylaxis — **Adults:** usual dosage 1 g IV or IM q 24 hr; in life-threatening infections, 2 g q 24 hr.

- Obtain specimen for culture and sensitivity tests before first dose.
- With large doses or prolonged therapy, monitor for superinfection.
- For IM use, when giving 2-g IM doses qd, divide dose equally and inject deeply into large muscle mass, such as gluteus maximus or lateral aspect of thigh.

CEFONICID SODIUM   55

DRUG / CLASS / CATEGORY	INDICATIONS / DOSAGES	KEY NURSING CONSIDERATIONS
cefoperazone sodium Cefobid *Third-generation cephalosporin* *Antibiotic* Preg. Risk Category: B	*Serious respiratory tract infections; intra-abdominal, gyn, and skin infections; bacteremia; and septicemia caused by susceptible organisms* — **Adults:** usual dosage 1 to 2 g q 12 hr IM or IV. In severe infections or infections caused by less sensitive organisms, total daily dosage or frequency may increase to 16 g/day in certain situations.	▪ Give doses of 4 g/day cautiously in hepatic disease or biliary obstruction. ▪ Obtain specimen for culture and sensitivity tests before first dose. ▪ With large doses or prolonged therapy, monitor for superinfection. ▪ Monitor PT regularly. Vitamin K promptly reverses bleeding. ▪ For IM use, inject deeply into large muscle mass.
cefotaxime sodium Claforan *Third-generation cephalosporin* *Antibiotic* Preg. Risk Category: B	*Periop prophylaxis in contaminated surgery* — **Adults:** 1 g IM or IV 30 to 60 min before surgery. For cesarean section, 1 g IM or IV as soon as umbilical cord clamped, then 1 g IM or IV 6 and 12 hr later. *Serious infection of lower respiratory and urinary tracts, CNS, skin, bone, and joints; gyn and intra-abdominal infections; bacteremia; and septicemia caused by susceptible organisms* — **Adults:** usual dose 1 g IV or IM q 6 to 8 hr. Up to 12 g daily can be given in life-threatening infections. **Children ≥ 50 kg:** usual adult dose, but don't exceed 12 g daily. **Children 1 mo to 12 yr weighing < 50 kg:** 50 to 180 mg/kg/day IM or IV in 4	▪ Obtain specimen for culture and sensitivity tests before first dose. ▪ **IV use:** Inject into large vein or into tubing of free-flowing IV solution over 3 to 5 min. For infusion, infuse over 20 to 30 min. ▪ For IM use, inject deeply into large muscle mass, such as gluteus maximus or lateral aspect of thigh. ▪ With large doses or prolonged therapy, monitor for superinfection. ▪ Advise to report adverse reactions promptly.

	to 6 divided doses. **Neonates to 1 wk:** 50 mg/kg IV q 12 hr. **Neonates 1 to 4 wk:** 50 mg/kg IV q 8 hr
cefotetan disodium Cefotan *Second-generation cephalosporin/cephamycin* *Antibiotic* Preg. Risk Category: B	*Serious UTI and lower respiratory tract infections and gyn, skin and skin-structure, intra-abdominal, and bone and joint infections caused by susceptible organisms* — **Adults:** 1 to 2 g IV or IM q 12 hr for 5 to 10 days. Up to 6 g daily in life-threatening infections. *Periop prophylaxis* — **Adults:** 1 to 2 g IV given once 30 to 60 min before surgery. In cesarean section, give dose as soon as umbilical cord clamped.	▪ Obtain specimen for culture and sensitivity tests before first dose. ▪ *IV use:* Reconstitute with sterile water for injection. Then drug may be mixed with 50 to 100 ml D₅W or 0.9% NaCl solution. ▪ With large doses or prolonged therapy, monitor for superinfection.
cefoxitin sodium Mefoxin *Second-generation cephalosporin/cephamycin* *Antibiotic* Preg. Risk Category: B	*Serious infections of respiratory and GU tracts; skin, soft-tissue, bone, and joint infections; bloodstream and intra-abdominal infections caused by susceptible organisms; periop prophylaxis* — **Adults:** 1 to 2 g q 6 to 8 hr in uncomplicated infections. Up to 12 g daily in life-threatening infections. **Children > 3 mo:** 80 to 160 mg/kg daily in 4 to 6 equally divided doses. Max 12 g daily. *Prophylactic use in surgery* — **Adults:** 2 g IM or IV 30 to 60 min before surgery, then 2 g IM or IV q 6 hr for 24 hr (72 hr after prosthetic arthroplasty). **Children ≥ 3 mo:**	▪ Obtain specimen for culture and sensitivity tests before first dose. ▪ *IV use:* For direct injection, inject into large vein or into tubing of free-flowing IV solution over 3 to 5 min. For intermittent infusion, add reconstituted drug to 50 or 100 ml D₅W or D₁₀W or 0.9% NaCl injection. Interrupt flow of primary IV solution during infusion. ▪ Assess IV site frequently. IV use is linked to thrombophlebitis. ▪ For IM use, reconstitute IM injection with 0.5% or 1% lidocaine hydrochloride (with-

(continued)

CEFOXITIN SODIUM   57

DRUG/CLASS/CATEGORY	INDICATIONS/DOSAGES	KEY NURSING CONSIDERATIONS
cefoxitin sodium *(continued)*	30 to 40 mg/kg IM or IV 30 to 60 min before surgery, then 30 to 40 mg/kg q 6 hr for 24 hr (72 hr after prosthetic arthroplasty).	out epinephrine) to minimize pain. Inject deeply into large muscle mass. ▪ With large doses or prolonged therapy, monitor for superinfection.
cefpodoxime proxetil Vantin *Second-generation cephalosporin* *Antibiotic* Preg. Risk Category: B	*Acute, community-acquired pneumonia caused by susceptible organisms* — **Adults and children ≥ 13 yr:** 200 mg PO q 12 hr for 14 days. *Acute bacterial exacerbation of chronic bronchitis caused by susceptible organisms* — **Adults and children ≥ 13 yr:** 200 mg PO q 12 hr for 10 days. *Uncomplicated UTI caused by E. coli, K. pneumoniae, P. mirabilis, or S. saprophyticus* — **Adults:** 100 mg PO q 12 hr for 7 days.	▪ Obtain specimen for culture and sensitivity tests before first dose. ▪ Keep oral suspension refrigerated. Shake well before measuring dose. ▪ Give with food to enhance absorption. ▪ Monitor for superinfection. ▪ May cause false-positive urine glucose results with copper sulfate tests (Clinitest). Glucose enzymatic tests (Clinistix, Tes-Tape) not affected.
cefprozil Cefzil *Second-generation cephalosporin* *Antibiotic* Preg. Risk Category: B	*Pharyngitis or tonsillitis caused by S. pyogenes* — **Adults and children ≥ 13 yr:** 500 mg PO daily for at least 10 days. *Otitis media caused by S. pneumoniae, H. influenzae, and M. (Branhamella) catarrhalis* — **Infants and children 6 mo to 12 yr:** 15 mg/kg PO q 12 hr for 10 days. *Acute sinusitis caused by susceptible organisms* — **Adults and children ≥ 13 yr:**	▪ Obtain specimen for culture and sensitivity tests before first dose. ▪ Removed by hemodialysis; give after hemodialysis treatment is completed. ▪ Monitor for superinfection. ▪ Tell to shake suspension well before measuring dose. ▪ Instruct to notify doctor if rash develops.

250 to 500 mg PO q 12 hr for 10 days. **Children 6 mo to 12 yr:** 7.5 to 15 mg/kg PO q 12 hr for 10 days.

ceftazidime
Ceptaz, Fortaz, Tazicef, Tazidime
Third-generation cephalosporin
Antibiotic
Preg. Risk Category: B

Serious infections of lower respiratory and urinary tracts; gyn, intra-abdominal, CNS, and skin infections; bacteremia; and septicemia — **Adults and children ≥ 12 yr:** 1 g IV or IM q 8 to 12 hr; up to 6 g daily in life-threatening infections. **Children 1 mo to 12 yr:** 25 to 50 mg/kg IV q 8 hr (sodium carbonate formulation). **Neonates 0 to 4 wk:** 30 mg/kg IV q 12 hr (sodium carbonate formulation).

- Obtain specimen for culture and sensitivity tests before first dose.
- **IV use:** Read and follow instructions for reconstitution carefully.
- Removed by hemodialysis; give supplemental dose after each dialysis period, as ordered.
- For IM use, inject deeply into large muscle mass.
- With large doses or prolonged therapy, monitor for superinfection.

ceftibuten
Cedax
Second-generation cephalosporin
Antibiotic
Preg. Risk Category: B

Acute bacterial exacerbation of chronic bronchitis due to susceptible organisms — **Adults and children ≥ age 12:** 400 mg PO daily for 10 days.

Pharyngitis and tonsillitis due to S. pyogenes; acute bacterial otitis media due to H. influenzae, M. catarrhalis, or S. pyogenes — **Adults and children ≥ age 12:** 400 mg PO daily for 10 days. **Children < age 12:** 9 mg/kg PO daily for 10 days. **Children > 45 kg:** max dose 400 mg PO daily for 10 days.

- Obtain specimen for culture and sensitivity tests before giving first dose.
- Discontinue if allergic reaction suspected. Emergency treatment may be required.
- Consider possibility of pseudomembranous colitis in patients who develop diarrhea secondary to therapy. Obtain specimens for *C. difficile*, as ordered.
- Monitor patient for superinfection.

DRUG/CLASS/CATEGORY	INDICATIONS/DOSAGES	KEY NURSING CONSIDERATIONS
ceftizoxime sodium Cefizox *Third-generation cephalosporin* *Antibiotic* Preg. Risk Category: B	*Serious infections of lower respiratory and urinary tracts; gyn, intra-abdominal, bone, joint, and skin infections; bacteremia; septicemia; and meningitis caused by susceptible microorganisms* — **Adults:** usual dosage 1 to 2 g IV or IM q 8 to 12 hr. In life-threatening infections, up to 2 g q 4 hr. **Children > 6 mo:** 33 to 50 mg/kg IV q 6 to 8 hr. Serious infections: up to 200 mg/kg/day in divided doses. Don't exceed 12 g/day.	▪ Obtain specimen for culture and sensitivity tests before first dose. ▪ *IV use:* To reconstitute powder, add 5 ml sterile water to 500-mg vial, 10 ml to 1-g vial, or 20 ml to 2-g vial. Reconstitute piggyback vials with 50 to 100 ml 0.9% NaCl solution or D₅W. Shake well. ▪ For IM use, inject deeply into large muscle mass. Divide larger doses (2 g) and inject at two separate sites. ▪ Monitor for superinfection.
ceftriaxone sodium Rocephin *Third-generation cephalosporin* *Antibiotic* Preg. Risk Category: B	*Most infections caused by susceptible organisms* — **Adults:** 1 to 2 g IM or IV daily or bid depending on type and severity of infection. *Serious infections of lower respiratory and urinary tracts; gyn, bone, joint, intra-abdominal, and skin infections; bacteremia; septicemia; and Lyme disease caused by susceptible organisms* — **Adults and children > 12 yr:** 1 to 2 g IM or IV daily or in equally divided doses bid. Max 4 g/day. **Children ≤ 12 yr:** 50 to 75 mg/kg IM or IV, not to exceed 2 g/day, in divided doses q 12 hr. *Meningitis* — **Adults and children:** initially, 100 mg/kg IV or IV (not to exceed 4 g),	▪ Obtain specimen for culture and sensitivity tests before first dose. ▪ For IM use, inject deeply into large muscle mass. ▪ Monitor for superinfection. ▪ Commonly used in home antibiotic programs for outpatient treatment of serious infections, such as osteomyelitis.

cefuroxime axetil
Ceftin
cefuroxime sodium
Kefurox, Zinacef
Second-generation
cephalosporin
Antibiotic
Preg. Risk Category: B

thereafter, 100 mg/kg IM or IV, once daily or in divided doses q 12 hr, not to exceed 4 g, for 7 to 14 days.

Injectable form used for serious infections and for periop prophylaxis. Oral form used for otitis media, pharyngitis, tonsillitis, infections of urinary and lower respiratory tracts, and skin and skin-structure infections due to susceptible organisms — **Adults and children ≥ 12 yr:** usual dosage of cefuroxime sodium: 750 mg to 1.5 g IM or IV q 8 hr for 5 to 10 days. For life-threatening infections and less susceptible organisms, 1.5 g IM or IV q 6 hr; for bacterial meningitis, up to 3 g IV q 8 hr. Or, 250 to 500 mg of cefuroxime axetil PO q 12 hr. **Children and infants > 3 mo:** 50 to 100 mg/kg/day of cefuroxime sodium IM or IV in divided doses q 6 to 8 hr. Higher doses used for meningitis. Or, 125 mg of cefuroxime axetil PO q 12 hr; for bacterial meningitis, 200 to 240 mg/kg IV in divided doses q 6 to 8 hr.

Otitis media — **Children < 2 yr:** 125 mg PO q 12 hr. **Children ≥ 2 yr:** 250 mg PO q 12 hr. *Early Lyme disease caused by B. burgdorferi —* **Adults and children ≥ 13 yr:** 500 mg PO bid for 20 days.

- Obtain specimen for culture and sensitivity tests before first dose.
- **IV use:** For direct injection, inject into large vein or into tubing of free-flowing IV solution over 3 to 5 min.
- For IM doses, inject deeply into large muscle mass.
- Food enhances absorption of cefuroxime axetil.
- With large doses or prolonged therapy, monitor for superinfection, especially in high-risk patients.
- Advise to report pain at IV site.
- Tell to report adverse reactions promptly.

DRUG/CLASS/ CATEGORY	INDICATIONS/ DOSAGES	KEY NURSING CONSIDERATIONS
cephalexin hydrochloride Keftab **cephalexin monohydrate** Apo-Cephalex†, Bio-cef, Cefanex, C-Lexin, Keflex *First-generation cephalosporin Antibiotic* Preg. Risk Category: B	*Respiratory tract, GI tract, skin, soft-tissue, bone, and joint infections and otitis media caused by E. coli and other coliform bacteria, group A beta-hemolytic streptococci, Klebsiella, P. mirabilis, S. pneumoniae, and staphylococci —* **Adults:** 250 mg to 1 g PO q 6 hr. **Children:** 6 to 12 mg/kg PO q 6 hr (monohydrate only). Max 25 mg/kg q 6 hr.	• Ask about previous allergic reactions to cephalosporins or penicillin before giving first dose. • Obtain specimen for culture and sensitivity tests before first dose. • With large doses or prolonged therapy, monitor for superinfection. • Group A beta-hemolytic streptococcal infections should be treated for ≥ 10 days.
cephapirin sodium Cefadyl *First-generation cephalosporin Antibiotic* Preg. Risk Category: B	*Periop prophylaxis in contaminated or potentially contaminated surgery —* **Adults:** 1 to 2 g IM or IV 30 to 60 min before surgery; then 1 to 2 g IM or IV q 6 hr for 24 hr. May give additional doses during procedures > 2 hours. In cases where infection would be devastating, prophylaxis may continue for 3 to 5 days. *Serious infections of respiratory, GU, or GI tract; skin and soft-tissue infections; bone and joint infections (including osteomyelitis); septicemia; and endocarditis caused by susceptible organisms —* **Adults:** 500 mg to 1 g IM or IV q 4 to 6 hr. In life-threatening infections, up to 12 g/day. **Children**	• Obtain specimen for culture and sensitivity tests before first dose. • For IV infusion with Y-tubing, dilute 4-g vial with 40 ml of diluent. During cephapirin infusion, stop flow of other solution. • When giving IV, check frequently for vein irritation and phlebitis. Alternate injection sites if IV therapy lasts > 3 days. Use of small IV needles in larger available veins may be preferable. • For IM use, inject deeply into large muscle mass, such as gluteus maximus or lateral aspect of thigh. • Monitor for superinfection.

> 3 mo: 10 to 20 mg/kg IV or IM q 6 hr; dose depends on age, weight, and severity of infection.

cephradine
Velosef
First-generation cephalosporin
Antibiotic
Preg. Risk Category: B

Serious infections of respiratory, GI, or GU tract; skin and soft-tissue infections; bone and joint infections; septicemia; endocarditis; otitis media caused by susceptible organisms; periop prophylaxis — **Adults:** 250 to 500 mg PO q 6 hr. **Children > 9 mo:** 25 to 50 mg/kg PO daily in divided doses.

Otitis media — **Children:** 75 to 100 mg/kg PO daily. Don't exceed 4 g daily. Any patient, regardless of age and weight, may receive doses up to 1 g qid for severe or chronic infections.

- Obtain specimen for culture and sensitivity tests before first dose.
- Group A beta-hemolytic streptococcal infections should be treated for ≥ 10 days.
- With large doses or prolonged therapy, monitor for superinfection, especially in high-risk patients.
- Tell to take with food or milk.
- Instruct to shake oral suspension well before measuring dose.
- Advise to report rash immediately.

cetirizine hydrochloride
Zyrtec
Selective H₁-receptor antagonist
Antihistamine agent
Preg. Risk Category: B

Seasonal allergic rhinitis, perennial allergic rhinitis, chronic urticaria — **Adults and children ≥ 12 yr:** 5 or 10 mg PO daily depending on symptom severity; 5 mg PO daily in renal or hepatic impairment.

Seasonal allergic rhinitis, perennial allergic rhinitis, chronic urticaria — **Children 6 to 11 yr:** 5 or 10 mg (1 or 2 tsp) PO qd depending on symptom severity.

- Not recommended for breast-feeding patients.
- Warn to avoid hazardous activities until CNS effects known.
- Advise to avoid alcohol and other CNS depressants.

CETIRIZINE HYDROCHLORIDE

†Canadian ‡Australian

DRUG / CLASS / CATEGORY

chloral hydrate
Aquachloral Supprettes, Dormel‡, Noctec, Novo-Chlorhidrate†
General CNS depressant
Sedative-hypnotic
Preg. Risk Category: C
Controlled Sub. Sched.: IV

INDICATIONS / DOSAGES

Sedation — **Adults:** 250 mg PO or PR tid after meals. **Children:** 8.3 mg/kg or 250 mg/m² PO or PR tid. Max daily dosage 500 mg tid.
Insomnia — **Adults:** 500 mg to 1 g PO or PR 15 to 30 min before bedtime. **Children:** 50 mg/kg or 1.5 g/m² PO or PR 15 to 30 min before bedtime. Max single dose 1 g.
Preop — **Adults:** 500 mg to 1 g PO or PR 30 min before surgery.
Premedication for EEG — **Children:** 20 to 25 mg/kg PO or PR.

KEY NURSING CONSIDERATIONS

- Note two strengths of oral liquid form. Double-check dose, especially when giving to children. Fatal overdoses have occurred.
- To minimize unpleasant taste and stomach irritation, dilute or give with liquid. Should be taken after meals.
- Take steps to prevent hoarding or self-overdosing by depressed, suicidal, or drug-dependent patients or those with history of drug abuse.
- Don't administer for 48 hours before fluorometric test, as ordered.
- Monitor BUN as ordered. Large dosage may raise BUN.

DRUG / CLASS / CATEGORY

chlorambucil
Leukeran
Alkylating agent
Antineoplastic
Preg. Risk Category: D

INDICATIONS / DOSAGES

Chronic lymphocytic leukemia; malignant lymphomas including lymphosarcoma, giant follicular lymphoma, and Hodgkin's disease — **Adults:** 0.1 to 0.2 mg/kg PO daily for 3 to 6 weeks; then adjusted for maintenance (usually 4 to 10 mg daily).

KEY NURSING CONSIDERATIONS

- Monitor CBC and serum uric acid level.
- If WBC count < 2,000/mm³ or granulocyte count < 1,000/mm³, follow institutional policy for infection control in immunocompromised patients.
- Avoid IM injections when platelet count < 100,000/mm³.

chloramphenicol

AK-Chlor, Chloromycetin Ophthalmic, Chloroptic, Chloroptic S.O.P., Chlorsig‡, Fenicol†, Isopto Fenicol†, Ophthoclor Ophthalmic, Pentamycetin†, Sopamycetin†

Dichloroacetic acid derivative

Antibiotic

Preg. Risk Category: NR

Surface bacterial infection involving conjunctiva or cornea — **Adults and children:** 1 or 2 drops of solution in eye q 3 to 6 hr or more often, if necessary. Or, small amount of ointment to lower conjunctival sac q 3 to 6 hr or more often, if necessary. Continued for at least 48 hr after eye appears normal.

- If chloramphenicol drops given qh and then tapered, follow closely to ensure adequate anterior chamber levels.
- Teach how to instill drops or apply ointment.
- Instruct to apply light finger pressure on lacrimal sac 1 min after drops instilled.

chloramphenicol

Chloromycetin Otic

Dichloroacetic acid derivative

Antibiotic

Preg. Risk Category: NR

External ear canal infection — **Adults and children:** 2 to 3 drops into ear canal tid.

- Watch for signs of superinfection or sore throat (early sign of toxicity).
- Reculture persistent drainage.

chlordiazepoxide

Libritabs

chlordiazepoxide hydrochloride

Librium, Novopoxide†

Benzodiazepine

Antianxiety agent/anticonvulsant/sedative-hypnotic

Preg. Risk Category: NR

Controlled Sub. Sched.: IV

Mild to moderate anxiety — **Adults:** 5 to 10 mg PO tid or qid. **Children > 6 yr:** 5 mg PO bid to qid. **Children > 6 yr:** 5 mg PO bid or tid.

Severe anxiety — **Adults:** 20 to 25 mg PO tid or qid. In geri patients, 5 mg bid to qid.

Withdrawal symptoms of acute alcoholism — **Adults:** 50 to 100 mg PO, IM, or IV; repeat in 2 to 4 hr prn. Max 300 mg daily.

Note: Parenteral form not recommended in children < 12 yr.

- **IV use:** Use 5 ml 0.9% NaCl solution or sterile water for injection as diluent; don't give packaged diluent. Administer over 1 min.
- When giving IV, be sure equipment for emergency airway management is available. Monitor respirations every 5 to 15 min and before each repeated IV dose.
- Injectable form comes in two types of ampules. Read directions carefully.
- Don't withdraw abruptly.

CHLORDIAZEPOXIDE HYDROCHLORIDE   65

†Canadian ‡Australian

DRUG/CLASS/CATEGORY	INDICATIONS/DOSAGES	KEY NURSING CONSIDERATIONS
chloroquine hydrochloride Aralen HCl, Chlorquin‡ **chloroquine phosphate** Aralen Phosphate, Chlorquin‡ **chloroquine sulfate** Nivaquine† *4-aminoquinoline* *Antimalarial/amebicide/anti-inflammatory* Preg. Risk Category: C	*Acute malarial attacks* — **Adults:** 600 mg (base) PO, then 300 mg at 6, 24, and 48 hr. Or 160 to 200 mg (base) IM initially; repeat in 6 hr prn. Switch to PO as soon as possible. **Children:** 10 mg (base)/kg PO, then 5 mg (base)/kg PO at 6, 24, and 48 hr (max < adult dose). Or 5 mg (base)/kg IM initially; repeated in 6 hr prn. Max 10 mg (base)/kg/24 hr. Switch to PO as soon as possible. *Malaria prophylaxis* — **Adults and children:** 5 mg (base)/kg PO (max 300 mg) weekly (begun 2 wk before exposure and continued for 4 to 6 wk after.) If treatment begins after exposure, initial dose doubled in 2 divided doses PO q 6 hr.	▪ Monitor for possible overdose, which can quickly lead to toxic symptoms. Children extremely susceptible to toxicity. ▪ Baseline and periodic ophthalmic and automatic exams needed. ▪ Monitor CBCs and liver function studies. ▪ Advise to take immediately before or after meals on same day each week. ▪ Tell to report adverse reactions promptly. ▪ Instruct to avoid exposure to sunlight.
chlorothiazide Chlotride‡, Diurigen, Diuril **chlorothiazide sodium** Diuril Sodium *Thiazide diuretic* *Diuretic/antihypertensive* Preg. Risk Category: C	*Edema, hypertension* — **Adults:** 500 mg to 1 g PO or IV daily or bid. *Diuresis, hypertension* — **Children 6 mo to 12 yr:** 10 to 20 mg/kg PO daily or in 2 divided doses; max 1,000 mg/day in children > 2 yr; in children < 2 yr, max dose is 375 mg/day. **Children < 6 mo:** up to 30 mg/kg PO daily in 2 divided doses.	▪ To prevent nocturia, give ordered doses in morning and early afternoon. ▪ Administer oral form with food. ▪ *IV use:* Reconstitute 500 mg with 18 ml of sterile water for injection. Inject directly into vein, through free-flowing IV line or intermittent infusion device. ▪ Never inject IM or SC. Avoid IV infiltration. ▪ Watch for signs of hypokalemia. Monitor serum creatinine, BUN, uric acid, calcium, and glucose levels

chlorpheniramine maleate

Aller-Chlor L, Chlor-Trimeton, Novopheniram‡, Teldrin

Propylamine-derivative antihistamine

Antihistamine (H_1-receptor antagonist)

Preg. Risk Category: B

Rhinitis, allergy symptoms — **Adults:** 4 mg PO q 4 to 6 hr, not to exceed 24 mg/day; or 8 to 12 mg timed-release PO q 8 to 12 hr, not to exceed 24 mg daily. Or, 5 to 20 mg IM, IV, or SC as single dose. Max 40 mg/24 hr. **Children 6 to 12 yr:** 2 mg PO q 4 to 6 hr, not to exceed 12 mg/day. Alternatively, may give 8 mg timed-release PO hs. **Children 2 to 6 yr:** 1 mg PO q 4 to 6 hr, not to exceed 4 mg daily.

- **IV use:** Available in 10-mg/ml ampules. Don't give 100 mg/ml strength IV. Drug compatible with most IV solutions. Check with pharmacist before mixing with IV solutions to verify specific compatibilities. Give injection over 1 min.
- If symptoms occur during or after parenteral dose, discontinue drug.

chlorpromazine hydrochloride

Chlorpromanyl-5†, Chlorpromanyl-20†, Chlorpromanyl-40†, Ormazine, Thorazine

Aliphatic phenothiazine

Antipsychotic/antiemetic

Preg. Risk Category: NR

Psychosis — **Adults:** 25 to 75 mg PO qd in 2 to 4 divided doses. Increase by 20 to 50 mg twice weekly until symptoms controlled. May need up to 800 mg daily. Or, 25 to 50 mg IM q 1 to 4 hr, prn. IM doses gradually increased over several days to max 400 mg q 4 to 6 hr. Switch to PO doses as possible. **Children ≥ 6 mo:** 0.55 mg/kg PO q 4 to 6 hr or IM q 6 to 8 hr; or 1.1 mg/kg PR q 6 to 8 hr. Max IM dose in children < 5 yr or < 22.7 kg: 40 mg. Max IM dose in children 5 to 12 yr or 22.7 to 45.5 kg: 75 mg.

Nausea and vomiting — **Adults:** 10 to 25 mg PO q 4 to 6 hr, prn; or 50 to 100 mg PR q 6 to 8 hr, prn; or 25 to 50 mg IM q 3 to 4 hr prn. **Children ≥ 6 mo:** 0.55 mg/kg q 4 to 6 hr; or IM q 6 to 8 hr; or 1.1 mg/kg PR q 6 to 8 hr. Max IM dose in children < 5 yr or < 22.7 kg: 40 mg. Max IM dose in children 5 to 12 yr or 22.7 to 45.5 kg: 75 mg.

- Obtain baseline BP before starting therapy and monitor BP regularly. Watch for orthostatic hypotension, especially with parenteral use. Monitor BP before and after IM administration; keep patient supine 1 hr afterward and instruct to get up slowly.
- Monitor for tardive dyskinesia, which may follow prolonged use (up to months or years later) and may disappear spontaneously or persist for life despite drug discontinuation.
- Watch for signs of neuroleptic malignant syndrome.
- Acute dystonic reactions may be treated with diphenhydramine.

CHLORPROMAZINE HYDROCHLORIDE 67

†Canadian ‡Australian

DRUG/CLASS/ CATEGORY	INDICATIONS/ DOSAGES	KEY NURSING CONSIDERATIONS
chlorthalidone Apo-Chlorthalidone†, Hygroton, Novo-Thalidone†, Thalitone, Uridont *Thiazide-like diuretic Diuretic/antihypertensive* Preg. Risk Category: B	*Edema, hypertension* — **Adults:** initially, 25 to 100 mg PO daily, or up to 200 mg PO on alternate days. **Children:** 2 mg/kg or 60 mg/ m² PO 3 times weekly.	▪ To prevent nocturia, give in morning. ▪ Monitor I&O, weight, BP, electrolytes, glucose creatinine, BUN, and uric acid. ▪ Watch for signs of hypokalemia. ▪ Don't confuse various brands.
cholestyramine Cholybar, Prevalite, Questran, Questran Light *Anion exchange resin Antilipemic/bile acid sequestrant* Preg. Risk Category: NR	*Primary hyperlipidemia or pruritus caused by partial bile obstruction; adjunct for reduction of elevated serum cholesterol in primary hypercholesterolemia* — **Adults:** 4 g PO daily or bid. Maintenance: 8 to 16 g daily divided into 2 doses. Max 24 g daily.	▪ Monitor serum cholesterol and triglyceride levels regularly. ▪ If patient also receiving cardiac glycoside, monitor serum cardiac glycoside levels. ▪ Don't give in dry form. ▪ Monitor bowel habits. Encourage diet high in fiber and fluids.
choline magnesium trisalicylate (choline salicylate and magnesium salicylate) Tricosal, Trilisate *Salicylate Nonnarcotic analgesic/antipyretic/anti-inflammatory* Preg. Risk Category: C	*Rheumatoid arthritis (RA) and other inflammatory conditions* — **Adults:** initially, 1.5 to 2.5 g PO daily as single dose or in 2 or 3 divided doses. Adjust dosage according to response. Maintenance: 1 to 4.5 g daily. *Juvenile RA* — **Children:** 60 to 110 mg/kg/ day PO in divided doses (q 6 to 8 hr). *Mild to moderate pain and fever* — **Adults:** 2 to 3 g PO daily in divided doses q 4 to 6 hr. **Children ≤37 kg:** 25 mg/kg PO bid. **Children >37 kg:** 2,250 mg/day.	▪ Monitor Hgb levels and PT in long-term or high-dose therapy. ▪ Monitor serum salicylate in long-term therapy. In arthritis, therapeutic level is 10 to 30 mg/100 ml.

choline salicylate
Arthropan, Teejel†
Salicylate
Nonnarcotic analgesic/antipyretic/anti-inflammatory
Preg. Risk Category: NR

Rheumatoid arthritis, osteoarthritis, mild to moderate pain or fever — **Adults and children > 12 yr:** ½ to 1 tsp (435 to 870 mg) PO q 4 hr, prn. If tolerated and needed, increase to 2 tsp. Not to exceed 8 tsp daily.

Relief of pain from inflamed gums — **Adults and children > 2 yr:** apply 1 cm of gel to affected area q 3 to 4 hr and hs, prn.

- Don't give to children or teenagers with chickenpox or flu-like illness.
- Febrile, dehydrated children can develop toxicity rapidly.
- Monitor serum salicylate levels in long-term therapy.
- Monitor Hgb and PT in patients receiving long-term treatment with large doses.

---

ciclopirox olamine
Loprox
N-hydroxypyridinone derivative
Topical antifungal
Preg. Risk Category: B

Tinea pedis, cruris, corporis, and versicolor; cutaneous candidiasis — **Adults and children > 10 yr:** massage gently into affected and surrounding areas bid, in morning and evening for 2 to 4 wk.

- Don't use occlusive dressings.
- Avoid drug contact with eyes.
- If hypersensitivity occurs, advise to discontinue treatment and notify doctor.
- Tell patient to continue using drug for prescribed period even if symptoms improve.

---

cidofovir
Vistide
Nucleotide analogue
Antiviral
Preg. Risk Category: C

CMV retinitis in patients with AIDS — **Adults:** initially, 5 mg/kg IV infused over 1 hr once weekly for 2 consecutive wk, then maintenance dosage of 5 mg/kg IV infused over 1 hr once q 2 wk. Must give probenecid and prehydration with 0.9% NaCl solution IV concomitantly (may reduce potential for nephrotoxicity).

- Give 1 L 0.9% NaCl, usually over 1 to 2 hr, immediately before each infusion.
- Monitor eye exam periodically.
- To prepare for infusion, transfer dose to bag containing 100 ml 0.9% NaCl.
- Mutagenic: prepare drug by following facility protocols.
- If drug contacts skin, wash mucous membranes and flush thoroughly with water.

DRUG / CLASS / CATEGORY	INDICATIONS / DOSAGES	KEY NURSING CONSIDERATIONS
cimetidine Tagamet, Tagamet HB, Tagamet HCl, Tagamet Tiltab *Histamine₂-receptor antagonist* *Antiulcer agent* Preg. Risk Category: B	*Duodenal ulcer (short-term treatment and maintenance)* — **Adults and children ≥ 16 yr:** 800 mg PO hs. Alternatively, 400 mg PO bid or 300 mg PO with meals and hs. Maintenance therapy: 400 mg hs. Parenteral therapy: 300 mg diluted to 20 ml by IV push over at least 5 min q 6 hr; or 300 mg diluted in 50 ml D₅W or other compatible IV solution by IV infusion over 15 to 20 min q 6 hr; or 300 mg IM q 6 hr (no dilution necessary). Max 2,400 mg daily prn. Alternatively, 900 mg/day (37.5 mg/hr) IV diluted in 100 to 1,000 ml by continuous IV infusion. *Active benign gastric ulceration* — **Adults:** 800 mg PO hs, or 300 mg PO qid (with meals and hs) for up to 6 wk. *Gastroesophageal reflux disease* — **Adults:** 800 mg PO bid or 400 mg PO qid before meals and hs for up to 12 wk.	• **IV use:** Dilute IV solutions with 0.9% NaCl solution, D₅W and D₁₀W (and combinations of these), lact Ringer's solution, or 5% sodium bicarbonate injection. Don't dilute with sterile water for injection. • Don't infuse IV too rapidly; bradycardia may occur. Some authorities recommend infusing over at least 30 min to reduce risk of adverse cardiac effects. Sometimes given as continuous IV infusion. Use infusion pump if given in total volume of 250 ml over 24 hr or less. • Identify tablet strength when obtaining drug history. • Schedule dose at end of hemodialysis treatment. • Up to 10-g overdose can occur without adverse reactions.
ciprofloxacin Cipro, Cipro IV, Ciproxin‡ *Fluroquinolone antibiotic* *Antibiotic* Preg. Risk Category: C	*Mild to moderate UTI caused by susceptible organisms* — **Adults:** 250 mg PO or 200 mg IV q 12 hr. *Severe or complicated UTI or mild to moderate bone, joint, skin, or skin structure infections caused by susceptible organisms* — **Adults:** 500 mg PO or 400 mg IV q 12 hr.	• Obtain specimen for culture and sensitivity tests before first dose. • Give oral form 2 hr after meal or 2 hr before or after taking antacids, sucralfate, or products that contain iron. • **IV use:** Infuse slowly (over 1 hr) into large vein.

Chronic bacterial prostatitis caused by E. coli *or* P. mirabilis — **Adults: 500 mg PO q 12 hr for 28 days.**

- Instruct to avoid excessive artificial ultraviolet light and to stop drug and call doctor if phototoxicity occurs.
- Encourage high fluid intake to avoid crystalluria.
- Tell to take on empty stomach.

---

ciprofloxacin hydrochloride
Cloxan
Fluoroquinolone
Antibacterial agent
Preg. Risk Category: C

Corneal ulcers caused by susceptible organisms — **Adults and children >12 yr:** 2 drops in affected eye q 15 min for 1st 6 hr, then 2 drops q 30 min for remainder of the 1st day. On day 2, 2 drops qh. On days 3 to 14, 2 drops q 4 hr.
Bacterial conjunctivitis caused by susceptible organisms — **Adults and children >12 yr:** 1 or 2 drops in affected eye q 2 hr *while awake* for 1st 2 days. Then 1 or 2 drops q 4 hr *while awake* for next 5 days.

- Discontinue at first sign of hypersensitivity and notify doctor.
- Prolonged use may result in superinfection.
- Teach how to instill drops.
- Instruct to apply light finger pressure on lacrimal sac for 1 min after drops instilled.

---

cisapride
Propulsid
Serotonin-4 receptor agonist
GI prokinetic agent
Preg. Risk Category: C

Symptoms of nocturnal heartburn caused by gastroesophageal reflux disease — **Adults:** initially, 10 mg PO qid 15 min before meals and hs. If response inadequate, increase to 20 mg qid.

- Use cautiously in breast-feeding patient.
- Protect 20-mg tablets from light; protect all products from moisture.
- Remind to avoid alcohol and sedatives while on this drug.

DRUG / CLASS / CATEGORY	INDICATIONS / DOSAGES	KEY NURSING CONSIDERATIONS
cisplatin (cis-platinum, CDDP) Platamine‡, Platinol, Platinol AQ *Alkylating agent* *Antineoplastic* Preg. Risk Category: D	*Adjunctive therapy in metastatic testicular cancer* — **Adults:** 20 mg/m² IV qd for 5 days. Repeated q 3 wk for 3 cycles or longer. *Adjunctive therapy in metastatic ovarian cancer* — **Adults:** 100 mg/m² IV; repeated q 4 weeks. Or 75 to 100 mg/m² IV once q 4 wk in combination with cyclophosphamide. *Advanced bladder cancer* — **Adults:** 50 to 70 mg/m² IV q 3 to 4 wk. Patients who have received other antineoplastic agents or radiation should receive 50 mg/m² q 4 wk.	• Monitor CBC, electrolyte levels, platelet count, and renal function studies. • Hydrate patient with 0.9% NaCl before giving drug. Maintain urine output of ≥ 100 ml/hr for 4 hr before therapy and for 24 hr after therapy. • Parenteral form associated with carcinogenic, mutagenic, and teratogenic risks for personnel. • Do not use needles or IV administration sets that contain aluminum. • Administer antiemetics, as ordered.
cladribine (2-chlorodeoxyadenosine, CdA) Leustatin *Purine nucleoside analogue* *Antineoplastic* Preg. Risk Category: D	*Active hairy cell leukemia* — **Adults:** 0.09 mg/kg daily by continuous IV infusion for 7 days.	• *IV use:* For a 24-hour infusion, add the calculated dose to a 500-ml infusion bag of 0.9% NaCl for injection. Don't use dextrose solutions. • Because of the risk of hyperuricemia from tumor lysis, administer allopurinol, as ordered, during therapy. • Monitor hematologic function closely. • Fever is common during the 1st month of therapy.

clarithromycin
Biaxin
Macrolide
Antibiotic
Preg. Risk Category: C

Pharyngitis or tonsillitis caused by S. pyogenes — **Adults:** 250 mg PO q 12 hr for 10 days. **Children:** 15 mg/kg/day PO in divided doses q 12 hr for 10 days.
Acute maxillary sinusitis caused by S. pneumoniae, H. influenzae, or M. (Branhamella) catarrhalis — **Adults:** 500 mg PO q 12 hr for 14 days. **Children:** 15 mg/kg/day PO in divided doses q 12 hr for 10 days.
M. avium complex disease in HIV infection — **Adults:** 500 mg PO q 12 hr, in combination with other antimycobacterial drugs, for life. **Children:** 7.5 mg/kg PO (max of 500 mg) q 12 hr, in combination with other antimycobacterial drugs, for life.
H. pylori infection — **Adults:** 500 mg PO q 8 hr for 14 days with omeprazole 40 mg PO each morning. Continue omeprazole (20 mg PO each morning) for total of 28 days.

- Obtain specimen for culture and sensitivity tests before first dose.
- May cause overgrowth of nonsusceptible bacteria or fungi. Monitor for superinfection.
- May take with or without food. Instruct not to refrigerate suspension.
- Advise to report persistent adverse reactions.

clemastine fumarate
Tavist, Tavist-1
Ethanolamine-derivative
antihistamine
Antihistamine (H₁-receptor antagonist)
Preg. Risk Category: C

Rhinitis, allergy symptoms — **Adults and children ≥ 12 yr:** 1.34 mg PO q 12 hr, or 2.68 mg PO qd to tid pm. Don't exceed 8.04 mg/day. **Children 6 to 12 yr:** 0.67 to 1.34 mg PO bid. Don't exceed 4.02 mg/day.

- Monitor blood counts during long-term therapy, as ordered; observe for blood dyscrasias.
- Instruct not to drink alcohol and to avoid activities that require alertness until CNS effects known.
- Tell to report tolerance to drug.

CLEMASTINE FUMARATE 73

DRUG / CLASS / CATEGORY	INDICATIONS / DOSAGES	KEY NURSING CONSIDERATIONS
clindamycin hydrochloride Cleocin HCl, Dalacin C†‡ **clindamycin palmitate hydrochloride** Cleocin Pediatric, Dalacin C Palmitate†‡ **clindamycin phosphate** Cleocin Phosphate, Cleocin T, Dalacin C†‡ *Lincomycin derivative Antibiotic* Preg. Risk Category: B	*Infections caused by sensitive aerobic and anaerobic organisms* — **Adults:** 150 to 450 mg PO q 6 hr; or 300 to 600 mg IM or IV q 6, 8, or 12 hr. **Children >1 mo:** 8 to 20 mg/kg PO daily in divided doses q 6 to 8 hr; or 20 to 40 mg/kg IM or IV daily in divided doses q 6 or 8 hr. *Endocarditis prophylaxis for dental procedures in patients allergic to penicillin* — **Adults:** initially, 300 mg PO 1 hr before procedure; then 150 mg 6 hr later. **Children:** initially, 10 mg/kg PO 1 hr before procedure; then half of initial dose 6 hr later. *Pelvic inflammatory disease* — **Adults:** 900 mg IV q 8 hr in conjunction with gentamicin. Continue at least 48 hr after symptoms improve; then switch to oral clindamycin 450 mg 5 times daily for total course of 10 to 14 days.	■ Obtain culture and sensitivity tests before first dose. ■ *IV use:* Check IV site daily for phlebitis and irritation. For infusion, dilute each 300 mg in 50 ml solution, and give no faster than 30 mg/min (over 10 to 60 min). Never give undiluted as bolus. ■ For IM use, inject deeply. Rotate sites. Doses > 600 mg per injection not recommended. ■ Observe for signs of superinfection. ■ Don't give opioid antidiarrheals to treat drug-induced diarrhea; may prolong and worsen diarrhea.
clindamycin phosphate Cleocin T Gel, Lotion, Solution; Cleocin Vaginal Cream *Lincomycin derivative Antibiotic* Preg. Risk Category: B	*Inflammatory acne vulgaris* — **Adults and adolescents:** apply to skin bid, morning and evening. *Bacterial vaginosis* — **Adults:** 1 applicatorful intravaginally hs for 7 consecutive days.	■ Drug can cause excessive dryness. ■ Warn to avoid too-frequent washing of affected area. Tell patient to cover entire affected area but avoid contact with eyes, nose, mouth, and other mucous membranes. ■ Warn not to smoke while applying topical solution.

clofazimine

Lamprene

Substituted iminophenazine dye

Leprostatic

Preg. Risk Category: C

Dapsone-resistant leprosy (Hansen's disease) — **Adults:** 100 mg PO daily in combination with other antileprotics for 3 yr. Then, clofazimine alone, 100 mg daily.

Erythema nodosum leprosum — **Adults:** 100 to 200 mg PO daily for up to 3 mo.

- Report colic, burning abdominal pain, or other GI symptoms to doctor.
- Warn that drug may temporarily discolor skin, body fluids, and excrement pink to brownish black.

clomipramine hydrochloride

Anafranil

Tricyclic antidepressant

Antiobsessional agent

Preg. Risk Category: C

Obsessive-compulsive disorder — **Adults:** initially, 25 mg PO daily with meals, gradually increased to 100 mg daily in divided doses during first 2 wk. Thereafter, increase to max 250 mg daily in divided doses with meals, prn. After titration, total daily dosage may be given hs. **Children and adolescents:** initially, 25 mg PO daily with meals, gradually increased over first 2 wk to daily max 3 mg/kg or 100 mg PO in divided doses, whichever is smaller. Max daily dosage 3 mg/kg or 200 mg, whichever is smaller; may be given hs after titration. Periodic reassessment and adjustment necessary.

- Should be gradually discontinued several days before surgery.
- Adverse anticholinergic effects can occur rapidly.
- Advise to use sunblock, wear protective clothing, and avoid prolonged exposure to strong sunlight.
- Don't withdraw abruptly.

clonazepam

Klonopin

Benzodiazepine

Anticonvulsant

Preg. Risk Category: NR

Controlled Sub. Sched.: IV

Lennox-Gastaut syndrome; atypical absence seizures; akinetic and myoclonic seizures — **Adults:** initially, not to exceed 1.5 mg PO in 3 divided doses. May increase by 0.5 to 1 mg q 3 days until seizures controlled. If given in unequal doses, give largest dose hs. Max recommended daily dosage 20 mg. **Children ≤10 yr or**

- Never withdraw suddenly because seizures may worsen. Monitor for oversedation. Call doctor at once if adverse reactions develop.
- Monitor blood drug levels. Therapeutic level 20 to 80 ng/ml.

(continued)

CLONAZEPAM 75

†Canadian ‡Australian

DRUG / CLASS / CATEGORY	INDICATIONS / DOSAGES	KEY NURSING CONSIDERATIONS
clonazepam *(continued)*	**30 kg:** initially, 0.01 to 0.03 mg/kg PO daily (not to exceed 0.05 mg/kg daily), in 2 or 3 divided doses. Increase by 0.25 to 0.5 mg q third day to max maintenance dosage: 0.1 to 0.2 mg/kg daily as needed.	• Withdrawal symptoms resemble those of barbiturates.
clonidine Catapres-TTS **clonidine hydrochloride** Catapres, Dixarit‡ *Centrally acting adrenergic agent* Antihypertensive Preg. Risk Category: C	*Essential and renal hypertension* — **Adults:** initially, 0.1 mg PO bid; then increase by 0.1 to 0.2 mg daily on weekly basis. Usual range 0.2 to 0.8 mg daily in divided doses. Infrequently, dosages up to 2.4 mg daily used. Or, as transdermal patch applied to nonhairy area of intact skin on upper arm or torso q 7 days, starting with 0.1-mg system and titrated with another 0.1-mg or larger system	• May be given to lower BP rapidly in some hypertensive emergencies. • Monitor BP and pulse frequently. • Remove transdermal patch before defibrillation to prevent arcing. • Observe for tolerance to therapeutic effects; may necessitate increased dosage. Transdermal effects may take 2 to 3 days to become apparent. Oral therapy may have to continue in interim.
clorazepate dipotassium Apo-Clorazepate†, Gen-XENE, Novoclopate†, Tranxene, Tranxene-SD, Tranxene-T-Tab *Benzodiazepine* Antianxiety agent/anticonvulsant/sedative-hypnotic	*Acute alcohol withdrawal* — **Adults:** day 1: 30 mg PO initially, then 30 to 60 mg PO in divided doses; day 2: 45 to 90 mg PO in divided doses; day 3: 22.5 to 45 mg PO in divided doses; day 4: 15 to 30 mg PO in divided doses; then gradually reduce dosage to 7.5 to 15 mg daily. Max recommended daily dosage 90 mg. *Adjunct in partial seizure disorder* — **Adults and children > 12 yr:** Max recommended	• Reduce dosage in elderly or debilitated patients. • Monitor liver, renal, and hematopoietic function studies periodically, as ordered, with repeated or prolonged therapy. • Possibility of abuse and addiction exists. Don't withdraw abruptly after prolonged use; withdrawal symptoms may occur. • Not recommended for children < 9 yr.

Preg. Risk Category: D
Controlled Sub. Sched.: IV

initial dosage 7.5 mg PO tid. Increase no more than 7.5 mg/wk to max 90 mg daily. **Children 9 to 12 yr:** max recommended initial dosage 7.5 mg PO bid. Increase no more than 7.5 mg/wk, to max 60 mg daily.

- Instruct to avoid alcohol.
- Tell to avoid activities requiring alertness until CNS effects known.

---

clotrimazole
Canestent, Gyne-Lotrimin, Lotrimin, Mycelex, Mycelex-7, Mycelex-G, Mycelex-OTC

Synthetic imidazole derivative

Antifungal

Preg. Risk Category: B

Superficial fungal infections — **Adults and children:** apply thinly and massage into affected and surrounding area, morning and evening, for 2 to 4 wk. If no improvement occurs after 4 wk, patient should be reevaluated.

Vulvovaginal candidiasis — **Adults:** two 100-mg vaginal tablets inserted daily hs for 7 days, or one 500-mg vaginal tablet daily hs for 1 day; or 1 applicatorful vaginal cream daily hs for 7 days.

Oropharyngeal candidiasis treatment — **Adults and children ≥ 3 yr:** dissolve lozenge over 15 to 30 min in mouth 5 times daily for 14 days.

Prevention of oropharyngeal candidiasis in immunocompromised patients — **Adults and children:** dissolve lozenge over 15 to 30 min in mouth tid for duration of chemotherapy or until steroid reduced to maintenance levels.

- Report irritation or sensitivity; discontinue if irritation occurs and notify doctor.
- Warn not to use occlusive wrappings or dressings.
- Ensure that patient understands that frequent or persistent yeast infections may be symptom of more serious medical problem.

DRUG/CLASS/ CATEGORY	INDICATIONS/ DOSAGES	KEY NURSING CONSIDERATIONS
clozapine Clozaril *Tricyclic dibenzodiazepine derivative* *Antipsychotic* Preg. Risk Category: B	*Schizophrenia in severely ill patients unresponsive to other therapies* — **Adults:** initially, 12.5 mg PO qd or bid, titrated upward at 25 to 50 mg daily (if tolerated) to 300 to 450 mg daily by end of 2 wk. Individual dosage based on clinical response, patient tolerance, and adverse reactions. Don't increase subsequent dosage more than once or twice weekly, and don't exceed 100 mg. Many patients respond to dosage of 300 to 600 mg daily, but some may need up to 900 mg. Don't exceed 900 mg daily.	▪ Poses significant risk of agranulocytosis. ▪ Ensure that weekly WBC counts and blood tests are done. ▪ Monitor closely for signs of infection. Protective isolation may be needed. ▪ Must be withdrawn gradually over 1 to 2 wk. Monitor closely for recurrence of psychotic symptoms. ▪ No more than 1-wk supply of drug should be dispensed. ▪ May cause seizures or transient fevers.
codeine phosphate Paveral† **codeine sulfate** *Opioid* *Analgesic/antitussive* Preg. Risk Category: C Controlled Sub. Sched.: II	*Mild to moderate pain* — **Adults:** 15 to 60 mg PO or 15 to 60 mg (phosphate) SC, IM, or IV q 4 to 6 hr, prn. **Children > 1 yr:** 0.5 mg/kg PO, SC, or IM q 4 hr, prn. *Nonproductive cough* — **Adults:** 10 to 20 mg PO q 4 to 6 hr. Max 120 mg/day. **Children 6 to 12 yr:** 5 to 10 mg PO q 4 to 6 hr. Max 60 mg/day. **Children 2 to 6 yr:** 2.5 to 5 mg PO q 4 to 6 hr. Don't exceed 30 mg/day.	▪ **IV use:** Give by very slow direct injection into large vein. ▪ Don't mix with other solutions. ▪ For full analgesic effect, administer before patient has intense pain. ▪ An antitussive, not for use when cough is beneficial or is crucial diagnostic sign (as after thoracic surgery). ▪ Monitor respiratory and circulatory status.
colchicine Colchicine MR‡, Colgout‡, Colsalide, Novocolchicine†	*Prevention of acute gout attacks as prophylactic or maintenance therapy* — **Adults:** 0.5 or 0.6 mg PO daily. Dosage and its frequency	▪ Obtain baseline lab studies before and during therapy. ▪ **IV use:** Give by slow IV push over 2 to 5 min.

Colchicum autumnale *alkaloid* *Antigout agent* Preg. Risk Category: C (oral), D (IV)	may vary with severity and frequency of attacks. *Prevention of gout attacks in patients undergoing surgery* — **Adults:** 0.5 to 0.6 mg PO tid 3 days before and 3 days after surgery. *Acute gout, acute gouty arthritis* — **Adults:** 0.5 to 1.3 mg PO, then 0.5 or 0.6 mg q 1 to 2 hr until relief, nausea, vomiting, or diarrhea ensues; or max dosage of 8 mg reached. Or, 2 mg IV, followed by 0.5 mg IV q 6 hr prn. 24 hr max (one course of treatment) 4 mg.	• Do not administer IM or SC. • Give with meals to reduce GI effects. • Monitor I&O, and keep output at 2,000 ml daily. • First sign of acute overdose may be GI symptoms.
colestipol hydrochloride Colestid *Anion exchange resin* *Antilipemic* Preg. Risk Category: NR	*Primary hypercholesterolemia* — **Adults:** granules: 5 to 30 g PO qd or in divided doses; tab: 2 to 16 g/day given once or in divided doses.	• Monitor serum cholesterol and triglyceride levels regularly. • Monitor bowel habits. • Don't administer in dry form. Encourage diet high in fiber and fluids. • In patient also receiving cardiac glycoside, monitor serum levels of that drug.
corticotropin [adrenocorticotropic hormone, ACTH] ACTH, Acthar **repository corticotropin** Acthar Gel (H.P.)†, ACTH Gel, H.P. Acthar Gel	*Diagnostic test of adrenocortical function* — **Adults:** 40 units IV infusion q 12 hr for 48 hr; or IM q 12 hr for 1 to 2 days; or 10 to 25 units aqueous form in 500 ml of D_5W over 8 hr, between blood samplings. Individual dosages generally vary with adrenal glands' sensitivity to stimulation and with specific disease. Infants and younger	• **IV use:** Use only aqueous form IV. Dilute in 500 ml D_5W and infuse over 8 hr. • If using gel, warm to room temp, draw into large needle, and give slowly as deep IM injection with 21G or 22G needle. • Unusual stress may call for additional use of rapidly acting corticosteroids. *(continued)*

†Canadian ‡Australian

DRUG/CLASS/ CATEGORY	INDICATIONS/ DOSAGES	KEY NURSING CONSIDERATIONS
corticotropin *(continued)* *Anterior pituitary hormone* *Diagnostic aid/replacement* *hormone/multiple sclerosis* *and nonsuppurative thy-* *roiditis treatment* Preg. Risk Category: C	children require larger doses per kg. *For therapeutic use* — **Adults:** 40 units aqueous form SC or IM in 4 divided doses; or 40 to 80 units q 24 to 72 hr (repository form).	• May mask signs of chronic disease and decrease host resistance and ability to lo- calize infection. • Record weight changes, fluid exchange, and resting BP until minimal effective dosage reached.
cortisone acetate Cortate‡, Cortone Acetate *Glucocorticoid/mineralocor-* *ticoid* *Anti-inflammatory/replace-* *ment therapy* Preg. Risk Category: C	*Adrenal insufficiency, allergy, inflamma-* *tion* — **Adults:** 25 to 300 mg PO or 20 to 300 mg IM daily. Dosages highly individual- ized, depending on disease severity.	• To reduce GI irritation, give with milk or food. • For better results and less toxicity, give once-daily dose in morning. • IM route produces slow onset of action. • Monitor serum electrolyte, blood glucose, and fluid imbalances.
co-trimoxazole **(sulfamethoxazole-** **trimethoprim)** Apo-Sulfatrim†, Bactrim DS, Septra, SMZ-TMP, Sul- fatrim *Sulfonamide and folate an-* *tagonist* *Antibiotic*	*Shigellosis or UTI caused by susceptible* *strains of E. coli, Proteus (indole positive or* *negative), Klebsiella, or Enterobacter* — **Adults:** 160 mg trimethoprim/800 mg sul- famethoxazole (double-strength tab) PO q 12 hr for 10 to 14 days in UTI and for 5 days in shigellosis. For uncomplicated cysti- tis or acute urethral syndrome, one double- strength tab q 12 hr for 3 days. If indicated, IV infusion given: 8 to 10 mg/kg/day in 2 to	• Dosage for mg/kg/day based on trimetho- prim component. • Obtain specimen for culture and sensitivity tests before first dose. • Adverse reactions, especially hypersensi- tivity reactions, rash, and fever, are more common in AIDS patients. • Promptly report rash, sore throat, fever, or mouth sores (early signs of blood dyscra- sia).

Preg. Risk Category: C
(contraindicated at term)

4 divided doses q 6, 8, or 12 hr for up to 14 days for severe UTI. Max 960 mg trimethoprim. **Children ≥ 2 mo:** 8 mg/kg/day PO, in 2 divided doses q 12 hr (10 days for UTI; 5 days for shigellosis). If indicated, IV infusion given: 8 to 10 mg/kg/day in 2 to 4 divided doses q 6, 8, or 12 hr. Don't exceed adult dose.

Chronic bronchitis and upper respiratory tract infections — **Adults:** 160 mg trimethoprim/800 mg sulfamethoxazole PO q 12 hr for 10 to 14 days.

UTI in men with prostatitis — **Adults:** 160 mg trimethoprim/800 mg sulfamethoxazole PO bid for 3 to 6 mo.

cromolyn sodium (sodium cromoglycate)
Crolom, Intal, Intal Aerosol Spray, Intal Nebulizer Solution, Nasalcrom
Chromone derivative
Mast cell stabilizer/antiasthmatic
Preg. Risk Category: B

Mild to moderate persistent asthma —
Adults and children ≥ 5 yr: 2 metered sprays using inhaler qid at regular intervals. Alternatively, 20 mg via nebulization qid at regular intervals.

Prevention and treatment of seasonal and perennial allergic rhinitis — **Adults and children > 5 yr:** 1 spray in each nostril tid or qid, up to 6 times daily.

Prevention of exercise-induced bronchospasm — **Adults and children ≥ 5 yr:** 2 metered sprays inhaled no more than 1 hr before anticipated exercise.

Conjunctivitis — **Adults and children ≥ 4 yr:** 1 to 2 drops in each eye 4 to 6 times daily at regular intervals.

- *IV use:* Dilute infusion in D$_5$W. Don't mix with other drugs or solutions. Infuse slowly over 60 to 90 min. Don't give by rapid infusion or bolus injection. Don't refrigerate. Use within 6 hr.
- Never administer IM.

- Except for ophthalmic solution, use only when acute asthma episode has been controlled, airway clear, and patient can breathe independently.
- Dissolve powder in capsules for oral dose in hot water, and further dilute with cold water before ingestion. Don't mix with fruit juice, milk, or food.
- Watch for recurrence of asthmatic symptoms when dosage decreased.

CROMOLYN SODIUM

81

DRUG/CLASS/CATEGORY	INDICATIONS/DOSAGES	KEY NURSING CONSIDERATIONS
cyanocobalamin (vitamin B$_{12}$) Anacobin†, Bedoz†, Crystamine, Crysti-12, Cyanoject **hydroxocobalamin (vitamin B$_{12}$)** Codroxomin, Hydrobexan, Hydro-Cobex, Hydro-Crysti-12, LA-12 *Water soluble vitamin Vitamin, nutritional supplement* Preg. Risk Category: NR	*Vitamin B$_{12}$ deficiency* — **Adults:** 30 mcg hydroxocobalamin IM daily for 5 to 10 days, depending on severity. Maintenance, 100 to 200 mcg IM q mo. **Children:** 1 to 5 mg hydroxocobalamin spread over ≥ 2 wk in doses of 100 mcg IM, depending on severity. Maintenance, 30 to 50 mcg/mo IM. *Pernicious anemia or vitamin B$_{12}$ malabsorption* — **Adults:** 100 mcg cyanocobalamin IM or SC qd for 6 to 7 days, then 100 mcg IM or SC q mo. **Children:** 30 to 50 mcg IM or SC qd over 2 or more wk; then 100 mcg IM or SC q mo for life. *Methylmalonic aciduria* — **Neonates:** 1,000 mcg cyanocobalamin IM daily.	▪ Use cautiously in anemic patients with co-existing cardiac, pulmonary, or hypertensive disease; and in patients with severe vitamin B$_{12}$–dependent deficiencies. ▪ Use cautiously in premature infants. ▪ Determine reticulocyte count, hematocrit, B$_{12}$, iron, and folate levels before therapy. ▪ Don't mix in same syringe with other drugs. ▪ Incompatible with many drugs and solutions. ▪ Closely monitor potassium levels for first 48 hr. ▪ Protect vitamin B$_{12}$ from light. Do not refrigerate or freeze. ▪ In pernicious anemia, stress need to return for monthly injections; anemia will recur if not treated monthly.
cyclobenzaprine hydrochloride Flexeril *Tricyclic antidepressant derivative Skeletal muscle relaxant* Preg. Risk Category: B	*Short-term treatment of muscle spasm* — **Adults:** 10 mg PO tid. Max 60 mg daily; max duration of treatment 2 to 3 wk.	▪ Be alert for nausea, headache, and malaise, which may occur with abrupt withdrawal after long-term use. ▪ Watch for symptoms of overdose, including cardiac toxicity. Notify doctor immediately and have physostigmine available.

Diagnostic procedures requiring mydriasis and cycloplegia — **Adults:** 1 or 2 drops of 0.5%, 1%, or 2% solution instilled into eyes followed by 1 or 2 drops in 5 to 10 min, if needed. **Children:** 1 drop of 0.5%, 1%, or 2% solution instilled into each eye, followed in 5 to 10 min with 1 drop 0.5% or 1% solution.

- Physostigmine is antidote of choice.
- Teach how to instill drug.
- Warn to avoid hazardous activities until temporary blurring subsides.

cyclopentolate hydrochloride
AK-Pentolate, Cyclogyl
Anticholinergic agent
Cycloplegic, mydriatic
Preg. Risk Category: NR

Breast and ovarian cancers; Hodgkin's disease; chronic lymphocytic leukemia; chronic myelocytic leukemia; acute lymphoblastic leukemia; acute myelocytic and monocytic leukemia; neuroblastoma; retinoblastoma; malignant lymphoma; multiple myeloma; mycosis fungoides; sarcoma — **Adults and children:** initially, 40 to 50 mg/kg IV in divided doses over 2 to 5 days. Or, 10 to 15 mg/kg IV q 7 to 10 days, 3 to 5 mg/kg IV twice weekly, or 1 to 5 mg/kg PO daily, depending on patient tolerance. Subsequent dosages adjusted according to response.
Minimal change nephrotic syndrome in children — **Children:** 2.5 to 3 mg/kg PO qd for 60 to 90 days.

- Parenteral form drug associated with carcinogenic, mutagenic, and teratogenic risks for personnel.
- After reconstitution, administer by direct IV injection or infusion. For IV infusion, dilute with compatible solution such as D_5W.
- Don't give drug at bedtime; may increase the possibility of cystitis. If cystitis occurs, discontinue drug and notify doctor. Mesna may be given to lower the incidence and severity of bladder toxicity.
- Monitor serum uric acid level.
- Encourage voiding q 1 to 2 hr while awake and drinking ≥3 L fluid daily.

cyclophosphamide
Cycloblastin‡, Cytoxan, Cytoxan Lyophilized, Endoxan-Asta‡, Neosar, Procytox†
Alkylating agent
Antineoplastic
Preg. Risk Category: D

Adjunctive treatment in pulmonary or extrapulmonary TB — **Adults:** initially, 250 mg PO q 12 hr for 2 wk; then, if blood levels < 25 to 30 mcg/ml and no toxicity has de-

- Obtain specimen for culture and sensitivity tests before therapy begins and periodically thereafter to detect possible resistance.

(continued)

cycloserine
Seromycin
Isoxizolidone/d-alanine analogue

DRUG / CLASS / CATEGORY	INDICATIONS / DOSAGES	KEY NURSING CONSIDERATIONS
cycloserine *(continued)* *Antitubercular agent* Preg. Risk Category: C	veloped, increase to 250 mg q 8 hr for 2 wk. If optimum blood levels still not achieved and no toxicity has developed, increase to 250 mg q 6 hr. Max 1 g/day. If CNS toxicity occurs, discontinue drug for 1 wk, then resume at 250 mg daily for 2 wk. If no serious toxic effects occur, increase dosage in 250-mg increments q 10 days until blood level of 25 to 30 mcg/ml reached.	• Observe for psychotic symptoms, hallucinations, and possible suicidal tendencies. • Administer pyridoxine, anticonvulsants, tranquilizers, or sedatives, as ordered, to relieve adverse reactions. • Monitor serum cycloserine levels, hematologic tests, and renal and liver function studies periodically as ordered.
cyclosporine (cyclosporin) Neoral, Sandimmun†, Sandimmune *Polypeptide antibiotic Immunosuppressant* Preg. Risk Category: C	*Prophylaxis of organ rejection in kidney, liver, or heart transplantation —* **Adults and children:** 15 mg/kg PO 4 to 12 hr before transplantation and continued qd postop for 1 to 2 wk. Then dosage reduced 5% each wk to maintenance level of 5 to 10 mg/kg/day. Or, 5 to 6 mg/kg IV concentrate 4 to 12 hr before transplantation. Postop, dosage repeated qd until patient can tolerate oral form.	• To increase palatability of oral solutions, mix with whole milk or fruit juice. Use glass container. • *IV use:* Administer cyclosporine IV concentrate at ⅓ oral dose and dilute before use. Dilute each ml of concentrate in 20 to 100 ml of D₅W or 0.9% NaCl for injection immediately before administration; infuse over 2 to 6 hr. • Monitor cyclosporine blood levels, BUN, liver function tests, and serum creatinine levels.
cytarabine (ara-C, cytosine arabinoside)	*Acute nonlymphocytic leukemia, acute lymphocytic leukemia, blast phase of chronic myelocytic leukemia —* **Adults and children:** 100 mg/m² daily by continuous IV in-	• Give antiemetic before administering. • Parenteral form associated with carcinogenic, mutagenic, and teratogenic risks for personnel.

Alexant, Cytosart, Cytosar-U
Antimetabolite
Antineoplastic
Preg. Risk Category: D

fusion or 100 mg/m^2 IV q 12 hr. Given for 7 days and repeated q 2 weeks. For maintenance, 1 mg/kg SC once or twice a week. **Meningeal leukemia — Adults and children:** highly variable from 5 mg/m^2 to 75 mg/m^2 intrathecally. Frequency also varies from once a day for 4 days to once q 4 days.

- For IV infusion, dilute using 0.9% NaCl for injection or D$_5$W.
- For intrathecal administration, use preservative-free 0.9% NaCl.
- Maintain high fluid intake and give allopurinol to avoid urate nephropathy.
- Monitor uric acid level, hepatic and renal function studies, and CBC.
- Assess patients for neurotoxicity.

cytomegalovirus immune globulin (human), intravenous (CMV-IGIV)
CytoGam
Immune globulin
Immune serum
Preg. Risk Category: C

To attenuate primary CMV disease in seronegative patients who received a kidney from CMV seropositive donor — **Adults:** administered IV based on time after transplantation: within 72 hr — 150 mg/kg; 2 wk after — 100 mg/kg; 4 wk after — 100 mg/kg; 6 wk after — 100 mg/kg; 8 wk after — 100 mg/kg; 12 wk after — 50 mg/kg; 16 wk after — 50 mg/kg. Initial dose given at 15 mg/kg/hr. Increased to 30 mg/kg/hr after 30 min if no untoward reactions occur, then to 60 mg/kg/hr after another 30 min if no reactions. Volume max 75 ml/hr. Subsequent doses may be given at 15 mg/kg/hr for 15 min, increasing q 15 min in steps to 60 mg/kg/hr.

- *IV use:* Administer through separate IV line with constant infusion pump. If unable to administer through separate line, piggyback into preexisting line. Do not dilute more than 1:2 with diluent.
- Begin infusion within 6 hr of entering vial; finish within 12 hr.
- Monitor vital signs ↑osely.
- For anaphylaxis or drop in BP, stop infusion, notify the doctor, and be prepared to administer CPR and such drugs as diphenhydramine and epinephrine.
- Refrigerate at 36° to 46° F (2° to 8° C).

CYTOMEGALOVIRUS IMMUNE GLOBULIN

85

DRUG/CLASS/ CATEGORY	INDICATIONS/ DOSAGES	KEY NURSING CONSIDERATIONS
D-penicillamine Cuprimine, Depen, D-Penamine† *Chelating agent* *Anti-inflammatory* Preg. Risk Category: NR	*Wilson's disease* — **Adults and children:** 250 mg PO qid 30 to 60 min before meals. Adjust dosage to achieve urinary copper excretion of 0.5 to 1 mg daily. *Cystinuria* — **Adults:** 250 mg to 1 g PO qid before meals. Adjust dosage to urinary cystine excretion < 100 mg daily when no calculi present or 100 to 200 mg daily when no calculi present. Max 4 g daily. **Children:** 30 mg/kg PO daily, divided qid before meals. Dosage adjusted to achieve urinary cystine excretion < 100 mg daily when renal calculi present, or 100 to 200 mg qd with no calculi. *Rheumatoid arthritis* — **Adults:** initially, 125 to 250 mg PO daily, with increases of 125 to 250 mg q 1 to 3 months, if necessary. Max 1.5 g daily.	▪ Give dose on empty stomach, preferably 1 hr before or 3 hr after meals. ▪ If patient has skin reaction, give antihistamines as prescribed. ▪ Report rash and fever to doctor immediately. ▪ Monitor CBC and renal and hepatic function q 2 wk for 1st 6 mo, then monthly, as ordered. Monitor urinalysis regularly for protein loss. ▪ Withhold drug and notify doctor if WBC count < 3,500/mm³ or platelet count < 100,000/mm³. Progressive decline in platelet or WBC count in 3 successive blood tests may necessitate temporary discontinuation. ▪ Patient should receive supplemental pyridoxine daily.
dacarbazine (DTIC) DTIC†, DTIC-Dome *Alkylating agent (cell cycle–phase nonspecific)* *Antineoplastic* Preg. Risk Category: C	*Metastatic malignant melanoma* — **Adults:** 2 to 4.5 mg/kg IV daily for 10 days; repeated q 4 wk as tolerated. Or 250 mg/m² IV daily for 5 days, repeated at 3-wk intervals. *Hodgkin's disease* — **Adults:** 150 mg/m² IV daily (in combination with other agents) for 5 days, repeated q 4 wk; or 375 mg/m² IV on 1st day of combination, repeated q 15 days.	▪ Avoid extravasation during infusion. If IV solution infiltrates, discontinue immediately, apply ice to area for 24 to 48 hr, and notify doctor. ▪ To prevent bleeding, avoid all IM injections when platelet count < 100,000/mm³. ▪ Toxicity often accompanied therapeutic effects. Monitor CBC and platelet count.

dactinomycin (actinomycin D)

Cosmegen

Antibiotic antineoplastic (cell cycle–phase non-specific)

Antineoplastic

Preg. Risk Category: C

Dosage and indications vary. Check treatment protocol with doctor.

Sarcoma, trophoblastic tumors in women, testicular cancer — **Adults:** 500 mcg (0.5 mg) IV daily for 5 days. Max 15 mcg/kg/day, or 400 to 600 mcg/m²/day for 5 days. After bone marrow recovery, may repeat course.

Wilms' tumor, rhabdomyosarcoma, Ewing's sarcoma — **Children:** 10 to 15 mcg/kg or 450 mcg/m²/day IV for 5 days. Max 500 mcg/day. Or 2.5 mg/m² IV in equally divided daily doses over 7 days. After bone marrow recovery, may repeat course.

- **IV use:** Give by direct injection into vein or through tubing of free-flowing IV solution of 0.9% NaCl for injection or D₅W.
- For IV infusion, dilute with up to 50 ml of D₅W or 0.9% NaCl for injection; infuse over 15 min.
- Vesicant; if extravasation occurs, severe tissue necrosis may result. If infiltration occurs, apply cold compresses and notify doctor.
- If skin contact occurs, irrigate with water for ≥ 15 min.
- Monitor CBC, platelet counts, and renal and hepatic functions, as ordered. Observe for stomatitis, diarrhea, and leukopenia.

dalteparin sodium

Fragmin

Low-molecular-weight heparin

Anticoagulant

Preg. Risk Category: B

Prophylaxis against DVT in patients undergoing abdominal surgery who are at risk for thromboembolic complications — **Adults:** 2,500 IU SC daily, starting 1 to 2 hr before surgery and repeated qd for 5 to 10 days postop.

- Have patient assume sitting or supine position when administering. Give SC injection deeply. Rotate sites daily.
- Not interchangeable (unit for unit) with unfractionated heparin or other low-molecular-weight heparin.
- Periodic, routine CBCs and fecal occult blood tests recommended. Regular monitoring of PT or activated PTT not required.
- Monitor closely for thrombocytopenia.
- Should be discontinued if thromboembolic event occurs despite dalteparin prophylaxis.

DALTEPARIN SODIUM 87

DRUG/CLASS/ CATEGORY	INDICATIONS/ DOSAGES	KEY NURSING CONSIDERATIONS
danaparoid sodium Orgaran *Glycosaminoglycan Anticoagulant/antithrombotic* Preg. Risk Category: B	*Prophylaxis against postop DVT in patients undergoing elective hip replacement surgery* — **Adults:** 750 anti-Xa units SC bid starting 1 to 4 hr preop, and then not sooner than 2 hr after surgery. Treatment continued for 7 to 10 days postop or until risk of DVT diminished.	• Never give IM. To administer, have patient lie down. Give SC injection deeply. Don't rub afterward. • Not interchangeable (unit for unit) with heparin or low-molecular-weight heparin. • Routine CBCs and fecal occult blood tests recommended during therapy. • Has little effect on PT, PTT, fibrinolytic activity, and bleeding time. • Monitor Hct and BP closely; decrease in either may signal hemorrhage. • If serious bleeding occurs, stop drug and transfuse blood products as ordered.
danazol Cyclomen, Danocrine *Androgen Antiestrogen/androgen* Preg. Risk Category: X	*Mild endometriosis* — **Women:** initially, 100 to 200 mg PO bid uninterrupted for 3 to 6 mo; may continue for 9 mo. Subsequent dosage based on patient response. *Moderate to severe endometriosis* — **Women:** 400 mg PO bid uninterrupted for 3 to 6 mo; may continue for 9 mo. *Fibrocystic breast disease* — **Women:** 100 to 400 mg PO daily in 2 divided doses uninterrupted for 2 to 6 mo.	• Unless contraindicated, instruct to use with diet high in calories and protein. • Monitor closely for virilization signs. Some androgenic effects, such as voice deepening, may not be reversible on drug discontinuation. • Periodic dosage decreases or gradual drug withdrawal preferred.

dantrolene sodium

Dantrium
Hydantoin derivative
Skeletal muscle relaxant
Preg. Risk Category: NR

Spasticity and sequelae secondary to severe chronic disorders (such as multiple sclerosis, cerebral palsy, spinal cord injury, CVA) — **Adults:** 25 mg PO daily. Increase gradually in 25-mg increments, up to 100 mg bid to qid, to max 400 mg daily. **Children:** initially, 0.5 mg/kg PO bid; increase to tid, then qid. Increase as needed by 0.5 mg/kg daily to 3 mg/kg bid to qid, to max 100 mg qid.

- Watch for hepatitis (fever and jaundice), severe diarrhea, severe weakness, and sensitivity reactions (fever and skin eruptions). Withhold dose and notify doctor if these occur.
- Prepare oral suspension for single dose by dissolving capsule contents in juice or other liquid.
- Obtain liver function tests at beginning of therapy.

dapsone

Avlosulfon†, Dapsone 100‡
Synthetic sulfone
Antileprotic/antimalarial
Preg. Risk Category: C

All forms of leprosy (Hansen's disease) — **Adults:** 100 mg PO daily, indefinitely; give with rifampin 600 mg PO daily for 6 mo.
Children: 1.4 mg/kg PO daily for min 3 yr.
Dermatitis herpetiformis — **Adults:** 50 mg PO daily; increase to 300 mg daily as prn.

- Monitor for signs and symptoms of erythema nodosum reaction (malaise, fever, painful inflammatory induration in skin and mucosa, iritis, neuritis).
- Be prepared to reduce or stop drug with decreased Hgb, or RBC or WBC count.
- If generalized, diffuse dermatitis occurs, notify doctor.
- Administer antihistamines as ordered to combat allergic dermatitis.

daunorubicin hydrochloride

Cerubidin†, Cerubidine
Antibiotic antineoplastic (cell-phase nonspecific)
Antineoplastic
Preg. Risk Category: D

Dosage and indications vary.
Remission induction in acute nonlymphocytic (myelogenous, monocytic, erythroid) leukemia — **Adults:** in combination, 30 to 45 mg/m2/day IV on days 1, 2, and 3 of 1st course and on days 1 and 2 of subsequent courses with cytarabine infusions.

- Take preventive measures (including adequate hydration) before treatment starts.
- **IV use:** Withdraw into syringe containing 10 to 15 ml of 0.9% NaCl for injection. Inject into tubing of free-flowing IV solution of D_5W or 0.9% NaCl for injection over 2 to 3 min. Or, dilute in 50 ml of 0.9% NaCl for *(continued)*

DAUNORUBICIN HYDROCHLORIDE 89

†Canadian ‡Australian

DRUG / CLASS / CATEGORY	INDICATIONS / DOSAGES	KEY NURSING CONSIDERATIONS
daunorubicin hydrochloride *(continued)*	*Remission induction in acute lymphocytic leukemia* — **Adults:** in combination, 45 mg/m²/day IV on days 1, 2, and 3 of 1st course. **Children ≥ 2 yr:** 25 mg/m² IV on day 1 wk, for up to 6 wk, if needed. **Children < 2 yr or BSA < 0.5 m²:** dose calculated based on body weight (1 mg/kg).	injection, and infuse over 10 to 15 min, or dilute in 100 ml and infuse over 30 to 45 min. Vesicant; if extravasation occurs, stop infusion immediately, apply ice for 24 to 48 hr, and notify doctor. - Monitor CBC, liver function tests, and pulse as ordered; monitor ECG q month during therapy. Monitor for nausea and vomiting, which may last 24 to 48 hr. - Stop drug and notify doctor if signs of heart failure or cardiomyopathy develop.
demeclocycline hydrochloride Declomycin, Ledermycin‡ *Tetracycline antibiotic Antibiotic* Preg. Risk Category: D	*Infections caused by susceptible gram-pos and gram-neg organisms,* Rickettsiae, M. pneumoniae, C. trachomatis; *psittacosis; granuloma inguinale* — **Adults:** 150 mg PO q 6 hr or 300 mg PO q 12 hr. **Children > 8 yr:** 6 to 12 mg/kg PO daily in divided doses q 6 to 12 hr. *Gonorrhea* — **Adults:** initially, 600 mg PO; then 300 mg PO q 12 hr for 4 days (total 3 g).	- Obtain specimen for culture and sensitivity tests before first dose. - Don't expose to light or heat; store in tightly capped container. - Monitor for superinfection. - Check tongue for signs of candidal infection. Stress good oral hygiene.
desipramine hydrochloride Norpramin, Pertofran‡	*Depression* — **Adults:** 100 to 200 mg PO daily in divided doses, increased to max 300 mg daily. Or give entire dosage hs. **Elderly**	- Record mood changes. Monitor for suicidal tendencies, and allow only min drug supply.

Pertofrane
Dibenzazepine tricyclic antidepressant
Antidepressant
Preg. Risk Category: NR

and adolescents: 25 to 100 mg PO daily in divided doses, increased gradually to max 150 mg daily if needed.

- Produces fewer anticholinergic effects than other TCAs. Adverse anticholinergic effects can occur rapidly.
- Should be gradually discontinued several days before surgery.

desmopressin acetate
DDAVP, Minirin‡, Stimate
Posterior pituitary hormone
Antidiuretic/hemostatic
Preg. Risk Category: B

Nonnephrogenic diabetes insipidus, temporary polyuria and polydipsia with pituitary trauma — **Adults:** 0.1 to 0.4 ml intranasally qd in 1 to 3 doses. Adjust am and pm doses separately for adequate diurnal rhythm of water turnover. Or, give injectable form 0.5 to 1 ml IV or SC qd, usually in 2 divided doses. **Children 3 mo to 12 yr:** 0.05 to 0.3 ml intranasally qd in 1 or 2 doses.

- Overdose may cause oxytocic or vasopressor activity. Withhold drug and notify doctor.
- Intranasal use can cause changes in nasal mucosa resulting in erratic, unreliable absorption. Report worsening condition to doctor; may prescribe injectable DDAVP.
- Adjust fluid intake to reduce risk of water intoxication and sodium depletion, especially in children and elderly patients.

desonide
DesOwen, Tridesilon
Topical adrenocorticoid
Anti-inflammatory
Preg. Risk Category: C

Inflammation associated with corticosteroid-responsive dermatoses — **Adults and children:** clean area; apply sparingly bid to qid.

- Gently wash skin before applying. Rub medication in gently, leaving thin coat. Don't apply near eyes, mucous membranes, or in ear canal.
- Notify doctor if skin infection, striae, atrophy, or fever develops.
- If antifungal agents or antibiotics used concomitantly, stop drug until infection controlled, as ordered.
- Systemic absorption likely with use of occlusive dressings, prolonged treatment, or extensive body-surface treatment. Watch for symptoms.

DESONIDE 91

DRUG / CLASS / CATEGORY	INDICATIONS / DOSAGES	KEY NURSING CONSIDERATIONS
dexamethasone Decadron, Hexadrol **dexamethasone acetate** Dalalone D.P., Decadron-LA, Dexasone-LA **dexamethasone sodium phosphate** Dalalone, Decadron Phosphate, Dexasone *Glucocorticoid* *Anti-inflammatory/immunosuppressant* Preg. Risk Category: C	*Cerebral edema* — **Adults:** initially, 10 mg (phosphate) IV; then 4 to 6 mg IM q 6 hr until symptoms subside (usually 2 to 4 days); then taper over 5 to 7 days. *Inflammatory conditions, allergic reactions, neoplasias* — **Adults:** 0.75 to 9 mg/day PO or 0.5 to 9 mg/day (phosphate) IM; or 4 to 16 mg (acetate) IM into joint or soft tissue q 1 to 3 wk; or 0.8 to 1.6 mg (acetate) into lesions q 1 to 3 wk. *Shock* — **Adults:** 1 to 6 mg/kg (phosphate) IV as single dose; or 40 mg IV q 2 to 6 hr, prn; continue only until patient stabilized.	▪ For better results and less toxicity, give once-daily dose in morning with food. ▪ Inspect skin for petechiae. ▪ Monitor weight, BP, serum electrolytes, and blood glucose. ▪ Watch for depression or psychotic episodes, especially with high-dose therapy. ▪ *IV use:* When giving as direct injection, inject undiluted over at least 1 min.
dexamethasone sodium phosphate inhalation Decadron Phosphate Respihaler *Glucocorticoid* *Anti-inflammatory/antiasthmatic* Preg. Risk Category: C	*Persistent asthma* — **Adults:** initially, 3 inhalations tid or qid. Decrease as needed and tolerated; most patients respond to 2 inhalations bid. Max 12 inhalations daily. **Children:** 2 inhalations tid or qid. Decrease as needed and tolerated; most patients respond to 2 inhalations bid. Max 8 inhalations daily.	▪ Taper oral therapy slowly as ordered. Instruct to report symptoms associated with corticosteroid withdrawal (fatigue, weakness, arthralgia, orthostatic hypotension, dyspnea). ▪ Spacer device helps to ensure delivery of proper dose and decrease local (oral) adverse effects. ▪ Check mucous membranes frequently for signs of fungal infection.

dexamethasone
Aeroseb-Dex, Decaderm, Decaspray

dexamethasone sodium phosphate
Decadron Cream
Corticosteroid
Anti-inflammatory
Preg. Risk Category: C

Inflammation associated with corticosteroid-responsive dermatoses — **Adults and children:** clean area; apply sparingly tid to qid. For aerosol use on scalp, shake can gently and apply to dry scalp after shampooing. Slide applicator tube under hair to touch scalp. Spray (about 2 sec) while moving tube to all affected areas, keeping it under the hair and in contact with scalp. Spot-spray inadequately covered areas. Don't massage drug into scalp or spray forehead or near eyes.

- Gently wash skin before applying. Rub in gently, leaving thin coat. Don't apply near eyes, mucous membranes, or in ear canal.
- Notify doctor if skin infection, striae, atrophy, or fever develops.
- When using aerosol around face, cover patient's eyes and warn against inhaling spray. To avoid freezing tissues, don't spray > 1 to 2 sec or closer than 6" (15 cm).
- Continue treatment for several days after lesions clear, as ordered.

dexamethasone
Maxidex Ophthalmic Suspension

dexamethasone sodium phosphate
Decadron Phosphate Ophthalmic, Maxidex Ophthalmic
Corticosteroid
Ophthalmic anti-inflammatory
Preg. Risk Category: C

Uveitis; iridocyclitis; inflammatory conditions of eyelids, conjunctiva, cornea, anterior or segment of globe; corneal injury from chemical or thermal burns, or penetration of foreign bodies; allergic conjunctivitis; suppression of graft rejection after keratoplasty — **Adults and children:** 1 to 2 drops susp or sol or 1.25 to 2.5 cm oint into conjunctival sac. In severe disease, drops may be used hourly, tapering to discontinuation as condition improves. In mild conditions, drops may be used up to 6 times daily or oint applied tid or qid. As condition improves, dosage tapered to bid, then qd.

- Use cautiously in patients with corneal abrasions that may be infected (especially with herpes).
- Glaucoma medications may need to be increased.
- Monitor for corneal ulceration.
- Tell to shake suspension well before use.
- Teach how to administer drug.
- Warn to stop drug and call doctor if visual acuity changes or visual field diminishes.
- Treatment may extend from days to weeks.

DEXAMETHASONE SODIUM PHOSPHATE 93

DRUG / CLASS / CATEGORY	INDICATIONS / DOSAGES	KEY NURSING CONSIDERATIONS
dextroampheta-mine sulfate Dexedrine, Dexedrine Spansule, Oxydess II, Robese, Spancap #1 *Amphetamine* CNS stimulant/short-term adjunctive anorexigenic/ sympathomimetic amine Preg. Risk Category: C Controlled Sub. Sched.: II	*Narcolepsy —* **Adults:** 5 to 60 mg PO daily in divided doses. **Children 6 to 12 yr:** 5 mg PO daily, with 5-mg increments wkly, prn. **Children ≥ 12 yr:** 10 mg PO daily, with 10-mg increments wkly, prn. Give first dose on awakening; additional doses (one or two) at intervals of 4 to 6 hr. *Short-term adjunct in exogenous obesity —* **Adults and children ≥ 12 yr:** 5 to 30 mg PO qd in divided doses 30 to 60 min before meals. Or, one 10- or 15-mg sust-release cap qd in morning. *Attention deficit disorder with hyper-activity —* **Children 3 to 5 yr:** 2.5 mg PO daily, with 2.5-mg increments wkly, prn. **Children ≥ 6 yr:** 5 mg PO qd or bid, with 5-mg increments wkly, prn.	• Not to be used to prevent fatigue. • Make sure obese patient is on weight-reduction program. • If tolerance to anorexigenic effect develops, discontinue drug and notify doctor. • Advise to avoid activities requiring alertness until CNS effects known. • Instruct to report excessive stimulation. • Fatigue may occur as drug wears off.
dextrose (d-glucose) *Carbohydrate* TPN component/caloric/ fluid volume replacement Preg. Risk Category: C	*Fluid replacement and caloric supplementation —* **Adults and children:** dosage varies. Peripheral IV infusion of 2.5% to 10% sol or central IV infusion of 20% sol for minimal fluid needs. 25% sol for acute hypoglycemia in neonates or infants. 50% sol for insulin-induced hypoglycemia. Sol of 10% to 70% diluted in admixtures, for TPN given through central vein.	• **IV use:** Control infusion rate carefully; max rate 0.5 g/kg/hr. Use infusion pump when infusing with amino acids for TPN. • Use central veins to infuse dextrose solutions with conc > 10%. • Monitor serum glucose carefully. • Never stop hypertonic solutions abruptly. • Monitor I&O and weight carefully. • Check vital signs frequently.

diazepam

Apo-Diazepam†, Diazemuls†, Intensol, T-Quil, Valium, Zetran

Benzodiazepine

Antianxiety agent/skeletal muscle relaxant/amnesic agent/anticonvulsant/sedative-hypnotic

Preg. Risk Category: D

Controlled Sub. Sched.: IV

Anxiety — Adults: 2 to 10 mg PO 2 to 4 times qd, or 15 to 30 mg ext-release cap PO qd. Or, 2 to 2.5 mg once or twice qd; increased gradually. **Children ≥ 6 mo:** 1 to 2.5 mg PO 3 or 4 times qd, increased gradually p.r.n.

Muscle spasm — Adults: 2 to 10 mg PO 2 to 4 times qd or 15 to 30 mg ext-release cap qd. Or, 5 to 10 mg IM or IV initially, then 5 to 10 mg IM or IV q 3 to 4 hr, prn. **Children > 30 days to 5 yr:** 1 to 2 mg IM or IV slowly, repeated q 3 to 4 hr, prn. **Children ≥ 5 yr:** 5 to 10 mg IM or IV q 3 to 4 hr, prn.

Status epilepticus and severe recurrent seizures — Adults: 5 to 10 mg IV (preferred) or IM. Repeat q 10 to 15 min, prn, to max 30 mg. Repeat q 2 to 4 hr p.r.n. **Children > 30 days to 5 yr:** 0.2 to 0.5 mg IV slowly q 2 to 5 min to max 5 mg. Repeat q 2 to 4 hr, prn. **Children ≥ 5 yr:** 1 mg IV q 2 to 5 min to max 10 mg. Repeat q 2 to 4 hr, prn.

- Monitor respirations q 5 to 15 min and before each repeated IV dose. Have emergency resuscitation equipment and oxygen at bedside.
- Don't mix injectable form with other drugs.
- Don't store parenteral solution in plastic syringes.
- IV route most reliable parenteral route; IM use not recommended because absorption variable and injection painful.
- **IV use:** Give no faster than 5 mg/min. Check daily for phlebitis at injection site.
- Avoid extravasation. Don't inject into small veins.

diazepam

Hyperstat IV

Peripheral vasodilator

Antihypertensive

Preg. Risk Category: C

Hypertensive crisis — Adults and children: 1 to 3 mg/kg by IV bolus (to max 150 mg) q 5 to 15 min until adequate response occurs. Repeat at 4- to 24-hr intervals as needed.

- **IV use:** Monitor BP and ECG continuously. Keep patient supine during and 1 hr after infusion. Protect IV solutions from light.
- Avoid extravasation.
- Monitor fluid balance and blood glucose.

DRUG / CLASS / CATEGORY	INDICATIONS / DOSAGES	KEY NURSING CONSIDERATIONS
diclofenac potassium Cataflam **diclofenac sodium** Fenac†, Voltaren, Voltaren SR† Nonsteroidal anti-inflammatory Antiarthritic agent/anti-inflammatory Preg. Risk Category: B	*Ankylosing spondylitis* — **Adults:** 25 mg PO qid (and hs, prn). *Osteoarthritis* — **Adults:** 50 mg PO bid or tid, or 75 mg PO bid (sodium form only). *Rheumatoid arthritis* — **Adults:** 50 mg PO tid or qid. Or, 75 mg PO bid (sodium form only) or 50 to 100 mg PR hs as substitute for last PO dose of day. Max 225 mg qd. *Analgesia and primary dysmenorrhea* — **Adults:** 50 mg PO tid (potassium form only).	• Can decrease renal blood flow and lead to reversible renal impairment. Monitor patient closely. • Monitor serum transaminase periodically during therapy. • May mask symptoms of infection. • To minimize GI distress, instruct to take with milk or meals. • Advise not to crush, chew, or break enteric-coated tablets.
dicyclomine hydrochloride Antispas, Bemote, Bentyl, Neoquess, Spasmoban† Anticholinergic Antimuscarinic/GI antispasmodic Preg. Risk Category: B	*Irritable bowel syndrome and other functional GI disorders* — **Adults:** initially, 20 mg PO qid, increased to 40 mg PO qid, or 20 mg IM q 4 to 6 hr.	• Don't give SC or IV. • Give 30 min to 1 hr before meals and hs. Bedtime dose can be larger; administer at least 2 hr after last meal. • Monitor vital signs and urine output. • Prepare to adjust dosage according to patient's needs and response, as ordered.
didanosine (ddI) Videx Purine analogue Antiviral agent Preg. Risk Category: B	*Treatment of HIV infection when antiretroviral therapy warranted* — **Adults ≥ 60 kg:** 200 mg (tab) PO q 12 hr, or 250 mg buff powder PO q 12 hr. **Adults < 60 kg:** 125 mg (tab) PO q 12 hr; or 167 mg buff powder PO q 12 hr. **Children:** 120 mg/m² PO q 12 hr.	• Administer on empty stomach. • Pediatric powder for oral sol must be prepared by pharmacist before dispensing. • Associated with high incidence of diarrhea. • Don't use fruit juice or other acidic beverages to dissolve powder.

- Don't give to children or teenagers with chickenpox or flu-like illness due to risk for Reye's syndrome.
- Advise to take with water, milk, or meals.

diflunisal
Dolobid

Mild to moderate pain, osteoarthritis, rheumatoid arthritis — **Adults:** 500 to 1,000 mg PO daily in 2 divided doses, usually q 12 hr. Max 1,500 mg daily. **Adults > 65 yr:** half of usual adult dose.

Nonsteroidal anti-inflammatory, salicylic acid derivative
Nonnarcotic analgesic/antipyretic/anti-inflammatory
Preg. Risk Category: C

digoxin
Digoxin, Lanoxicaps, Lanoxin, Novodigoxin†

Cardiac glycoside
Antiarrhythmic/inotropic
Preg. Risk Category: C

Heart failure, PSVT, atrial fibrillation and flutter — **Adults:** loading dose 0.5 to 1 mg IV or PO in divided doses over 24 hr; maintenance dosage 0.125 to 0.5 mg IV or PO daily (average: 0.25 mg). **Adults > 65 yr:** 0.125 mg PO daily as maintenance dose. **Premature neonates:** loading dose 0.015 to 0.025 mg/kg IV in 3 divided doses over 24 hr; maintenance: 0.01 mg/kg daily, divided q 12 hr. **Neonates:** loading dose 0.025 to 0.035 mg/kg PO, divided q 8 hr over 24 hr; IV loading dose 0.02 to 0.03 mg/kg; maintenance: 0.01 mg/kg daily, divided q 12 hr. **Children 1 mo to 2 yr:** loading dose 0.035 to 0.06 mg/kg PO in three divided doses over 24 hr; IV loading dose 0.03 to 0.05 mg/kg; maintenance: 0.01 to 0.02 mg/kg PO daily, divided q 12 hr. **Children > 2 yr:** loading dose 0.02 to 0.04 mg/kg PO daily; IV loading dose divided q 8 hr over 24 hr; maintenance: 0.015 to 0.035 mg/kg; maintenance: 0.012 mg/kg PO daily, divided q 12 hr.

- Before therapy, obtain baseline data (apical pulse, HR, BP, and electrolytes) and ask about use of cardiac glycosides within previous 2 to 3 wk.
- Before administering, take apical-radial pulse for full minute. Record and report significant changes. If changes occur, check BP and obtain ECG.
- Excessive slowing of pulse (≤ 60) may signal digitalis toxicity. Withhold drug and notify doctor.
- *IV use:* Infuse slowly over at least 5 min.
- Encourage consumption of potassium-rich foods.
- Smaller doses given in impaired renal function or to frail patients.

DIGOXIN   97

DRUG/CLASS/ CATEGORY	INDICATIONS/ DOSAGES	KEY NURSING CONSIDERATIONS
digoxin immune FAB (ovine) Digibind *Antibody fragment Cardiac glycoside antidote* Preg. Risk Category: C	*Potentially life-threatening digoxin or digitoxin intoxication —* **Adults and children:** IV dosage varies according to amount of digoxin or digitoxin to be neutralized. Each vial binds about 0.5 mg of digoxin or digitoxin. Avg dosage 6 vials (228 mg). However, if toxicity resulted from acute digoxin ingestion and neither serum digoxin level nor estimated ingestion amount known, 20 vials (760 mg) required. See pkg insert for complete, specific dosage instructions.	• Use only for life-threatening overdose in shock or cardiac arrest; with ventricular arrhythmias, progressive bradycardia, or 2nd- or 3rd-degree AV block not responsive to atropine. • **IV use:** Reconstitute 38-mg vial with 4 ml sterile water for injection. Gently roll vial to dissolve powder. Reconstituted solution contains 9.5 mg/ml. May give by direct injection if cardiac arrest seems imminent. Alternatively, dilute with 0.9% NaCl for injection to appropriate volume and give by intermittent infusion over 30 min through 0.22-micron membrane filter. • Monitor serum potassium closely. • Interferes with digitalis immunoassay measurements; standard serum digoxin levels misleading until drug cleared from body (about 2 days).
dihydroergotamine mesylate D.H.E. 45, Dihydergot‡ *Ergot alkaloid Vasoconstrictor* Preg. Risk Category: X	*To prevent or abort vascular or migraine headache —* **Adults:** 1 mg IM or IV. Repeat q 1 to 2 hr, prn, to total of 2 mg IV or 3 mg IM per attack. Max wkly dosage 6 mg.	• Most effective when used at first sign of migraine or soon after onset. • **IV use:** Directly inject solution into vein over 3 min. • Be alert for ergotamine rebound. • Protect ampules from heat and light.

diltiazem hydrochloride

Apo-Diltiaz†, Cardizem, Cardizem CD, Cardizem SR, Vasocardol Sr‡
Vasocardol Sr‡
Calcium channel blocker
Antianginal
Preg. Risk Category: C

Vasospastic angina (Prinzmetal's [variant] angina) and classic chronic stable angina pectoris — **Adults:** 30 mg PO tid or qid before meals and hs. Increase gradually to max 360 mg/day in divided doses. Alternatively, 120 or 180 mg (ext-release cap). Titrate as needed and tolerated to max 480 mg daily.
Hypertension — **Adults:** 60 to 120 mg PO bid (sust-release). Titrate to effect. Max recommended dosage 360 mg/day. Alternatively, 180 to 240 mg daily (ext-release) initially. Adjust dosage as necessary.
Atrial fibrillation or flutter; PSVT — **Adults:** 0.25 mg/kg as IV bolus injection over 2 min. If response inadequate, 0.35 mg/kg IV after 15 min followed with continuous infusion of 10 mg/hr. Some patients respond well to rates of 5 mg/hr; max dose 15 mg/hr.

- *IV use:* Infusions longer than 24 hr not recommended.
- Monitor BP and HR during initiation of therapy and dosage adjustments.
- If systolic BP < 90 or HR < 60, withhold dose and notify doctor.
- Tell to avoid hazardous activities during initiation of therapy.
- Advise that SL nitroglycerin may be taken concomitantly prn if anginal symptoms acute.

dimenhydrinate

Dimetabs, Dinate, Dommanate, Dramamine, Nauseatol†
Nauseatol†
Ethanolamine-derivative antihistamine
Antihistamine (H₁-receptor antagonist)/antiemetic/antivertigo agent
Preg. Risk Category: B

Prevention and treatment of motion sickness — **Adults and children ≥ 12 yr:** 50 to 100 mg PO q 4 to 6 hr; 50 mg IM, prn; or 50 mg IV diluted in 10 ml NaCl for injection, injected over 2 min. Max 400 mg daily. **Children 6 to 12 yr:** 25 to 50 mg PO q 6 to 8 hr, not to exceed 150 mg PO q 6 to 8 hr. **Children 2 to 6 yr:** 12.5 to 25 mg PO q 6 to 8 hr, not to exceed 75 mg in 24 hr. **Children > 2 yr:** 1.25 mg/kg or 37.5 mg/m² IM qid. Max 300 mg daily.

- Most IV products contain benzyl alcohol, associated with fatal "gasping syndrome" in premature and low-birth-weight infants.
- May mask symptoms of ototoxicity, brain tumor, or intestinal obstruction.
- *IV use:* Before giving, dilute each ml of drug with 10 ml sterile water for injection, D₅W, or 0.9% NaCl for injection. Give by direct injection over not less than 2 min.
- Avoid mixing parenteral preparation with other drugs.

DIMENHYDRINATE 99

†Canadian ‡Australian

DRUG/CLASS/ CATEGORY	INDICATIONS/ DOSAGES	KEY NURSING CONSIDERATIONS
dinoprostone Prepidil, Prostin E₂ *Prostaglandin* *Oxytocic* Preg. Risk Category: C	*To abort 2nd-trimester pregnancy; to evacuate uterus in missed abortion, intrauterine fetal deaths up to 28 wk of gestation, or benign hydatidiform mole* — **Adults:** 20-mg supp inserted high into posterior vag fornix. Repeat q 3 to 5 hr until abortion complete. *Ripening of unfavorable cervix in pregnant patients at or near term* — **Adults:** gel contents of 1 syringe given intravaginally; if cervix unfavorable after 6 hr, repeat. Don't give > 1.5 mg within 24-hr period.	• After administration, have patient remain supine for 10 min. • When used as abortifacient, may pretreat patient with antiemetic and antidiarrheal agent. • Treat dinoprostone-induced fever with water or alcohol sponging and increased fluid intake, not with aspirin. • Abortion should be complete within 30 hr when suppository used.
diphenhydramine hydrochloride Allerdryl†, Benadryl, Hydramine, Nytol Maximum Strength, Sominex Formula 2 *Ethanolamine-derivative antihistamine* *Antihistamine/antiemetic/ antivertigo agent/antitussive/sedative-hypnotic/antidyskinetic (anticholinergic)* Preg. Risk Category: B	*Rhinitis, allergy symptoms, motion sickness, Parkinson's disease* — **Adults and children ≥ 12 yr:** 25 to 50 mg PO tid or qid; or 10 to 50 mg deep IM or IV. Max IM or IV dosage 400 mg daily. **Children < 12 yr:** 5 mg/kg qd PO, deep IM, or IV in divided doses qid. Max 300 mg daily. *Sedation* — **Adults:** 25 to 50 mg PO, or deep IM, prn. *Nonproductive cough* — **Adults:** 25 mg PO q 4 to 6 hr (max 150 mg daily). **Children 6 to 12 yr:** 12.5 mg PO q 4 to 6 hr (max 75 mg daily). **Children 2 to 6 yr:** 6.25 mg PO q 4 to 6 hr (max 25 mg/day).	• Children < 12 yr should use only as directed by doctor. • Alternate injection sites to prevent irritation. Administer IM injection deeply into large muscle. • Instruct to take with food or milk to reduce GI distress. • Tell to take 30 min before travel to prevent motion sickness. • Advise to take with food or milk. • Instruct to use sunscreen and to avoid overexposure to sunlight.

diphtheria and tetanus toxoids, adsorbed *Toxoid* *Diphtheria and tetanus prophylaxis agent* Preg. Risk Category: C	*Primary immunization* — **Adults and children ≥ 7 yr:** adult strength; 0.5 ml IM 4 to 8 wk apart for 2 doses and 3rd dose 6 to 12 mo after 2nd dose. Booster — 0.5 ml IM q 10 yr. **Infants 6 wk to 1 yr:** ped strength; 0.5 ml IM ≥ 4 wk apart for 3 doses. Give booster dose 6 to 12 mo after 3rd inj. **Children 1 to 6 yr:** ped strength; 0.5 ml IM ≥ 4 wk apart for 2 doses. Give booster dosage 6 to 12 mo after 2nd inj. If final immunizing dose given after 7th birthday, use adult strength.	• Obtain history of allergies and reaction to immunization. • Before injection, verify strength (ped or adult) of toxoid to use. • Keep epinephrine 1:1,000 available to treat anaphylaxis. • Give in site not recently used for vaccines or toxoids.
diphtheria and tetanus toxoids and whole-cell pertussis vaccine (DTP, DPT) DTwP, Tri-Immunol **diphtheria and tetanus toxoids and acellular pertussis vaccine** Acel-Imune, DTaP, Tripedia *Combination toxoid and vaccine* *Diphtheria, tetanus, and pertussis prophylaxis agent* Preg. Risk Category: C	*Primary immunization* — **Children 6 wk to 6 yr:** 0.5 ml IM 4 to 8 wk apart for 3 doses and 4th dose 1 yr later. Booster—0.5 ml IM when starting school, unless 4th dose in series administered after 4th birthday; then, booster not necessary at time of school entrance. Not advised for adults or children > 6 yr. Products containing acellular pertussis vaccine may now be used for any dose in DTP immunization.	• Obtain history of allergies and reaction to immunization. • Keep epinephrine 1:1,000 available to treat anaphylaxis. • Shake before using. Refrigerate. • Administer only by deep IM injection, preferably in thigh or deltoid muscle. Don't give SC. • Acellular vaccine may be associated with lower incidence of local pain and fever.

DRUG/CLASS/ CATEGORY	INDICATIONS/ DOSAGES	KEY NURSING CONSIDERATIONS
dipivefrin Propine *Sympathomimetic agent* *Antiglaucoma agent* Preg. Risk Category: B	*IOP reduction in chronic open-angle glaucoma* — **Adults:** for initial glaucoma therapy, 1 drop of 0.1% sol q 12 hr. Adjust dosage based on patient response as determined by tonometric readings.	• Often used concomitantly with other antiglaucoma drugs. • May cause fewer adverse reactions than conventional epinephrine therapy.
dipyridamole IV Persantine, Persantin‡, Persantine *Pyrimidine analogue* *Coronary vasodilator/* *platelet aggregation* *inhibitor* Preg. Risk Category: B	*Inhibition of platelet adhesion in prosthetic heart valves* — **Adults:** 75 to 100 mg PO qid. *Alternative to exercise in CAD evaluation during thallium (²⁰¹Tl) myocardial perfusion scintigraphy* — **Adults:** 0.57 mg/kg as IV infusion at constant rate over 4 min (0.142 mg/kg/min). *Acute coronary insufficiency* — **Adults:** 10 mg IV or IM.	• If patient develops GI distress, give 1 hr before meals or with meals. • **IV use:** If using as diagnostic agent, dilute in 0.45% or 0.9% NaCl solution or D₅W in at least 1:2 ratio for total volume of 20 to 50 ml. Inject ²⁰¹Tl within 5 min after completing dipyridamole infusion. • Observe for adverse reactions. • Observe for signs of bleeding.
dirithromycin Dynabac *Macrolide* *Antibiotic* Preg. Risk Category: C	*Acute bacterial exacerbations of chronic bronchitis or secondary bacterial infection of acute bronchitis due to M. catarrhalis or S. pneumoniae; uncomplicated skin and skin-structure infections due to S. aureus (methicillin-susceptible strains)* — **Adults and children ≥ 12 yr:** 500 mg PO qd for 7 days. *Community-acquired pneumonia due to L. pneumophila, M. pneumoniae, or S. pneumoniae* — **Adults and children ≥ 12 yr:** 500 mg PO qd for 14 days.	• Obtain culture and sensitivity results to ensure organism is sensitive to drug. Not recommended for empiric use. • Don't use in patients with known, suspected, or potential bacteremias. • Administer with food or within 1 hr of food intake. • Monitor for superinfection. • Safety in children < 12 yr not established.

disopyramide
Rythmodan†
disopyramide phosphate
Norpace, Norpace CR, Rythmodan LA†
Pyridine derivative antiarrhythmic
Antiarrhythmic
Preg. Risk Category: C

Ventricular tachycardia and ventricular arrhythmias thought to be life-threatening —
Adults > 50 kg: 150 mg q 6 hr with conventional capsules or 300 mg q 12 hr with ext-release prep. **Adults 50 kg or less:** highly individualized. **Children < 1 yr:** 10 to 30 mg/kg PO qd. **Children 1 to 4 yr:** 10 to 20 mg/kg PO qd. **Children 4 to 12 yr:** 10 to 15 mg/kg PO qd. **Children 12 to 18 yr:** 6 to 15 mg/kg PO qd. For pediatric dosages, divide into equal amounts and give q 6 hr.

- Check apical pulse before administering. Notify doctor if < 60 or > 120.
- Discontinue if heart block develops, QRS complex widens by more than 25%, or QT interval lengthens by more than 25% above baseline; also notify doctor.
- Watch for recurrence of arrhythmias and check for adverse reactions; notify doctor if any occurs.
- Correct electrolyte abnormalities before therapy begins, as ordered.

disulfiram
Antabuse
Aldehyde dehydrogenase inhibitor
Alcoholic deterrent
Preg. Risk Category: NR

Adjunct in management of chronic alcoholism — **Adults:** 250 to 500 mg PO as single dose in morning for 1 to 2 wk or in evening if drowsiness occurs. Maintenance dosage 125 to 500 mg PO daily (avg dosage 250 mg) until permanent self-control established. Treatment may continue for months or years.

- Use only under close medical and nursing supervision. Never administer until patient has abstained from alcohol for ≥ 12 hr. Patient should clearly understand consequences of drug and give permission for its use. Use only in patients who are cooperative, well motivated, and receiving supportive psychiatric therapy.
- Complete physical exam and lab studies, including CBC, SMA-12, and transaminase level, should precede therapy and be repeated regularly, as ordered.

DRUG / CLASS / CATEGORY	INDICATIONS / DOSAGES	KEY NURSING CONSIDERATIONS
dobutamine hydrochloride Dobutrex *Adrenergic, beta₁ agonist* *Inotropic agent* Preg. Risk Category: B	*To increase cardiac output in short-term treatment of cardiac decompensation caused by depressed contractility, such as during refractory heart failure, and as adjunct in cardiac surgery —* **Adults:** 2.5 to 10 mcg/kg/min IV infusion. Rates up to 40 mcg/kg/min may be needed (rare).	▪ Administer after cardiac glycoside. ▪ Continuously monitor ECG, BP, PCWP, cardiac condition, and urine output. ▪ Before starting therapy, correct hypovolemia with plasma volume expanders, as ordered. ▪ *IV use:* Give through large vein. Use infusion pump. Avoid extravasation. ▪ Dilute concentrate for injection before administration. Don't exceed maximum concentration of 5 mg/ml.
docetaxel Taxotere *Taxoid* *Antineoplastic agent* Preg. Risk Category: D	*Treatment of patients with locally advanced or metastatic breast cancer who have progressed during anthracycline-based therapy or have relapsed during anthracycline-based adjuvant therapy —* **Adults:** 60 to 100 mg/m² IV over 1 hr q 3 wk.	▪ Monitor liver function studies. ▪ Premedicate with oral corticosteroids, such as dexamethasone 16 mg PO (8 mg bid) daily for 5 days starting 1 day before docetaxel administration. ▪ Wear gloves during preparation and administration. If solution contacts skin, wash immediately and thoroughly with soap and water. Mark all waste materials with CHEMOTHERAPY HAZARD labels. ▪ Bone marrow toxicity most frequent and dose-limiting toxic effect. Frequent blood count monitoring necessary during therapy. ▪ Monitor for hypersensitivity reactions.

docusate calcium
Dioctocal, Surfak
docusate sodium
Colace, Doxinate, Genasoft
Surfactant
Emollient laxative
Preg. Risk Category: C

Stool softener — **Adults and children > 12 yr:** 50 to 500 mg PO qd until bowel movements normal. **Children < 3 yr:** 10 to 40 mg docusate sodium PO qd. **Children 3 to 6 yr:** 20 to 60 mg docusate sodium PO qd. **Children 6 to 12 yr:** 40 to 120 mg docusate sodium PO qd.

- Give liquid in milk, fruit juice, or infant formula to mask bitter taste.
- Before administering, determine if patient has adequate fluid intake, exercise, and diet.
- Teach about dietary sources of bulk.
- Instruct to use only occasionally and not for > 1 wk without doctor's knowledge.

donepezil hydrochloride
Aricept
Acetylcholinesterase inhibitor
CNS agent for Alzheimer's disease
Preg. Risk Category: C

Mild to moderate dementia of Alzheimer's type — **Adults:** initially, 5 mg PO hs. After 4 to 6 wk, may increase to 10 mg qd.

- Monitor for symptoms of active or occult GI bleeding.

dopamine hydrochloride
Intropin, Revimine†
Adrenergic
Inotropic, vasopressor
Preg. Risk Category: C

To treat shock and correct hemodynamic imbalances; to improve perfusion to vital organs; to increase cardiac output; to correct hypotension — **Adults:** initially, 1 to 5 mcg/kg/min by IV infusion. Titrate dosage to desired hemodynamic or renal response; may increase infusion by 1 to 4 mcg/kg/min at 10- to 30-min intervals.

- If volume deficit exists, replace fluid before giving drug.
- Frequently monitor ECG, BP, cardiac output, CVP, PCWP, pulse rate, urine output, and color and temp of extremities.
- *IV use:* Don't mix with alkaline solutions. Use central line or large vein to minimize risk of extravasation.

DRUG/CLASS/ CATEGORY	INDICATIONS/ DOSAGES	KEY NURSING CONSIDERATIONS
dorzolamide hydrochloride Trusopt *Sulfonamide* *Antiglaucoma agent* Preg. Risk Category: C	*Treatment of increased IOP in patients with ocular hypertension or open-angle glaucoma* — **Adults:** 1 drop in conjunctival sac of affected eye tid.	• If patient receiving > 1 topical ophth drug, administer drugs ≥ 10 min apart.
doxazosin mesylate Cardura *Alpha-adrenergic blocker* *Antihypertensive* Preg. Risk Category: C	*Essential hypertension* — **Adults:** 1 mg PO qd, and determine effect on standing and supine BP at 2 to 6 hr and 24 hr after dosing. If necessary, increase to 2 mg daily. Titrate slowly. May increase to 4 mg qd, then 8 mg. Max 16 mg. *Benign prostatic hyperplasia* — **Adults:** initially, 1 mg PO qd in morning or evening; may increase to 2 mg and, thereafter, 4 mg and 8 mg qd, as needed. Recommended titration interval 1 to 2 wk.	• Monitor BP closely. • If syncope occurs, place patient in recumbent position and treat supportively. Transient hypotensive response doesn't contraindicate continued therapy. • Orthostatic hypotension most common after first dose but also can occur during dosage adjustment or interruption of therapy.
doxepin hydrochloride Deptran‡, Novo-Doxepin†, Sinequan, Triadapin† *Tricyclic antidepressant* *Antidepressant* Preg. Risk Category: NR	*Depression or anxiety* — **Adults:** initially, 25 to 75 mg PO daily in divided doses to max 300 mg daily. Alternatively, give entire maintenance dosage qd with max 150 mg PO.	• Record mood changes. Monitor patient for suicidal tendencies, and allow only minimal drug supply. • Discontinue gradually several days before surgery. • Dilute oral concentrate with 120 ml (4 oz) of water, milk, or juice (not grape juice).

doxorubicin hydrochloride

Adriamycin†, Adriamycin PFS, Adriamycin RDF, Rubex

Antineoplastic antibiotic (cell cycle-phase nonspecific)

Antineoplastic
Preg. Risk Category: D

Dosage and indications vary. Check treatment protocol with doctor.

Bladder, breast, lung, ovarian, stomach, and thyroid cancers; Hodgkin's disease; acute lymphoblastic and myeloblastic leukemia; Wilms' tumor; neuroblastoma; lymphoma; sarcoma — **Adults:** 60 to 75 mg/m² IV as single dose q 3 wk; or 30 mg/m² IV in single daily dose, days 1 to 3 of 4-wk cycle. Alternatively, 20 mg/m² IV once weekly. Max cumulative dosage 550 mg/m².

- Never give IM or SC.
- Cardiac function studies (including ECG) should be performed before treatment and periodically throughout.
- May be given concomitantly with doxorubicin if accumulated doxorubicin dose has reached 300 mg/m².
- Don't place IV line over joints or in extremities with poor venous or lymphatic drainage. If extravasation occurs, discontinue and apply ice for 24 to 48 hr, and notify doctor. Monitor area closely. Early consultation with plastic surgeon may be advisable.
- If vein streaking occurs, slow administration rate. If welts occur, stop administration and report to doctor.
- Monitor CBC and hepatic function tests, as ordered; monitor ECG monthly. If tachycardia develops, be prepared to stop drug or slow infusion rate and notify doctor.
- If signs of heart failure develop, stop drug and notify doctor. In many cases, heart failure can be prevented by limiting cumulative dosage to 550 mg/m² (400 mg/m² when patient also receiving or has received cyclophosphamide or radiation therapy to cardiac area).

DRUG / CLASS / CATEGORY	INDICATIONS / DOSAGES	KEY NURSING CONSIDERATIONS
doxycycline calcium Vibramycin **doxycycline hyclate** Doryx, Doxy-Caps, Doxycin†, Monodox, Vibramycin **doxycycline hydrochloride** Cyclidox†, Doryx†, Doxylin†; Vibramycin‡, Vibra-Tabs 50‡ **doxycycline monohydrate** Monodox, Vibramycin *Tetracycline* *Antibiotic* Preg. Risk Category: D	*Infections caused by susceptible gram-pos and gram-neg organisms* Rickettsiae, M. pneumoniae, C. trachomatis, *and* B. burgdorferi *(Lyme disease); psittacosis; granuloma inguinale* — **Adults and children > 8 yr weighing ≥ 45 kg:** 100 mg PO q 12 hr on first day, then 100 mg PO daily; or 200 mg IV on first day in 1 or 2 infusions, then 100 to 200 mg IV daily. **Children > 8 yr weighing < 45 kg:** 4.4 mg/kg PO or IV daily, in divided doses q 12 hr on first day; then 2.2 to 4.4 mg/kg daily in 1 or 2 divided doses. Give IV infusion slowly (minimum 1 hr). Infusion must be completed within 12 hr (within 6 hr in lact Ringer's solution or dextrose 5% in lact Ringer's solution). *Uncomplicated urethral, endocervical, or rectal infections caused by* C. trachomatis *or* U. urealyticum — **Adults:** 100 mg PO bid for at least 7 days (10 days for epididymitis). *Pelvic inflammatory disease* — **Adults:** 100 mg IV q 12 hr and continued for at least 2 days after symptomatic improvement; thereafter, 100 mg PO q 12 hr for total course of 14 days.	• Obtain specimen for culture and sensitivity tests before first dose. • Check expiration date. Outdated or deteriorated tetracyclines have associated with reversible nephrotoxicity (Fanconi's syndrome). • Administer with milk or food if adverse GI reactions develop. • Don't expose to light or heat. Protect from sunlight during infusion. • Check tongue for signs of fungal infection. Stress good oral hygiene

dronabinol (delta-9-tetrahydro-cannabinol)
Marinol
Cannabinoid
Antiemetic/appetite stimulant
Preg. Risk Category: C
Controlled Sub. Sched.: II

Nausea and vomiting associated with cancer chemotherapy — **Adults:** 5 mg/m² PO 1 to 3 hr before chemotherapy. Then same dose q 2 to 4 hr after chemotherapy for total of 4 to 6 doses per day. If needed, increase in 2.5-mg/m² increments to max 15 mg/m² per dose.
Anorexia and weight loss in patients with AIDS — **Adults:** 2.5 mg PO bid before lunch and dinner. If unable to tolerate, decrease dose to 2.5 mg PO, given as single dose daily in evening or hs. May gradually increase to max 20 mg/day.

- Principal active substance in *Cannabis sativa* (marijuana); can produce physical and psychological dependence and has high abuse potential.
- CNS effects intensify at higher dosages.
- Effects may persist for days after treatment ends.

---

e

econazole nitrate
Ecostatin†, Spectazole
Synthetic imidazole derivative
Antifungal
Preg. Risk Category: C

Tinea pedis, tinea cruris, tinea corporis, tinea versicolor; cutaneous candidiasis — **Adults and children:** rub into affected areas qd for ≥ 2 wk.
Cutaneous candidiasis — **Adults and children:** rub into affected areas bid.

- Clean affected area before applying.
- Don't use occlusive dressings.

---

enalaprilat
Vasotec IV
enalapril maleate
Amprace‡, Renitec‡, Vasotec

Hypertension — **Adults:** if patient not on diuretics, initially 5 mg PO qd, then adjust according to response. Usual dosage range 10 to 40 mg daily as single dose or 2 divided doses. Alternatively, 1.25 mg IV infusion q 6 hr over 5 min. For patient on diuretics,

- Monitor potassium intake and serum potassium.
- Monitor CBC with differential.
- **IV use:** Inject slowly over at least 5 min, or dilute in 50 ml compatible solution and infuse over 15 min.

(continued)

ENALAPRILAT 109

†Canadian ‡Australian

DRUG/CLASS/CATEGORY	INDICATIONS/DOSAGES	KEY NURSING CONSIDERATIONS
enalaprilat *(continued)* ACE inhibitor *Antihypertensive* Preg. Risk Category: C (D in 2nd and 3rd trimesters)	initially 2.5 mg PO qd. Alternatively, 0.625 mg IV over 5 min; repeat in 1 hr if needed, then 1.25 mg IV q 6 hr. *To switch from IV to oral therapy* — **Adults:** initially, 5 mg PO qd; if patient was receiving 0.625 mg IV q 6 hr, then 2.5 mg PO qd. Adjust dosage to response. *To convert from oral to IV therapy* — **Adults:** 1.25 mg IV over 5 min q 6 hr.	▪ Monitor BP response. ▪ Advise to report adverse reactions. ▪ Advise caution in hot weather and during repositioning or exercise to avoid lightheadedness and syncope.
enoxaparin sodium Lovenox *Low-molecular-weight heparin* *Anticoagulant* Preg. Risk Category: B	*To prevent pulmonary embolism and DVT after hip or knee replacement surgery* — **Adults:** 30 mg SC q 12 hr for 7 to 10 days. Give initial dose between 12 and 24 hr postop if hemostasis established.	▪ Never administer IM. Don't massage after SC injection. Watch for signs of bleeding at site. Rotate sites and keep record. ▪ Don't expel gas bubble from syringe before injection. ▪ Avoid excessive IM injections of other drugs. If possible, don't give any IM injections. ▪ Regularly inspect for bleeding gums, bruises, petechiae, nosebleeds, melena, tarry stools, hematuria, and hematemesis.
ephedrine sulfate Vicks Vatronol Nose Drops *Adrenergic* *Bronchodilator/nasal decongestant* Preg. Risk Category: NR	*Nasal congestion* — **Adults and children:** 2 to 3 drops of 0.5% sol into each nostril. Don't use more frequently than q 4 hr.	▪ Don't exceed recommended dosage. ▪ Instruct to use only when needed.

epinephrine (adrenaline)

Adrenalin, Bronkaid Mist, Bronkaid Mistometer†, Primatene Mist

epinephrine bitartrate

AsthmaHaler, Broniten Mist, Bronkaid Mist Suspension, Medihaler-Epi

epinephrine hydrochloride

Adrenalin Chloride, Asthma-Nefrin†, Epi-Pen, Epi-Pen Jr., Racepinephrine, Sus-Phrine, Vaponefrine

Adrenergic

Bronchodilator/vasopressor/cardiac stimulant

Preg. Risk Category: C

Bronchospasm, hypersensitivity reactions, anaphylaxis — **Adults:** 0.1 to 0.5 ml of 1:1,000 SC or IM. Repeat q 10 to 15 min, prn. Or, 0.1 to 0.25 ml of 1:1,000 IV slowly over 5 to 10 min. **Children:** 0.01 ml (10 mcg) of 1:1,000/kg SC; repeat q 20 min to 4 hr, prn. Or, 0.004 to 0.005 ml/kg of 1:200 (Sus-Phrine) SC; repeat q 8 to 12 hr, prn.

Acute asthmatic attacks — **Adults and children ≥ 4 yr:** 160 to 250 mcg (metered aerosol), equiv to 1 inhalation, repeated once if necessary after at least 1 min; don't give subsequent doses for at least 3 hr. Or, 1% (1:100) solution epinephrine or 2.25% solution racepinephrine by hand-bulb nebulizer as 1 to 3 deep inhalations, repeated q 3 hr prn.

To restore cardiac rhythm in cardiac arrest — **Adults:** usual dose 0.5 to 1 mg IV. May repeat q 3 to 5 min prn. Higher-dose epinephrine may be used: 3 to 5 mg (approx 0.1 mg/kg) repeated q 3 to 5 min. **Children:** usual dose 0.01 mg/kg (0.1 ml/kg 1:10,000 injection) IV. Usual initial dose through ET tube 0.1 ml/kg (0.1 ml/kg 1:1,000 injection) diluted in 1 to 2 ml 0.45% or 0.9% NaCl solution. Subsequent IV or intratracheal doses 0.1 to 0.2 mg/kg (0.1 to 0.2 ml/kg of 1:1,000 injection). May repeat q 3 to 5 min.

- Drug of choice in emergency treatment of acute anaphylactic reactions.
- ***IV use:*** Don't mix with alkaline solutions.
- When giving IV, monitor BP, HR, and ECG when therapy starts and frequently thereafter.
- Avoid IM inj of parenteral suspension into buttocks. Gas gangrene may occur.
- Massage site after IM injection.
- Observe closely for adverse reactions. Notify doctor if these develop.
- If > 1 inhalation ordered, tell patient to wait at least 2 min before repeating procedure.
- If patient also uses steroid inhaler, instruct to use bronchodilator first, then wait about 5 min before using steroid.
- Patient with history of acute hypersensitivity reactions may need to learn how to self-inject drug at home.

DRUG/CLASS/ CATEGORY	INDICATIONS/ DOSAGES	KEY NURSING CONSIDERATIONS
epinephrine hydrochloride Epifrin, Glaucon **epinephryl borate** Epinal, Eppy/N *Adrenergic* *Topical anesthetic (adjunct)/topical antihemorrhagic/antiglaucoma agent* Preg. Risk Category: C	*Open-angle glaucoma* — **Adults:** 1 or 2 drops 1% or 2% sol qd or bid. Adjust dosage according to tonometric readings.	• Can be injected into anterior chamber to produce rapid mydriasis during cataract removal, or can be used to control local bleeding during surgery. • Don't substitute one salt if another ordered; these salts not interchangeable. • Monitor BP and other vital signs. • Apply light finger pressure on lacrimal sac for 1 min after drops instilled. Don't touch dropper tip to eye or surrounding tissues.
epinephrine hydrochloride Adrenalin Chloride *Adrenergic* *Topical anesthetic (adjunct)/topical antihemorrhagic*	*Nasal congestion, local superficial bleeding* — **Adults and children ≥ 6 yr:** instill 1 or 2 drops of sol.	• Instruct to use only when needed and not to exceed recommended dosage.
epoetin alfa (erythropoietin) Epogen, Procrit *Glycoprotein* *Anti-anemic agent* Preg. Risk Category: C	*Anemia due to reduced production of endogenous erythropoietin caused by end-stage renal disease* — **Adults:** dosage individualized. Starting dose 50 to 100 units/kg IV 3 times weekly. (Can use SC or IV route in nondialysis patients with chronic renal failure or patients receiving continuous peri-	• Monitor BP before therapy starts. BP may rise, especially when Hct level increases in early part of therapy. Monitor blood count, as ordered. Hct may rise and cause excessive clotting. • **IV use:** Give by direct injection without dilution. Solution contains no preservatives.

Discard unused portion. Don't mix with other drugs.

- When used in HIV-infected patients, be prepared to individualize dosage based on response. Dosage recommendations are for patients with endogenous erythropoietin levels of 500 units/L or less and cumulative zidovudine doses of 4.2 g/wk or less.
- Patient should receive iron supplementation starting no later than when treatment starts and continuing throughout therapy. Response depends on amount of endogenous erythropoietin in plasma. Patients with 500 units/L or more usually have transfusion-dependent anemia and probably won't respond. Those with levels < 500 units/L usually respond well.

toneal dialysis). Reduce dosage when target Hct reached or if Hct rises > 4 points in any 2-wk period. Increase dosage if Hct doesn't increase by 5 to 6 points after 8 wk of therapy. Maintenance dosage highly individualized. *Adjunctive treatment of HIV-infected patients with anemia secondary to zidovudine therapy* — **Adults:** 100 units/kg IV or SC 3 times weekly for 8 wk or until target Hgb level reached. If response unsatisfactory after 8 wk, may increase dose by 50 to 100 units/kg IV or SC 3 times weekly. After 4 to 8 wk, may increase dosage further in increments of 50 to 100 units/kg 3 times weekly, to max 300 units/kg IV or SC 3 times weekly. *Anemia secondary to cancer chemotherapy* — **Adults:** 150 units/kg SC 3 times weekly for 8 wk or until target Hgb level reached.

ergotamine tartrate

Ergodryl Mono‡, Ergomar, Ergostat, Gynergent, Medihaler Ergotamine
Ergot alkaloid
Vasoconstrictor
Preg. Risk Category: X

Vascular or migraine headache — **Adults:** initially, 2 mg PO or SL, then 1 to 2 mg PO q hr or SL q ½ hr, to max 6 mg daily and 10 mg weekly. Alternatively, aerosol inhaler: 1 spray (360 mcg) initially, repeated q 5 min prn to max of 6 sprays (2.16 mg) per 24 hr or 15 sprays (5.4 mg) per wk.

- Most effective when used during prodromal stage of headache or as soon as possible after onset.
- Obtain accurate dietary history to determine if headache onset associated with certain foods.
- Be alert for ergotamine rebound.
- With long-term use, instruct to check for and report coldness in extremities or tingling in fingers and toes.

ERGOTAMINE TARTRATE   113

DRUG/CLASS/CATEGORY	INDICATIONS/DOSAGES	KEY NURSING CONSIDERATIONS
erythromycin base E-Mycin, Eramycin, ERYC, Robimycin **erythromycin estolate** Ilosone, Ilosone pulvules **erythromycin ethylsuccinate** EryPed, EryPed 200 **erythromycin lactobionate** Erythrocin **erythromycin stearate** Erythrocin Stearate *Antibiotic* Preg. Risk Category: B	*Acute PID caused by N. gonorrhoeae* — **Adults:** 500 mg IV (gluc. or lacto.) q 6 hr for 3 days, then 250 mg (base, estolate, stear.) or 400 mg (ethyl.) PO q 6 hr for 7 days. *Endocarditis prophylaxis for dental procedures in patients allergic to penicillin* — **Adults:** 800 mg (ethyl.) or 1 g (stearate) PO 1½ to 2 hr before; then 400 mg (ethyl.) or 500 mg (stearate) PO 6 hr later. **Children:** 20 mg/kg (ethyl., stearate) PO 1½ to 2 hr before procedure; half amount 6 hr later. *Mild to mod. severe respiratory tract, skin, and soft-tissue infections* — **Adults:** 250 to 500 mg (base, estolate, stearate) PO q 6 hr; or 400 to 800 mg (ethyl.) PO q 6 hr; or 15 to 20 mg/kg IV daily (gluc. lacto.) continuous inf or divided doses q 6 hr for 10 days. **Children:** 30 to 50 mg/kg (oral salts) PO qd, divided doses q 6 hr; or 15 to 20 mg/kg IV qd, divided doses q 4 to 6 hr for 10 days.	• Obtain urine specimen for culture and sensitivity tests before first dose. • Monitor hepatic function. • When giving suspension, note concentration. • *IV use:* Reconstitute according to manufacturer's directions and dilute each 250 mg in at least 100 ml 0.9% NaCl solution. Infuse over 1 hr. • Don't give erythromycin lactobionate with other drugs. • Monitor for superinfection. • For best absorption, instruct to take oral form with full glass of water 1 hr before or 2 hr after meals. May take with food if GI upset occurs. Coated tablets may be taken with meals. Caution not to drink fruit juice with drug and not to swallow chewable tablets whole. • Instruct to report adverse reactions.
erythromycin Akne-mycin, Erycette, Ery-Derm, EryGel, Ery-Sol† *Erythromycin* *Topical antibiotic* Preg. Risk Category: C	*Inflammatory acne vulgaris* — **Adults and children:** apply in thin film to affected areas bid.	• Wash, rinse, and dry affected areas before application. • Prolonged use may be necessary when treating acne vulgaris; may result in overgrowth of nonsusceptible organisms.

erythromycin

Ilotycin Ophthalmic Ointment

Erythromycin

Ophthalmic antibiotic

Preg. Risk Category: NR

Acute and chronic conjunctivitis, trachoma, other eye infections — **Adults and children:** 1-cm ribbon applied directly to infected eye up to 6 times daily.

Prophylaxis of ophthalmia neonatorum due to N. gonorrhoeae or C. trachomatis — **Neonates:** ribbon of oint approx 1 cm long applied in lower conjunctival sac of each eye shortly after birth.

- For prophylaxis of ophthalmia neonatorum, apply ≤ 1 hr after birth. Used in neonates born either by vag delivery or cesarean section. Gently massage eyelids for 1 min to spread ointment.
- For use only when sensitivity studies show drug effective against infecting organisms.
- Store at room temp in tightly closed, light-resistant container.

esmolol hydrochloride

Brevibloc

Beta1-adrenergic blocker

Antiarrhythmic

Preg. Risk Category: C

SVT; to control ventricular rate in atrial fibrillation or flutter in periop, postop, or other emergent circumstances; noncompensatory sinus tachycardia when HR requires specific interventions — **Adults:** loading dose: 500 mcg/kg/min by IV infusion over 1 min, then 4-min maintenance infusion of 50 mcg/kg/min. If no adequate response in 5 min, repeat loading dose and follow with maintenance infusion of 100 mcg/kg/min for 4 min. Repeat loading dose and increase maintenance infusion by 50-mcg/kg/min increments. Max maintenance infusion for tachycardia 200 mcg/kg/min.

Periop and postop tachycardia or hypertension — **Adults:** for periop treatment of tachycardia or hypertension, 80 mg (approximately 1 mg/kg) IV bolus over 30 sec, followed by 150 mcg/kg/min IV infusion, if needed. Adjust rate as needed to max 300 mcg/kg/min.

- **IV use:** Don't give by IV push; use infusion control device. May use 10-mg/ml single-dose vials without diluting, but always dilute injection concentrate (250 mg/ml) to max concentration of 10 mg/ml before infusion. Remove 20 ml from 500 ml of D₅W, lact Ringer's solution, or 0.45% or 0.9% NaCl solution, and add two ampules esmolol (final concentration 10 mg/ml).
- Solutions incompatible with diazepam, furosemide, sodium bicarbonate, and thiopental sodium.
- Monitor ECG and BP continuously during infusion; hypotension possible.
- Hypotension can usually be reversed within 30 min by decreasing dose or, if necessary, stopping infusion. Notify doctor.
- Instruct to report adverse reactions promptly.

ESMOLOL HYDROCHLORIDE   115

†Canadian ‡Australian

DRUG/CLASS/ CATEGORY	INDICATIONS/ DOSAGES	KEY NURSING CONSIDERATIONS
estazolam ProSom *Benzodiazepine Hypnotic* Preg. Risk Category: X Controlled Sub. Sched.: IV	*Insomnia* — **Adults:** 1 mg PO hs. Some patients may require 2 mg. **Elderly patients:** 1 mg PO hs. Use higher doses with extreme care.	▪ Monitor liver and renal functions and CBC. ▪ Caution not to perform activities that require mental alertness or physical coordination. ▪ Warn that additive depressant effects can occur if alcohol consumed during therapy.
esterified estrogens Estratab, Menest, Neo-Estrone† *Estrogen Estrogen replacement/anti-neoplastic* Preg. Risk Category: X	*Inoperable prostate cancer* — **Men:** 1.25 to 2.5 mg PO tid. *Breast cancer* — **Men and postmenopausal women:** 10 mg PO tid for 3 or more mo. *Female hypogonadism* — **Women:** 2.5 to 7.5 mg daily in divided doses in cycles of 20 days on, 10 days off. *Female castration, primary ovarian failure* — **Women:** 1.25 mg daily in cycles of 3 wk on, 1 wk off. Adjust for symptoms.	▪ Should discontinue at least 1 mo before procedures associated with prolonged immobilization or thromboembolism. ▪ Warn to immediately report adverse reactions. ▪ Tell diabetic to report elevated blood glucose. ▪ Teach how to perform routine breast self-exam.
estradiol (oestradiol) Climara, Estrace, Estraderm **estradiol cypionate** depGynogen, Depo-Estradiol, E-Cypionate, Estrofem **estradiol valerate (oestradiol valerate)** Climara Patch, Delestrogen,	*Vasomotor menopause symptoms, female hypogonadism, female castration, primary ovarian failure* — **Adults:** 1 to 2 mg PO (estradiol) daily in cycles of 21 days on and 7 days off, or cycles of 5 days on and 2 days off; or 1 transdermal system (Estraderm) delivering 0.05 mg/24 hr, or as system (Climara) delivering either 0.05 mg/ 24 hr or 0.1 mg/24 hr and applied q wk in	▪ Ensure that patient undergoes physical exam before and during therapy. ▪ Ask patient about allergies, especially to foods or plants. ▪ Never give IV. ▪ Apply transdermal patch to clean, dry, hairless, intact skin on abdomen or buttocks. Don't apply to areas where clothing can loosen patch.

Dioval, Estradiol L.A., Estra-L 20, Estra-L 40, Estraval, Femogex, Gynogen LA, LAE, Menaval, Primogyn Depot‡
polyestradiol phosphate
Estradurin
Estrogen
Estrogen replacement/antineoplastic
Preg. Risk Category: X

cycles of 3 wk on and 1 wk off. Alternatively, 1 to 5 mg (cypionate) IM q 3 to 4 wk, or 10 to 20 mg (valerate) IM q 4 wk, prn.
Palliative treatment of advanced, inoperable breast cancer — **Men and postmenopausal women:** 10 mg PO (estradiol) tid for 3 mo.
Palliative treatment of advanced inoperable prostate cancer — **Men:** 30 mg (valerate) IM q 1 to 2 wk, or 1 to 2 mg PO (estradiol) tid. Polyestradiol phosphate injection: 40 mg IM q 2 to 4 wk.

- Rotate application sites.
- Warn to immediately report adverse reactions.
- Tell diabetic to report elevated blood glucose.

estrogens, conjugated (estrogenic substances, conjugated; oestrogens, conjugated)
C.E.S.†, Premarin, Premarin Intravenous
Estrogen
Estrogen replacement/antineoplastic/antiosteoporotic
Preg. Risk Category: X

Abnormal uterine bleeding (hormonal imbalance) — **Women:** 25 mg IV or IM, repeated in 6 to 12 hr as needed.
Female castration, primary ovarian failure — **Women:** 1.25 mg PO daily in cycles of 3 wk on and 1 wk off.
Osteoporosis — **Postmenopausal women:** 0.625 mg PO daily in cyclic regimen (3 wk on, 1 wk off).

- Ensure that patient undergoes thorough physical exam before and during therapy. Periodically monitor serum lipid levels, BP, weight, and hepatic function.
- *IV use:* When giving by direct injection, administer slowly to avoid flushing reaction.
- When giving IM, inject deeply into large muscle. Rotate injection sites to prevent muscle atrophy.
- Warn to immediately report adverse reactions.
- Tell diabetic to report elevated blood glucose so that antidiabetic medication dosage can be adjusted.

†Canadian ‡Australian

DRUG/CLASS/ CATEGORY	INDICATIONS/ DOSAGES	KEY NURSING CONSIDERATIONS
estropipate (piperazine estrone sulfate) Ogen, OrthoEST *Estrogen* Estrogen replacement Preg. Risk Category: X	*Primary ovarian failure, female castration, female hypogonadism* — **Women:** 1.25 to 7.5 mg PO daily for first 3 wk, followed by rest period of 8 to 10 days. If bleeding does not occur by end of rest period, cycle repeated. *Vasomotor menopause symptoms* — **Women:** 0.625 mg to 5 mg PO daily in cyclic method of 3 wk on, 1 wk off. *Prevention of osteoporosis* — **Women:** 0.625 mg PO daily for 25 days of 31-day cycle.	• Ensure that patient undergoes thorough physical exam before therapy starts. Patients on long-term therapy should have exams yearly. Periodically monitor serum lipid levels, BP, weight, and hepatic function. • Warn to immediately report adverse reactions. • Teach women how to perform routine breast self-exams.
ethacrynate sodium Sodium Edecrin **ethacrynic acid** Edecril,† Edecrin *Loop diuretic* Diuretic Preg. Risk Category: B	*Acute pulmonary edema* — **Adults:** 50 mg or 0.5 to 1 mg/kg IV. Usually only 1 dose necessary, though 2nd dose may be required. *Edema* — **Adults:** 50 to 200 mg PO daily. Refractory cases may require up to 200 mg bid. **Children:** initial dose 25 mg PO, increased cautiously in 25-mg increments daily until desired effect achieved.	• **IV use:** Reconstitute vacuum vial with 50 ml D_5W or 0.9% NaCl solution. Give slowly through tubing of running infusion over several min. Discard unused sol after 24 hr. Don't use cloudy or opalescent solutions. • Don't give SC or IM. Don't mix with whole blood or its derivatives. • If dose > 1 IV necessary, use new injection site to avoid thrombophlebitis. • Monitor I&O, weight, BP, serum electrolytes, and blood uric acid levels. • Watch for signs of hypokalemia. • Discontinue if severe diarrhea occurs.

ethambutol hydrochloride

Etibi†, Myambutol

Semisynthetic antitubercular

Antitubercular agent

Preg. Risk Category: C

Adjunctive treatment in pulmonary TB — **Adults and children > 13 yr:** Initial treatment for patients who haven't received previous antitubercular therapy, 15 mg/kg PO as single dose daily.

Retreatment: 25 mg/kg PO daily as single dose for 60 days (or until bacteriologic smears and cultures become negative) with at least one other antitubercular; then decrease to 15 mg/kg/day as single dose.

- Obtain AST and ALT levels before therapy and monitor levels q 3 to 4 wk.
- Always administer with other antituberculars to prevent development of resistant organisms.
- Urge to report adverse effects, especially blurred vision, red-green color blindness, or changes in urinary elimination.
- Reassure that visual disturbances should disappear several weeks to months after drug stopped.

ethinyl estradiol (ethinyloestradiol)

Estinyl, Feminone

Estrogen

Estrogen replacement/antineoplastic

Preg. Risk Category: X

Palliative treatment of metastatic breast cancer (at least 5 yr after menopause) — **Women:** 1 mg PO tid for at least 3 mo.

Female hypogonadism — **Women:** 0.05 mg PO qd to tid 2 wk per mo, followed by 2 wk of progesterone per mo; continued for 3 to 6 mo dosing cycles, followed by 2 mo off.

Vasomotor menopausal symptoms — **Women:** 0.02 to 0.05 mg PO daily for cycles of 3 wk on and 1 wk off.

Palliative treatment of metastatic inoperable prostate cancer — **Men:** 0.15 to 2 mg PO daily.

- Warn to immediately report adverse reactions.
- Tell diabetic to report elevated blood glucose.
- Explain to patient on cyclic therapy for postmenopausal symptoms that although withdrawal bleeding may occur during week off drug, fertility isn't restored.
- Teach women how to perform breast self-exams.

DRUG/CLASS/CATEGORY

ethinyl estradiol

monophasic: w/ desogestrel — Desogen; w/ ethynodiol diacetate — Demulen 1/35; w/ levonorgestrel — Nordette; w/ norethindrone — Genora 1/35; w/ norethindrone acetate — Loestrin 21 1/20; w/ norgestimate — Ortho Cyclen; w/ norgestrel — Ovral; w/ norethindrone acetate and ferrous fumarate — Loestrin Fe 1/20; *biphasic:* w/ norethindrone — Jenset-28; *triphasic:* w/ levonorgestrel — Triphasil; w/ norethindrone — Ortho-Novum 7/7/7; w/ norgestimate — Ortho Tri-Cyclen

mestranol

monophasic: w/ norethindrone — Genora 1/50; w/ norethynodrel — Enovid

Estrogen and progestin
Oral contraceptive
Preg. Risk Category: X

INDICATIONS/DOSAGES

Contraception — **Adults:** *Monophasic oral contraceptives* — 1 tab PO daily, starting on day 5 of menstrual cycle. With 20- and 21-tab pkg, new dosing cycle begins 7 days after last tab taken. With 28-tab pkg. dosage is 1 tab qd without interruption.

Biphasic oral contraceptives — 1 color tab PO daily for 10 days; then next color tab for 11 days. With 21-tab pkg, new dosing cycle begins 7 days after last tab taken. With 28-tab pkg, dosage is 1 tab daily without interruption.

Triphasic oral contraceptives — 1 tab PO daily in sequence specified by brand. With 21-tab pkg, new dosing cycle begins 7 days after last tab taken. With 28-tab pkg. dosage is 1 tab daily without interruption.

Endometriosis — **Adults:** 1 tab Enovid 5 mg or 10 mg PO daily for 2 wk starting on day 5 of menstrual cycle. Continue without interruption for 6 to 9 mo, increasing by 5 to 10 mg q 2 wk, up to 20 mg daily; up to 40 mg daily as needed and ordered if breakthrough bleeding occurs.

KEY NURSING CONSIDERATIONS

- Triphasic contraceptives may cause fewer adverse reactions, such as breakthrough bleeding and spotting.
- Monitor serum lipid levels, BP, weight, and hepatic function.
- Oral contraceptives affect many lab tests.
- Monitor blood glucose.
- Warn to immediately report adverse reactions.
- Advise of increased risks associated with simultaneous use of cigarettes and oral contraceptives.
- Instruct to take tablets at same time each day; nighttime dosing may reduce nausea and headaches.
- Advise to use additional method of birth control, such as condoms or diaphragm with spermicide, for first week of administration in initial cycle.
- Stress importance of Papanicolaou tests and annual gynecologic exams.

etidronate disodium

Didronel
Pyrophosphate analogue
Antihypercalcemic
Preg. Risk Category: C

Symptomatic Paget's disease of bone (osteitis deformans) — **Adults:** 5 to 10 mg/kg PO daily (not to exceed 6 mo of therapy) or 11 to 20 mg/kg PO daily (not to exceed 3 mo of therapy) in single dose 2 hr before meal with water or juice.

Heterotopic ossification after total hip replacement — **Adults:** 20 mg/kg PO daily for 1 mo before total hip replacement and for 3 mo afterward.

Malignancy-associated hypercalcemia — **Adults:** 7.5 mg/kg IV daily for 3 consecutive days; period of ≥ 7 days should elapse between courses of IV therapy. Maintenance dosage 20 mg/kg PO daily for 30 days, initiated day after last IV dosage. May use for max 90 days.

- *IV use:* Dilute daily dose in ≥ 250 ml 0.9% NaCl solution or D₅W, and infuse over ≥ 2 hr.
- Don't give with food, milk, or antacids; may reduce absorption.
- Some patients may receive IV drug for up to 7 days. Risk of hypokalemia increases after 3 days.
- Monitor renal function before and during therapy as ordered.
- To monitor effect, review serum alkaline phosphatase and urinary hydroxyproline excretion. Serum phosphate may rise, especially in patients receiving higher doses. Phosphate level usually returns to normal 2 to 4 wk after drug discontinued.

etodolac (ultradol)

Lodine
Nonsteroidal anti-inflammatory
Antiarthritic
Preg. Risk Category: C

Acute and chronic management of pain — **Adults:** 200 to 400 mg PO q 6 to 8 hr, prn, not to exceed 1,200 mg daily. For patients ≤ 60 kg, total daily dose shouldn't exceed 20 mg/kg.

- Can lead to reversible renal impairment.
- To minimize GI discomfort, instruct to take with milk or meals.
- Teach about signs and symptoms of GI bleeding, and tell to contact doctor immediately if any occurs.
- Advise to avoid alcoholic beverages or aspirin.

†Canadian ‡Australian

ETODOLAC 121

DRUG/CLASS/ CATEGORY	INDICATIONS/ DOSAGES	KEY NURSING CONSIDERATIONS
etoposide (VP-16) VePesid **etoposide phosphate** Etopophos *Podophyllotoxin (cell cycle– phase specific, G$_2$ and late S phase) Antineoplastic* Preg. Risk Category: D	*Testicular cancer* — **Adults:** 50 to 100 mg/m^2 IV on 5 consecutive days q 3 to 4 wk; or 100 mg/m^2 on days 1, 3, and 5 q 3 to 4 wk. *Small-cell carcinoma of lung* — **Adults:** 35 mg/m^2/day IV for 4 days; or 50 mg/m^2/day IV for 5 days. Oral dosage: twice IV dose, rounded to nearest 50 mg.	▪ Monitor BP q 15 min. If systolic pressure < 90, stop infusion and notify doctor. ▪ Have emergency drugs and equipment available in case of anaphylaxis. ▪ **IV use:** Give etoposide by slow IV infusion (over ≥ 30 min) to prevent severe hypotension. May give etoposide phosphate over 5 to 210 min. Don't administer etoposide through membrane-type in-line filter. ▪ Dilute etoposide for infusion in either D$_5$W or 0.9% NaCl solution to conc of 0.2 or 0.4 mg/ml. May give etoposide phosphate without further dilution, or may dilute to conc as low as 0.1 mg/ml in either D$_5$W or 0.9% NaCl.
etretinate Tegison *Retinoid Anti-inflammatory/dekeratinizing agent* Preg. Risk Category: X	*Severe recalcitrant psoriasis, including erythroderma and generalized pustular types in patients unresponsive to standard therapy* (topical tar plus UVB light, psoralens plus UVA light, systemic corticosteroids, and methotrexate) — **Adults:** initially, 0.75 to 1 mg/kg PO daily in divided doses. Max initial dosage 1.5 mg/kg daily. After initial response, maintenance 0.5 to 0.75 mg/kg daily.	▪ Don't give to women of childbearing age unless pregnancy excluded Therapy may begin on 2nd or 3rd day of next normal menstrual period. ▪ Monitor LFTs q 1 to 2 wk for 1st 1 to 2 mo of therapy, and q 1 to 3 mo thereafter. Stop if hepatotoxicity suspected. ▪ Monitor blood lipids q 1 to 2 wk. ▪ Monitor for pseudotumor cerebri. Check for papilledema.

famciclovir
Famvir
Synthetic acyclic guanine derivative
Antiviral
Preg. Risk Category: B

Acute herpes zoster infection (shingles) —
Adults: 500 mg PO q 8 hr for 7 days.
Recurrent episodes of genital herpes —
Adults: 125 mg PO bid for 5 days. Start as soon as symptoms occur.

- May take without regard to meals.
- Inform that drug won't cure genital herpes but can decrease symptom length and severity.
- Teach how to prevent spread of herpes infection.
- Urge to report early symptoms.

famotidine
Pepcid, Pepcid AC, Pepcidine‡
Histamine₂-receptor antagonist
Antiulcer agent
Preg. Risk Category: B

Duodenal ulcer (short-term treatment) —
Adults: Acute therapy: 40 mg PO qd hs or 20 mg PO bid. Maintenance therapy: 20 mg PO qd hs.
Benign gastric ulcer (short-term) —
Adults: 40 mg PO daily hs for 8 wk.
Gastroesophageal reflux disease (GERD) —
Adults: 20 mg PO bid up to 6 wk. For esophagitis caused by GERD, 20 to 40 mg bid up to 12 wk.
Prevention or treatment of heartburn —
Adults: 10 mg (Pepcid AC only) PO 1 hr before meals (prevention) or 10 mg (Pepcid AC only) PO with water for symptoms. Max 20 mg daily. Don't take daily for > 2 wk.

- *IV use:* To prepare injection, dilute 2 ml (20 mg) with compatible IV solution to total volume of 5 or 10 ml; inject over at least 2 min. Or, give by intermittent IV infusion. Dilute 20 mg (2 ml) in 100 ml compatible solution, and infuse over 15 to 30 min. Stable for 48 hr at room temp after dilution.
- Prescription drug most effective taken hs.
- With doctor's knowledge, allow to take antacids concomitantly, especially at start of therapy when pain severe.
- Urge to avoid cigarette smoking.

DRUG/CLASS/ CATEGORY	INDICATIONS/ DOSAGES	KEY NURSING CONSIDERATIONS
felodipine Agona, Agon SR‡, Plendil, Plendil ER‡, Renedil† *Calcium channel blocker* *Antihypertensive* Preg. Risk Category: C	*Hypertension* — **Adults:** initially, 5 mg PO daily. Adjust according to patient response, generally at intervals not less than 2 wk. Usual dose 5 to 10 mg daily; max recommended 20 mg daily. In elderly patients and impaired hepatic function, 5 mg PO daily; dosage adjusted as for adults. Max recommended 10 mg daily.	▪ Monitor BP for response. ▪ Monitor for peripheral edema. ▪ Tell to swallow tablets whole and not to crush or chew them. ▪ Teach to continue taking even when patient feels better and to check with doctor or pharmacist before taking other drugs, including OTC.
fenoprofen calcium Nalfon, Nalfon 200 *Nonsteroidal anti-inflammatory* *Non-narcotic* Preg. Risk Category: NR	*Rheumatoid arthritis and osteoarthritis* — **Adults:** 300 to 600 mg PO tid to qid. Max 3.2 g daily. *Mild to moderate pain* — **Adults:** 200 mg PO q 4 to 6 hr, prn. *Fever* — **Adults:** single PO doses up to 400 mg.	▪ May lead to reversible renal impairment. ▪ Inform that full therapeutic effect for arthritis may take 2 to 4 wk. ▪ Instruct to take 30 min before or 2 hr after meals. If adverse GI reactions occur, may be taken with milk or meals. ▪ Tell to contact doctor immediately GI bleeding occurs. ▪ Advise to avoid alcoholic beverages or aspirin.
fentanyl citrate Sublimaze **fentanyl transdermal system** Duragesic-25, Duragesic-50, Duragesic-75, Duragesic-100	*Preop* — **Adults:** 50 to 100 mcg IM 30 to 60 min before surgery. Or, 5 mcg/kg as oralet unit, 20 to 40 min prior to need. *Adjunct to general anesthetic* — **Adults:** Low-dose therapy, 2 mcg/kg IV. Moderate-dose therapy, 2 to 20 mcg/kg IV; then 25 to 100 mcg IV prn. High-dose therapy, 20 to	▪ Monitor circulatory and respiratory status and urinary function carefully. ▪ Keep narcotic antagonist and resuscitation equipment available when giving IV. ▪ Give before onset of intense pain. ▪ Periodically monitor postop vital signs and bladder function.

fentanyl transmucosal

Fentanyl Oralet
Opioid agonist
Analgesic/adjunct to anesthesia/anesthetic
Preg. Risk Category: C
Controlled Sub. Sched.: II

50 mcg/kg IV; then 25 mcg to half of initial loading dose IV, prn.

Adjunct to regional anesthesia — **Adults:** 50 to 100 mcg IM or IV over 1 to 2 min, prn.

Induction and maintenance of anesthesia —
Children 2 to 12 yr: 2 to 3 mcg/kg IV.

Postop — **Adults:** 50 to 100 mcg IM q 1 to 2 hr, prn.

Management of chronic pain — **Adults:** 1 transdermal system applied to upper torso skin area not irritated or irradiated. Start with 25-mcg/hr system; adjust dosage as needed and tolerated. May wear system for 72 hr; some may need applied q 48 hr.

- Remove foil overwrap of oralet just before administration. Have patient place oralet in mouth and suck (not chew or swallow) it.
- Remove oralet unit using handle after it's consumed, patient shows adequate effect, or patient shows signs of respiratory depression. Place any remaining portion in plastic overwrap and dispose accordingly for Schedule II drugs, or flush down toilet.
- Transdermal form not recommended for postop pain.

---

ferrous fumarate

Femiron, Feostat, Fumasorb, Fumerin, Novofumart†
Oral iron supplement
Hematinic
Preg. Risk Category: A

Iron deficiency — **Adults:** 50 to 100 mg elemental iron PO tid. **Children:** 4 to 6 mg/kg/day of elemental iron PO in 3 divided doses.

- GI upset may be related to dose. Between-meal doses preferable, but can be given with some foods. Enteric-coated products reduce GI upset but decrease amount of iron absorbed.
- Check for constipation; record color and amount of stools.
- Oral iron may turn stools black. Although harmless, could mask presence of melena.
- Monitor Hgb, Hct, and reticulocyte count.
- Combination products, such as Ferro-Sequels and Ferocyl, contain stool softeners, which help prevent constipation (common adverse reaction).

126

FERROUS FUM✓

†Canadian ✝Australian

DRUG/CLASS/ CATEGORY	INDICATIONS/ DOSAGES	KEY NURSING CONSIDERATIONS
ferrous gluconate Fergon, Fertinic†, Simron *Oral iron supplement* *Hematinic* Preg. Risk Category: A	*Iron deficiency* — **Adults:** 50 to 100 mg elemental iron PO tid. **Children:** 4 to 6 mg/kg/ day elemental iron PO in 3 divided doses.	• GI upset may be related to dose. Between-meal doses preferable, but can be given with some foods. Enteric-coated products reduce GI upset but decrease amount of iron absorbed. • Check for constipation; record color and amount of stools. • May turn stools black. Although harmless, could mask melena. • Monitor Hgb, Hct, and reticulocyte count.
ferrous sulfate Apo-Ferrous Sulfate†, Feosol, Feritard‡, Mol-Iron **ferrous sulfate, dried** Feosol *Oral iron supplement* *Hematinic* Preg. Risk Category: A	*Iron deficiency* — **Adults:** 50 to 100 mg elemental iron PO tid. **Children:** 4 to 6 mg/kg/day elemental iron PO in 3 divided doses.	• GI upset may be related to dose. Between-meal doses preferable, but can be given with some foods. Enteric-coated products reduce GI upset but decrease amount of iron absorbed. • Oral iron may turn stools black. Although harmless, could mask melena. • Monitor Hgb, Hct, and reticulocyte count, as ordered.

fexofenadine hydrochloride

Allegra

H_1-receptor antagonist

Antihistaminic agent

Preg. Risk Category: C

---

filgrastim (granulo-cyte colony-stimu-lating factor; G-CSF)

Neupogen

Biologic response modifier

Colony stimulating factor

Preg. Risk Category: C

Seasonal allergic rhinitis — **Adults and children ≥ 12 yr:** 60 mg PO bid; initially 60 mg PO qd in impaired renal function.

- Caution not to perform hazardous activities if drowsiness occurs.
- Instruct not to exceed prescribed dosage and to take only when needed.
- Use caution in breast-feeding women.

To decrease incidence of infection in patients with nonmyeloid malignant disease receiving myelosuppressive antineoplastic agents — **Adults and children:** 5 mcg/kg/day IV or SC as 1 dose given ≥ 24 hr after cytotoxic chemotherapy. May increase by 5 mcg/kg for each chemotherapy cycle depending on duration and severity of nadir of absolute neutrophil count (ANC).

To decrease incidence of infection in patients with nonmyeloid malignant disease receiving myelosuppressive antineoplastic agents followed by bone marrow transplantation — **Adults and children:** 10 mcg/kg/day IV or SC ≥ 24 hr after cytotoxic chemotherapy and bone marrow infusion. Adjust dosage according to neutrophil response.

Congenital neutropenia — **Adults:** 6 mcg/kg SC bid. Dosage adjusted to response.

- Obtain baseline CBC and platelet count before therapy, then twice weekly during therapy, as ordered.
- **IV use:** Dilute in 50 to 100 ml D_5W and give by intermittent infusion over 15 to 60 min or continuous infusion over 24 hr. If final conc will be 2 to 15 mcg/ml, add albumin at conc of 2 mg/ml (0.2%).
- Once dose withdrawn, don't reenter vial. Discard unused portion. Vials are for single-dose use and contain no preservatives.
- Refrigerate at 36° to 46° F (2° to 8° C). Don't freeze; avoid shaking. Store at room temp for max 6 hr; discard after 6 hr.
- Transiently increased neutrophil count common 1 or 2 days after therapy starts. Give daily for up to 2 wk or until ANC returns to 10,000/mm³ after expected chemotherapy-induced neutrophil nadir.

DRUG / CLASS / CATEGORY	INDICATIONS / DOSAGES	KEY NURSING CONSIDERATIONS
finasteride Proscar *Steroid (synthetic 4-azasteroid) derivative* *Androgen synthesis inhibitor* Preg. Risk Category: X	*Symptomatic benign prostatic hyperplasia (BPH)* — **Adults:** 5 mg PO daily.	• Before therapy, evaluate for conditions that might mimic BPH. • Monitor patients with large residual urine volume or severely diminished urine flow. May not be candidates for drug. • Evaluate sustained increases in serum prostate-specific antigen; could signal non-compliance. • More than 6 mo of therapy may be necessary to determine if patient responds to drug.
flecainide acetate Tambocor *Benzamide derivative local anesthetic* *Ventricular antiarrhythmic* Preg. Risk Category: C	*PSVT, paroxysmal atrial fibrillation or flutter in patients without structural heart disease; life-threatening ventricular arrhythmias, such as sustained ventricular tachycardia* — **Adults:** for PSVT, 50 mg PO q 12 hr. May increase in increments of 50 mg bid q 4 days until efficacy achieved. Max 300 mg/day. For life-threatening ventricular arrhythmias, 100 mg PO q 12 hr. Increase in increments of 50 mg bid q 4 days until efficacy achieved. Max 400 mg daily.	• Stress importance of taking drug exactly as prescribed. • Instruct to report adverse reactions promptly and to limit fluid and sodium intake.

floxuridine
FUDR
*Antimetabolite (cell cycle-
phase specific, S phase)*
Antineoplastic
Preg. Risk Category: D

GI adenocarcinoma metastatic to liver —
Adults: 0.1 to 0.6 mg/kg daily by intra-arterial infusion for 14 to 21 days or until toxicity
occurs; or 0.4 to 0.6 mg/kg daily into hepatic artery.

- Use infusion pump with intra-arterial infusions. Check line for bleeding, blockage,
displacement, or leakage.
- Monitor I&O, CBC, and renal and hepatic
function, as ordered.
- Provide diligent mouth care to help prevent stomatitis.
- Discontinue and notify doctor if WBC
count < 3,500/mm³ or if platelet count
< 100,000/mm³.
- Severe skin and adverse GI reactions ne-
cessitate discontinuation.

fluconazole
Diflucan
Bis-triazole derivative
Antifungal
Preg. Risk Category: C

*Oropharyngeal and esophageal candidia-
sis —* **Adults:** 200 mg PO or IV on first day,
then 100 mg qd. Continue for at least 2 wk
after symptoms resolve. **Children:** 6 mg/kg
on first day, then 3 mg/kg for at least 2 wk.
Vaginal candidiasis — **Adults:** 150 mg PO
as single dose.
Systemic candidiasis — **Adults:** Up to 400
mg PO or IV qd. Continue for at least 2 wk
after symptoms resolve.
Cryptococcal meningitis — **Adults:** 400 mg
PO or IV on first day, then 200 mg qd. Continue for 10 to 12 wk after CSF cultures
negative.

- *IV use:* Give by continuous infusion no
faster than 200 mg/hr. Use infusion pump.
To prevent air embolism, don't connect in
series with other infusions. Don't add other drugs to solution.
- Periodically monitor liver function during
prolonged therapy, as ordered.
- If mild rash occurs, monitor closely. If lesions progress, stop drug and notify doctor.
- Incidence of adverse reactions greater in
patients with HIV.

DRUG/CLASS/CATEGORY	INDICATIONS/DOSAGES	KEY NURSING CONSIDERATIONS
flucytosine (5-fluorocytosine, 5-FC) Ancobon, Ancotil *Fluorinated pyrimidine* *Antifungal* Preg. Risk Category: C	*Severe fungal infections caused by susceptible strains of* Candida *(including septicemia, endocarditis, UTIs, and pulmonary infections) and* Cryptococcus *(meningitis, pulmonary infection, and possible UTI)* — **Adults and children > 50 kg:** 50 to 150 mg/kg daily PO q 6 hr. **Adults and children < 50 kg:** 1.5 to 4.5 g/m²/day PO in 4 divided doses.	• Obtain hematologic tests and renal and liver function studies, as ordered. • Give capsules over 15 min to reduce adverse GI reactions. • Monitor fluid I&O; report marked change. • Instruct to report adverse reactions promptly. • Inform that therapeutic response may take weeks or months.
fludrocortisone acetate Florinef *Mineralocorticoid/glucocorticoid* *Mineralocorticoid replacement therapy* Preg. Risk Category: C	*Adrenal insufficiency (partial replacement), salt-losing adrenogenital syndrome* — **Adults:** 0.1 to 0.2 mg PO daily. Decrease to 0.05 mg daily if transient hypertension occurs. **Children:** 0.05 to 0.1 mg PO daily. *Postural hypotension in diabetic patients, orthostatic hypotension* — **Adults:** 0.1 to 0.4 mg PO daily.	• Used with cortisone or hydrocortisone in adrenal insufficiency. • Monitor BP and serum electrolytes. • Weigh patient daily; report sudden gain. • Unless contraindicated, give low-sodium diet that's high in potassium and protein. • Tell to report worsening symptoms, such as hypotension, weakness, cramping, and palpitations.
flumazenil Romazicon *Benzodiazepine antagonist* *Antidote* Preg. Risk Category: C	*Complete or partial reversal of sedative effects of benzodiazepines after anesthesia or short diagnostic procedures (conscious sedation)* — **Adults:** 0.2 mg IV over 15 sec. If patient doesn't reach desired LOC after 45 sec, repeat at 1-min intervals until total dose of 1 mg given (initial dose plus 4 additional doses).	*IV use:* Administer by direct injection or dilute with compatible solution. Discard unused drug that has been drawn into syringe or diluted within 24 hr. • Administer into IV line in large vein with free-flowing IV solution to minimize pain at injection site. Compatible solutions in-

tional doses), prn. Most patients respond after 0.6 to 1 mg. In case of resedation, may repeat after 20 min; however, don't give > 1 mg at one time and not > 3 mg/hr.

Suspected benzodiazepine overdose —
Adults: 0.2 mg IV over 30 sec. If patient doesn't reach desired LOC after 30 sec, 0.3 mg given over 30 sec. If poor response, 0.5 mg given over 30 sec; repeat 0.5-mg doses prn at 1-min intervals until total dose of 3 mg given. Most patients respond to total doses between 1 and 3 mg; rarely, patients who respond partially after 3 mg may require additional doses, up to 5 mg total. If patient doesn't respond in 5 min after receiving 5 mg, sedation unlikely to be caused by benzodiazepines. In case of resedation, may repeat dosage after 20 min; however, don't give > 1 mg at one time and not > 3 mg/hr.

clude D_5W, lact Ringer's injection, and 0.9% NaCl.

- Monitor patient closely for resedation that may occur after reversal of benzodiazepine effects (flumazenil's duration of action shorter than that of all benzodiazepines). Duration of monitoring period depends on which drug being reversed. Monitor closely after long-acting benzodiazepines, such as diazepam, or after high doses of short-acting benzodiazepines, such as 10 mg midazolam. In most cases, severe resedation unlikely in patients showing no signs of resedation 2 hr after 1-mg flumazenil.
- Tell to avoid alcohol, CNS depressants, and OTC drugs for 24 hours.
- Patient won't recall information given in postprocedure period; drug doesn't reverse amnesic effects of benzodiazepines.

---

flunisolide
AeroBid, AeroBid-M,
Nasalide (nasal inhalant)
Glucocorticoid
Anti-inflammatory/antiasthmatic
Preg. Risk Category: C

Persistent asthma — **Adults:** 2 inhalations (500 mcg) bid. Max total daily 2,000 mcg (8 inhalations/day). **Children 6 to 15 yr:** 2 inhalations (500 mcg) bid. Don't exceed 4 inhalations/day.

Seasonal or perennial rhinitis: **Adults:** 2 sprays (50 mcg) in each nostril bid. If needed, increase to 2 sprays in each nostril tid. **Children 6 to 14 yr:** 1 spray in each nostril tid or 2 sprays in each nostril bid.

- Withdraw slowly as ordered in patients who've received long-term oral corticosteroids.
- Warn that drug won't relieve emergency asthma attacks.
- If patient is using a bronchodilator, teach to use several minutes before flunisolide.
- Instruct to wait 1 min before repeating inhalation and to hold breath several seconds to enhance drug action.

FLUNISOLIDE 131

†Canadian ‡Australian

DRUG / CLASS / CATEGORY	INDICATIONS / DOSAGES	KEY NURSING CONSIDERATIONS
fluocinolone acetonide Fluocet, Fluonid, Flurosyn, Synalar, Synemol *Topical adrenocorticoid* *Anti-inflammatory* Preg. Risk Category: C	*Inflammation associated with cortico-steroid-responsive dermatoses* — **Adults and children:** apply cream, oint, or topical sol sparingly bid to qid. Rub in gently, leaving thin coat.	▪ Don't apply near eyes, mucous membranes, or in ear canal. ▪ Notify doctor if skin infection, striae, atrophy or fever develops. Remove occlusive dressing if fever develops. ▪ Watch for symptoms of systemic absorption. ▪ Solution on dry lesions may increase dryness, scaling, or pruritus; on denuded or fissured areas, may produce burning or stinging. If either persists, discontinue solution and notify doctor.
fluocinonide Lidemol†, Lidex, Lidex-E, Topsyn *Topical adrenocorticoid* *Anti-inflammatory* Preg. Risk Category: C	*Inflammation associated with cortico-steroid-responsive dermatoses* — **Adults and children:** clean area; apply cream, gel, oint, or topical sol sparingly bid or qid.	▪ Gently wash skin before applying. Rub in gently, leaving thin coat. When treating hairy sites, part hair and apply directly to lesion. Don't apply near eyes, mucous membranes, or in ear canal. ▪ Notify doctor if skin infection, striae, atrophy, or fever develops. ▪ Systemic absorption likely with use of occlusive dressings, prolonged treatment, or extensive body-surface treatment. Watch for symptoms. ▪ Continue treatment for several days after lesions clear, as ordered.

fluorescein sodium

Fluorescite, Fluor-I-Strip, Fluor-I-Strip A.T., Ful-Glo, Fluor-I-Strip Injections, Funduscein Injections

Dye

Diagnostic aid

Preg. Risk Category: C

Diagnostic aid in corneal abrasions and foreign bodies; fitting hard contact lenses; lacrimal patency; fundus photography; applanation tonometry — **Adults and children:** 1 or 2 drops 2% sol followed by irrigation; or strip moistened with sterile water, then conjunctiva or fornix touched with moistened tip, and eye flushed with irrigating sol. Patient should blink several times after application.

Retinal angiography — **Adults:** 5 ml of 10% sol (500 mg) or 3 ml of 25% sol (750 mg) rapidly injected into antecubital vein. **Children:** 7.5 mg/kg injected rapidly into antecubital vein.

- Always use aseptic technique. Easily contaminated by *P. aeruginosa.*
- **IV use:** Keep antihistamine, epinephrine, and O_2 available when giving parenterally. Avoid extravasation during injection.
- Use topical anesthetic as ordered before instilling to relieve burning and irritation.
- Never instill while patient is wearing soft contact lenses; fluorescein will ruin them.
- Defects appear green under normal light or bright yellow under cobalt blue light. Foreign bodies surrounded by green ring. Similar conjunctival lesions delineated in orange-yellow.

fluorometholone

Flarex, FML Forte, FML Liquifilm Ophthalmic

Corticosteroid

Ophthalmic anti-inflammatory

Preg. Risk Category: C

Inflammatory and allergic conditions of cornea, conjunctiva, sclera, anterior uvea — **Adults and children:** 1 to 2 drops instilled in conjunctival sac bid to qid. May give q 2 hr during 1st 1 to 2 days if needed. Alternatively, 1.25-cm ribbon of oint applied to conjunctival sac q 4 hr, decreased to 1 to 3 times daily as inflammation subsides.

- Not for long-term use.
- Shake well before using.
- Less likely to cause increased IOP with long-term use than other ophth anti-inflammatory drugs (except medrysone).
- Store in tightly covered, light-resistant container.

DRUG/CLASS/ CATEGORY	INDICATIONS/ DOSAGES	KEY NURSING CONSIDERATIONS
fluorouracil (5-fluorouracil, 5-FU) Adrucil, Efudex, Fluoroplex *Antimetabolite (cell cycle-phase specific, S phase)* *Antineoplastic* Preg. Risk Category: D (injection), X (topical)	*Colon, rectal, breast, stomach, and pancreatic cancers* — **Adults:** 12 mg/kg IV daily for 4 days; if no toxicity, 6 mg/kg on 6th, 8th, 10th, and 12th day; then single weekly maintenance dosage begun after toxicity from 1st course subsides. Max single dose 800 mg/day. *Palliative treatment of advanced colorectal cancer* — **Adults:** 425 mg/m² IV daily for 5 consecutive days. Given with 20 mg/m² of leucovorin IV. Repeat at 4-wk intervals for 2 additional courses; then repeat at intervals of 4 to 5 wk if tolerated. *Multiple actinic (solar) keratoses; superficial basal cell carcinoma* — **Adults:** apply cream or topical sol bid. Usual duration of treatment 2 to 6 wk.	• Toxicity may be delayed for 1 to 3 wk. • Use plastic IV containers to give continuous infusions. Don't refrigerate. Protect from sunlight. • Monitor CBC and platelet counts. Watch for ecchymoses, petechiae, easy bruising, and anemia. Monitor I&O, and renal and hepatic function tests. • Ingestion and systemic absorption of topical cream form may cause serious adverse reactions. Application to large ulcerated areas may cause systemic toxicity. • Watch for stomatitis or diarrhea (toxicity signs). Discontinue drug and notify doctor if diarrhea occurs. • Encourage diligent oral hygiene to prevent superinfection of denuded mucosa.
fluoxetine hydrochloride Prozac, Prozac-20‡ *Selective serotonin reuptake inhibitor* *Antidepressant* Preg. Risk Category: B	*Depression, obsessive-compulsive disorder* — **Adults:** initially, 20 mg PO in morning; increase dosage according to response. May give bid in morning and at noon. Gradually increase as needed and tolerated to 60 to 80 mg daily. *Treatment of binge-eating and vomiting behavior in moderate to severe bulimia nervosa* — **Adults:** 60 mg/day PO in morning.	• Warn to avoid hazardous activities until CNS effects known. • Tell to consult doctor before taking other medications and to avoid alcohol. • Instruct to avoid taking in afternoon because of possible nervousness and insomnia. • Advise to promptly report rash or hives, anxiety or nervousness, anorexia, or suspicion of pregnancy.

fluoxymesterone
Android-F, Halotestin

Androgen

Androgen replacement/anti-neoplastic

Preg. Risk Category: X
Controlled Sub. Sched.: III

Hypogonadism caused by testicular deficiency — **Adults:** 5 to 20 mg PO daily, in single dose or in 3 or 4 divided doses.

Delayed puberty — **Males:** 2.5 to 20 mg daily.

Palliation of breast cancer in women — **Adults:** 10 to 40 mg PO daily in 3 or 4 divided doses. All dosages individualized and reduced to minimum when effect noted.

- Instruct to take with food or meals if GI upset occurs.
- Tell women to report menstrual irregularities or irregular bleeding and stop drug.
- Urge female patient to report androgenic effects immediately.
- Watch for hypoglycemia in diabetics; check blood glucose.
- If liver function results abnormal, notify doctor; therapy should be stopped.

---

fluphenazine decanoate
Modecate†‡, Prolixin Decanoate

fluphenazine enanthate
Prolixin Enanthate

fluphenazine hydrochloride
Moditen HCl†, Permitil Concentrate, Prolixin, Prolixin Concentrate

Phenothiazine

Antipsychotic

Preg. Risk Category: NR

Psychotic disorders — **Adults:** initially, 0.5 to 10 mg HCl PO daily in divided doses q 6 to 8 hr; may increase cautiously to 20 mg. Higher doses (50 to 100 mg) have been given. Maintenance: 1 to 5 mg PO daily. For IM doses, give third or half of oral doses. Usual IM dose 1.25 mg. Use dosages above 10 mg/day with caution. Use lower dosages for elderly patients (1 to 2.5 mg daily). Alternatively, 12.5 to 25 mg of long-acting esters (decanoate or enanthate) IM or SC q 1 to 6 wk; maintenance: 25 to 100 mg, prn.

- Watch for neuroleptic malignant syndrome.
- Monitor therapy with bilirubin tests, CBC and liver function, and periodic renal function and ophthalmic tests as ordered.
- Check dosage order carefully.
- Dilute liquid concentrate with water, fruit juice, milk, or semisolid food.
- Oral liquid and parenteral forms can cause contact dermatitis.
- Withhold dose and notify doctor if patient develops symptoms of blood dyscrasia or persistent extrapyramidal reactions.
- Warn to avoid activities that require alertness and good psychomotor coordination until CNS effects known.
- Instruct to relieve dry mouth with sugarless gum or hard candy.
- Inform of possible urine discoloration.

FLUPHENAZINE HYDROCHLORIDE 135

†Canadian ‡Australian

DRUG/CLASS/ CATEGORY	INDICATIONS/ DOSAGES	KEY NURSING CONSIDERATIONS
flurazepam hydrochloride Apo-Flurazepam†, Dalmane, Novoflupam† *Benzodiazepine* *Sedative-hypnotic* Preg. Risk Category: X Controlled Sub. Sched.: IV	*Insomnia* — **Adults:** 15 to 30 mg PO hs. **Adults > age 65:** 15 mg PO hs.	• Check hepatic and renal function and CBC during long-term therapy. • Assess mental status before initiating. • Encourage to keep taking even if insomnia occurs on first night. • Instruct to avoid alcohol use. • Caution not to perform activities that require mental alertness or physical coordination. • Prevent hoarding or self-overdosing.
flurbiprofen Ansaid, Apo-Flurbiprofen†, Froben†, Froben SR† *Nonsteroidal anti-inflammatory/phenylalkanoic acid derivative* *Antiarthritic agent* Preg. Risk Category: B	*Rheumatoid arthritis and osteoarthritis* — **Adults:** 200 to 300 mg PO daily, divided bid, tid or qid. Where available, patients maintained on 200 mg daily may switch to one 200-mg ext-release cap PO daily, taken in evening after food.	• Tell to take with food, milk, or antacid if GI upset occurs. • Teach signs and symptoms of GI bleeding and tell to contact doctor immediately if they occur. • Advise to avoid alcohol and aspirin. • Tell patient taking ext-release capsules to swallow them whole.
flurbiprofen sodium Ocufen Liquifilm *Nonsteroidal anti-inflammatory* *Ophthalmic anti-inflammatory/antimiotic* Preg. Risk Category: C	*Inhibition of intraoperative miosis* — **Adults:** 1 drop instilled into affected eye approximately q ½ hr, beginning 2 hr before surgery. Total of 4 drops given.	• Wound healing may be delayed. • Alert doctor immediately if visual acuity decreases or visual field diminishes.

flutamide
Euflex†, Eulexin
Nonsteroidal antiandrogen
Antineoplastic
Preg. Risk Category: D

Metastatic prostate cancer (stage B_2, C, D_2) in combination with LH-releasing hormone analogues such as leuprolide acetate — **Adults:** 250 mg PO q 8 hr.

- Monitor liver function tests and CBC periodically, as ordered.
- Must be taken continuously with agent used for medical castration (such as leuprolide acetate) for full benefit of therapy.

fluticasone propionate
Cutivate
Corticosteroid
Topical anti-inflammatory
Preg. Risk Category: C

Inflammatory and pruritic manifestations associated with corticosteroid-responsive dermatoses — **Adults:** apply sparingly to affected area bid; rub in gently and completely.

- Don't mix with other bases or vehicles; may affect potency.
- One-time coverage of adult body requires 12 to 26 g. Don't use > 50 g wkly.
- Discontinue, as ordered, if local irritation or systemic infection, absorption, or hypersensitivity occurs.
- Absorption enhanced when applied to inflamed or damaged skin, eyelids, or scrotal area; lowest when applied to intact normal skin, palms, or soles.

fluticasone propionate
Flonase
Corticosteroid
Topical anti-inflammatory
Preg. Risk Category: C

Seasonal and perennial allergic rhinitis — **Adults:** initially, 2 sprays (50 mcg each spray) in each nostril qd. Alternatively, 1 spray in each nostril bid. After several days, may reduce dosage to 1 spray in each nostril daily. Max daily dosage 2 sprays in each nostril. **Children ≥ 12 yr:** initially, 1 spray (50 mcg) in each nostril qd. If no response or symptoms severe, increase to 2 sprays in each nostril. Depending on response, may decrease dosage to 1 spray in each nostril daily. Max daily dosage 2 sprays in each nostril.

- Don't use after recent nasal septal ulcers, nasal surgery, or nasal trauma until healing occurs.
- Monitor for signs of immediate hypersensitivity reactions or contact dermatitis after intranasal administration.
- Drug effectiveness depends on regular use.
- Tell to avoid exposure to persons with chickenpox or measles. If exposure occurs, tell to seek medical advice.

FLUTICASONE PROPIONATE 137

†Canadian ‡Australian

DRUG/CLASS/CATEGORY	INDICATIONS/DOSAGES	KEY NURSING CONSIDERATIONS
fluvastatin sodium Lescol Hydroxymethylglutaryl-coenzyme A (HMG-CoA) reductase inhibitor Cholesterol-lowering agent/antilipemic agent Preg. Risk Category: X	*Reduction of LDL and total cholesterol levels in patients with primary hypercholesterolemia (types IIa and IIb)* — **Adults:** initially, 20 mg PO hs. Increase as needed to max 40 mg daily.	• Should be initiated only after diet and other nonpharmacologic measures fail. • Liver function tests should be done when therapy starts and periodically thereafter. • Watch for signs of myositis. • Teach about proper dietary management, weight control, and exercise. • Warn to avoid alcohol and that drug contraindicated during pregnancy.
fluvoxamine maleate Luvox Selective serotonin reuptake inhibitor Anticompulsive agent Preg. Risk Category: C	*Obsessive-compulsive disorder* — **Adults:** initially, 50 mg PO daily in 50-mg increments q 4 to 7 days until max benefit achieved. Max 300 mg daily. Give total daily doses of more than 100 mg in 2 divided doses.	• Record mood changes. Monitor for suicidal tendencies, and allow only minimal drug supply. • Warn not to engage in hazardous activities until CNS effects known. • Tell to notify doctor allergic reaction occurs. • Advise not to discontinue until directed by doctor.
folic acid (vitamin B₉) Folvite, Novofolacid† Folic acid derivative Vitamin supplement Preg. Risk Category: NR	*Recommended daily allowance (RDA)* — **Neonates and infants to 6 mo:** 25 mcg. **Infants 6 mo to 1 yr:** 35 mcg. **Children 1 to 3 yr:** 50 mcg. **Children 4 to 6 yr:** 75 mcg. **Children 7 to 10 yr:** 100 mcg. **Children 11 to 14 yr:** 150 mcg. **Males ≥ 15 yr:** 200 mcg. **Females ≥ 15 yr:** 180 mcg. **Pregnant women:** 400 mcg. **Breast-feeding women**	• Don't mix with other medications in same syringe when giving IM. • Patients with small-bowel resections and intestinal malabsorption may require parenteral administration. • Protect from light and heat; store at room temp. • Monitor CBC to measure drug effectiveness.

- Patients undergoing renal dialysis are at risk for folate deficiency.
- Many drugs, such as oral contraceptives and alcohol, can cause folate deficiencies.
- Teach about dietary sources of folic acid, such as yeast, whole grains, leafy vegetables, beans, nuts, and fruit.
- Inform that overcooking and canning destroy folate.
- Should be taken only under medical supervision.

(1st 6 mo): 280 mcg. **Breast-feeding women (2nd 6 mo):** 260 mcg.

Megaloblastic or macrocytic anemia secondary to folic acid or other nutritional deficiency; hepatic disease, alcoholism, intestinal obstruction, excessive hemolysis — **Adults and children > 4 yr:** 0.4 mg to 1 mg PO, SC, or IM daily. After correction of anemia secondary to folic acid deficiency, proper diet and RDA supplements necessary to prevent recurrence. **Children < 4 yr:** up to 0.3 mg PO, SC, or IM daily. **Pregnant and breast-feeding women:** 0.8 mg PO, SC, or IM daily.

Prevention of megaloblastic anemia during pregnancy to prevent fetal damage — **Adults:** up to 1 mg PO, SC, or IM daily throughout pregnancy.

---

foscarnet sodium (phosphonoformic acid)
Foscavir
Pyrophosphate analogue
Antiviral agent
Preg. Risk Category: C

CMV retinitis in patients with AIDS
Adults: initially, 60 mg/kg IV as induction treatment in patients with normal renal function. Give IV over 1 hr q 8 hr for 2 to 3 wk, depending on clinical response. Follow with maintenance infusion of 90 to 120 mg/kg daily, given over 2 hr.

Mucocutaneous acyclovir resistant herpes simplex virus (HSV) infection — **Adults:** 40 mg/kg IV. Give IV infusion over 1 hr q 8 to 12 hr for 2 to 3 wk.

- **IV use:** Use infusion pump. To minimize renal toxicity, ensure adequate hydration before and during infusion.
- Can alter serum electrolytes; monitor levels. Assess for tetany and seizures associated with abnormal electrolyte levels.
- Monitor Hgb and Hct.
- Advise to report perioral tingling, numbness in extremities, and paresthesia.
- Instruct to alert nurse if discomfort occurs at IV insertion site.

FOSCARNET SODIUM 139

DRUG/CLASS/ CATEGORY	INDICATIONS/ DOSAGES	KEY NURSING CONSIDERATIONS
fosfomycin tromethamine Monurol *Phosphonic acid derivative* *Antibiotic* Preg. Risk Category: B	*Uncomplicated UTI (acute cystitis) in women caused by susceptible strains of E. coli and E. faecalis* — **Women > 18 yr:** 1 sachet PO mixed with cold water just before ingestion.	▪ Instruct about proper way to take. Advise to mix entire contents of single-dose sachet with 3 to 4 oz (½ cup) water; stir to dissolve, and drink immediately. Tell to notify doctor if symptoms don't improve in 2 to 3 days.
fosinopril sodium Monopril *ACE inhibitor* *Antihypertensive* Preg. Risk Category: C (D in 2nd and 3rd trimesters)	*Hypertension* — **Adults:** initially, 10 mg PO daily. Adjusted based on BP response at peak and trough levels. Usual dosage 20 to 40 mg, up to 80 mg daily. May be divided. *Heart failure* — **Adults:** initially, 10 mg PO qd. Increase over several wk to max 40 mg PO daily.	▪ Monitor potassium intake and serum potassium. ▪ Monitor CBC with differential. ▪ Monitor BP for effect. ▪ Advise to report signs or symptoms of infection. ▪ Instruct to use caution in hot weather and during exercise.
fosphenytoin sodium Cerebyx *Hydantoin derivative* *Anticonvulsant* Preg. Risk Category: D	*Status epilepticus* — **Adults:** 15 to 20 mg phenytoin sodium equiv (PE)/kg IV at 100 to 150 mg PE/min as loading dose; then 4 to 6 mg PE/kg/day IV as maintenance dose. (Phenytoin may be used instead of fosphenytoin as maintenance, using appropriate dose.) *Prevention and treatment of seizures during neurosurgery* — **Adults:** loading dose 10 to 20 mg PE/kg IM or IV at infusion rate not exceeding 150 mg PE/min. Maintenance dose: 4 to 6 mg PE/kg/day IV.	▪ Should always be prescribed and dispensed in phenytoin sodium equivalent units (PE). Don't adjust recommended doses when substituting fosphenytoin for phenytoin, and vice versa. ▪ Before IV infusion, dilute in 5% dextrose or 0.9% NaCl solution to concentration ranging from 1.5 to 25 mg PE/ml. ▪ Monitor ECG, BP, and respirations. ▪ Severe CV complications most common in elderly or gravely ill patients.

Short-term substitution for oral phenytoin — **Adult:** same total daily dosage equivalent as oral phenytoin sodium therapy as single daily dose IM or IV at infusion rate not exceeding 150 mg PE/min. May require more frequent dosing.

- If rash appears, discontinue and notify doctor.
- Abrupt withdrawal may trigger status epilepticus.
- Warn that sensory disturbances may occur with IV use.

---

furosemide
(frusemide†‡)
Apo-Furosemide†, Lasix, Myrosemide, Novosemide†, Urex‡
Loop diuretic
Diuretic/antihypertensive
Preg. Risk Category: C

Acute pulmonary edema — **Adults:** 40 mg IV injected slowly over 1 to 2 min; then 80 mg IV in 1 to ½ hr if needed.
Edema — **Adults:** 20 to 80 mg PO daily in morning, 2nd dose in 6 to 8 hr; carefully titrated up to 600 mg daily if needed. Or 20 to 40 mg IM or IV, increased by 20 mg q 2 hr until desired response achieved. Give IV dose slowly over 1 to 2 min. **Infants and children:** 2 mg/kg PO daily, increased by 1 to 2 mg/Kg in 6 to 8 hr if needed; carefully titrate to 6 mg/kg daily if needed.
Hypertension — **Adults:** 40 mg PO bid. Adjust dosage according to response.

- **IV use:** Give by direct injection over 1 to 2 min. Alternatively, dilute with D_5W, 0.9% NaCl solution, or lact Ringer's, and infuse no faster than 4 mg/min to avoid ototoxicity. Use prepared infusion solution within 24 hr.
- Can lead to profound water and electrolyte depletion. Monitor weight, BP, and HR routinely with chronic use and during rapid diuresis.
- If oliguria or azotemia develops or worsens, may need to discontinue.
- Monitor I&O, and serum electrolyte, BUN, blood uric acid, and CO_2 levels frequently.
- May be poorly absorbed orally in severe heart failure. May need to be given IV even if patient receiving other oral medications.

FUROSEMIDE

DRUG/CLASS/CATEGORY	INDICATIONS/DOSAGES	KEY NURSING CONSIDERATIONS
gabapentin Neurontin 1-aminomethyl cyclohexaneacetic acid Anticonvulsant Preg. Risk Category: C	*Adjunctive treatment of partial seizures with and without secondary generalization in adults with epilepsy* — **Adults:** initially 300 mg PO hs on day 1; 300 mg PO bid on day 2; then 300 mg PO tid on day 3. Increase as needed and tolerated to 1,800 mg daily in 3 divided doses. Dosages up to 3,600 mg daily have been well tolerated.	• Give first dose at bedtime to minimize drowsiness, dizziness, fatigue, and ataxia. • Discontinue or substitute alternative drug gradually, over at least 1 wk, as ordered. • Don't suddenly withdraw other anticonvulsants. • Warn to avoid driving and operating heavy machinery until CNS effects known.
ganciclovir Cytovene Synthetic nucleoside Antiviral agent Preg. Risk Category: C	*CMV retinitis in immunocompromised patients, including those with AIDS and normal renal function* — **Adults:** induction: 5 mg/kg IV q 12 hr for 14 to 21 days; maintenance: 5 mg/kg IV qd for 7 days each wk, or 6 mg/kg IV qd for 5 days each wk. Or, 1,000 mg PO tid with food; or 500 mg PO q 3 hr while awake (6 times daily). Adjust dosage for impaired renal function based on creatinine clearance. *Prevention of CMV disease in advanced HIV infection and normal renal function* — **Adults:** 1,000 mg PO tid with food. *Prevention of CMV disease in transplant recipients with normal renal function* — **Adults:** 5 mg/kg IV q 12 hr for 7 to 14 days, then 5 mg/kg qd for 7 days each wk, or 6 mg/kg qd for 5 days each wk.	• **IV use:** Give infusion at a constant rate over at least 1 hr. Too-rapid infusions cause increased toxicity. Use infusion pump. Don't give as bolus. • Solution alkaline; use caution when preparing. • Don't administer SC or IM. • Obtain neutrophil and platelet counts every 2 days during twice-daily dosing and at least weekly thereafter. • Dosage adjustment necessary if creatinine clearance < 70/ml.min. • Explain importance of adequate hydration during therapy. • Instruct to report adverse reactions promptly.

gemcitabine hydrochloride

Gemzar

Nucleoside analogue (cell cycle-phase specific, S and G_1 phase)

Antineoplastic

Preg. Risk Category: D

Locally advanced or metastatic adenocarcinoma of pancreas and patients treated previously with fluorouracil — **Adults:** 1,000 mg/m² IV over 30 min q wk ≤ 7 wk, unless toxicity occurs. Patients should be monitored before each dose with CBC (including differential) and platelet count. If bone marrow suppression detected, adjust therapy. Give full dose if absolute granulocyte count (AGC) ≥ 1,000/mm³ and platelet count ≥ 100,000/mm³. If AGC 500/mm³ to 999/mm³ or platelet count 50,000/mm³ to 99,999/mm³, give 75% of dose. Withhold dose if AGC < 500/mm³ or platelet count < 50,000/mm³. Follow treatment course of 7 wk with 1 wk rest. Subsequent dosage cycles consist of 1 infusion q wk for 3 of 4 consecutive wk. Base dosage adjustments for subsequent cycles on AGC and platelet count nadirs and degree of nonhematologic toxicity.

- Obtain baseline and periodic renal and hepatic lab tests, as ordered.
- *IV use:* Reconstitute at conc > 40 mg/ml not recommended. May further dilute resulting conc with 0.9% NaCl injection, to as low as 0.1 mg/ml, if needed. Solution should be clear to light straw-colored and free of particulates. Stable for 24 hr at room temp. Don't refrigerate reconstituted drug.
- Prolonging infusion time beyond 60 min or giving drug more frequently than once weekly may increase toxicity.
- Careful hematologic monitoring, especially of neutrophil and platelet counts, required.
- Monitor patient closely. Expect dosage modification according to toxicity and degree of myelosuppression. Age, gender, and presence of renal impairment may predispose to toxicity.

gemfibrozil

Lopid

Fibric acid derivative

Antilipemic

Preg. Risk Category: C

Types IV and V hyperlipidemia unresponsive to diet and other drugs; reduction of CAD risk in patients with type IIb hyperlipidemia who can't tolerate or are refractory to bile acid sequestrants or niacin — **Adults:** 1,200 mg PO daily in 2 divided doses, 30 min before morning and evening meals.

- Instruct to take ½ hr before breakfast and dinner.
- Teach proper dietary management of serum lipids.
- Advise to avoid driving and other potentially hazardous activities until CNS effects known.
- Tell to report signs of bile duct obstruction.

GEMFIBROZIL 143

†Canadian ‡Australian

DRUG / CLASS / CATEGORY	INDICATIONS / DOSAGES	KEY NURSING CONSIDERATIONS
gentamicin sulfate Cidomycin†, Garamycin, Gentamicin Sulfate ADD-Vantage, Jenamicin *Aminoglycoside* *Antibiotic* Preg. Risk Category: NR	*Serious infections caused by susceptible organisms* — **Adults:** 3 mg/kg qd in divided doses IM or IV infusion q 8 hr. For life-threatening infections, up to 5 mg/kg qd in 3 to 4 divided doses; reduce to 3 mg/kg qd as soon as indicated. **Children:** 2 to 2.5 mg/kg q 8 hr IM or by IV infusion. **Neonates > 1 wk or infants:** 7.5 mg/kg qd in divided doses q 8 hr. *Meningitis* — **Adults:** systemic therapy as above; or 4 to 8 mg intrathecally qd. **Children and infants > 3 mo:** systemic therapy as above; or 1 to 2 mg intrathecally qd. *Endocarditis prophylaxis for GI or GU procedure or surgery* — **Adults:** 1.5 mg/kg IM or IV 30 to 60 min before procedure or surgery. Max 80 mg. Repeat in 8 hr. **Children:** 2 mg/kg IM or IV 30 min before procedure or surgery. Max 80 mg. After 8 hr, give half of initial dose.	• Evaluate hearing before and during therapy. Notify doctor of tinnitus, vertigo, or hearing loss. • *IV use:* For intermittent IV infusion, dilute with 50 to 200 ml D₅W or 0.9% NaCl injection and infuse over 30 min to 2 hr. After completing infusion, flush line with 0.9% NaCl solution or D₅W. • Obtain blood for peak drug level 1 hr after IM injection and 30 min to 1 hr after IV infusion; for trough levels, draw blood just before next dose. Don't collect blood in heparinized tube. • Monitor renal function (output, specific gravity, urinalysis, BUN, creatinine, and creatinine clearance). Notify doctor of signs of decreasing renal function. • Drug given in combination with ampicillin (vancomycin in penicillin-allergic patients) for endocarditis prophylaxis.
gentamicin sulfate Garamycin, G-Myticin *Aminoglycoside* *Topical antibiotic* Preg. Risk Category: C	*Treatment and prophylaxis of superficial skin infections caused by susceptible bacteria* — **Adults and children > 1 yr:** rub in small amount gently tid or qid, with or without gauze dressing.	• Clean affected area before applying. Remove crusts before application for impetigo contagiosa. • Prolonged use may result in overgrowth of nonsusceptible organisms.

gentamicin sulfate

Garamycin Ophthalmic, Genoptic, Gentacidin, Gentak, Ocu-Mycin

Aminoglycoside
Ophthalmic antibiotic
Preg. Risk Category: C

External ocular infections (conjunctivitis, keratoconjunctivitis, corneal ulcers, blepharitis, blepharoconjunctivitis, meibomianitis, and dacryocystitis) caused by susceptible organisms, especially P. aeruginosa, Proteus, K. pneumoniae, E. coli, and other gram-neg organisms — **Adults and children:** 1 to 2 drops instilled in eye q 4 hr. In severe infections, up to 2 drops q hr. Alternatively, apply oint to lower conjunctival sac bid or tid.

- Have culture taken before giving drug. Therapy may begin before culture results known.
- Apply light finger pressure on lacrimal sac for 1 min after instilling drops.
- If ophth form given concomitantly with systemic form, monitor serum gentamicin levels.
- Solution not for injection into conjunctiva or anterior chamber of eye.
- Store away from heat.

glimepiride

Amaryl

Sulfonylurea
Antidiabetic
Preg. Risk Category: C

Adjunct to diet and exercise to lower blood glucose in type 2 diabetes mellitus when hyperglycemia can't be managed by diet and exercise alone — **Adults:** Initially, 1 to 2 mg PO qd with first main meal of day; usual maintenance: 1 to 4 mg PO qd. After reaching 2 mg, increase dosage in increments not exceeding 2 mg q 1 to 2 wk, based on blood glucose response. Max 8 mg/day.
Adjunct to insulin therapy in type 2 diabetes mellitus when hyperglycemia can't be managed by diet and exercise in conjunction with oral hypoglycemic agents — **Adults:** 8 mg PO qd with first main meal of day; used in combination with low-dose insulin.

- Monitor fasting blood glucose periodically to determine therapeutic response. Also monitor glycosylated Hgb, usually every 3 to 6 mo, to more precisely assess long-term glycemic control.
- Instruct to take with first meal of day.
- Advise that drug relieves symptoms but doesn't cure diabetes. Explain potential risks and advantages of drug and other treatment methods.
- Stress importance of adhering to diet and therapeutic regimen. Tell patient and family how and when to perform blood glucose self-monitoring, and teach how to recognize hyperglycemia and hypoglycemia.

DRUG / CLASS / CATEGORY	INDICATIONS / DOSAGES	KEY NURSING CONSIDERATIONS
glipizide Glucotrol, Glucotrol XL, Minidiab† *Sulfonylurea* *Antidiabetic* Preg. Risk Category: C	*Adjunct to diet to lower blood glucose in type 2 diabetes mellitus —* **Adults:** generally 5 mg PO daily. Usual maintenance: 10 to 15 mg. Max daily dose 40 mg. Divide doses above 15 mg, except when using ext-release tablets. For ext-release tablets, 5 mg PO daily. Titrate in 5-mg increments q 3 mo for glycemic control. Max daily dosage 20 mg. *To replace insulin therapy —* **Adults:** if insulin dosage > 20 units daily, start at usual dosage plus 50% of insulin. If insulin dosage < 20 units, may stop insulin on initiating glipizide.	• Give about 30 min before meals. • During increased stress, patient may need insulin therapy. • Patients switching from insulin therapy to oral antidiabetic require blood glucose monitoring at least three times daily before meals. • Instruct about disease, importance of adhering to diet and therapeutic regimen. Tell how and when to perform blood glucose self-monitoring, and teach recognition of hypoglycemia and hyperglycemia.
glucagon *Antihyperglycemic agent* *Antidiabetic/diagnostic agent* Preg. Risk Category: B	*Hypoglycemia —* **Adults and children > 20 kg:** 0.5 to 1 mg SC, IM, or IV; may repeat q 20 min for 2 doses, if necessary. In deep coma, also give glucose 10% to 50% IV. When patient responds, give more carbohydrate immediately. **Children ≤ 20 kg:** 0.025 mg SC, IM, or IV; may repeat within 25 min. In deep coma, also give glucose 10% to 50% IV. When patient responds, give more carbohydrate immediately. *Note:* May repeat in 15 min, if necessary. Must give IV glucose if patient fails to respond. When patient responds, must give	• *IV use:* Use only diluent supplied by manufacturer when preparing doses of 2 mg or less. For larger doses, dilute with sterile water for injection. • For IV drip infusion, use dextrose solution. • Arouse patient from coma as quickly as possible and give additional carbohydrates orally to prevent secondary hypoglycemic reactions. • Unstable hypoglycemic diabetics may not respond to glucagon; give dextrose IV instead as ordered.

- Instruct patient and family in proper glucagon administration and hypoglycemia recognition.

supplemental carbohydrate immediately.
Diagnostic aid for radiologic examination — **Adults:** 0.25 to 2 mg IV or IM before radiologic procedure.

glyburide
(glibenclamide)
DiaBeta, Euglucon†, Glynase PresTab, Micronase
Sulfonylurea
Antidiabetic agent
Preg. Risk Category: C

Adjunct to diet to lower blood glucose in type 2 diabetes — **Adults:** initially, 2.5 to 5 mg regular tabs PO qd with breakfast. In sensitive patients, start at 1.25 mg qd. Usual maintenance: 1.25 to 20 mg qd as single dose or in divided doses or may use micronized formulation. Initial dosage 1.5 to 3 mg qd. In sensitive patients, started at 0.75 mg qd. Usual maintenance: 0.75 to 12 mg/day. Patients receiving > 6 mg/day may respond better with bid dosing.
To replace insulin therapy — **Adults:** If insulin dosage > 40 units/day, may start at 5 mg daily plus 50% of insulin dose; if < 20 units/day, should receive 2.5 to 5 mg/day. If 20 to 40 units/day, should receive 5 mg/day. In all patients, substitute glyburide and discontinue insulin abruptly. For micronized tablets, if insulin dosage > 40 units/day, give 3 mg PO with 50% reduction in insulin; if 20 to 40 units/day, should receive 3 mg PO as single daily dose; if < 20 units/day, should receive 1.5 to 3 mg/day as single dose.

- Micronized glyburide not bioequivalent to regular glyburide tablets.
- Instruct about nature of disease, importance of adhering to diet, therapeutic regimen, weight reduction, exercise, and personal hygiene programs, and avoiding infection. Explain how and when to perform blood glucose self-monitoring and teach how to recognize and intervene for hypoglycemia and hyperglycemia.
- Instruct to report hypoglycemic episodes to doctor immediately.
- Teach to carry candy or other simple sugars to treat mild hypoglycemic episodes.
- Patients switching from insulin to oral antidiabetic require blood glucose monitoring at least tid before meals. May require hospitalization during transition.
- Caution not to change dosage without doctor's consent and to report abnormal blood or urine glucose results.

DRUG / CLASS / CATEGORY	INDICATIONS / DOSAGES	KEY NURSING CONSIDERATIONS
glycerin Fleet Babylax, Sani-Supp *Trihydric alcohol* *Laxative (osmotic)/lubricant* Preg. Risk Category: C	*Constipation* — **Adults and children ≥ 6 yr:** 2 to 3 g as rectal supp or 5 to 15 ml as enema. **Children 2 to 6 yr:** 1 to 1.7 g as rectal supp or 2 to 5 ml as enema.	• Used mainly to restablish normal toilet habits in laxative-dependent patients. • Advise to retain drug for at least 15 min. • Usually acts within 1 hr. Entire suppository need not melt to be effective. • Warn about adverse GI reactions.
goserelin acetate Zoladex *Synthetic decapeptide* *Luteinizing hormone-releasing hormone (LHRH; GnRH) analog* Preg. Risk Category: X (endometriosis); D (breast cancer)	*Endometriosis, palliative treatment of advanced prostate cancer* — **Adults:** 3.6 mg SC q 28 days into upper abdominal wall. For endometriosis, max duration of therapy 6 months. For prostate cancer, 10.8 mg SC q 12 wk into upper abdominal wall. *Palliative treatment of advanced breast cancer in pre- and perimenopausal women* — **Adults:** 3.6 mg SC q 28 days into upper abdominal wall.	• Before giving to female, rule out pregnancy. • Administer into upper abdominal wall. After cleaning area with alcohol swab and injecting local anesthetic, stretch skin with 1 hand while grasping barrel of syringe with other. Insert needle into subcutaneous fat; then change needle direction so it parallels abdominal wall. Push needle in until hub touches skin; then withdraw about 1 cm before depressing plunger completely. • Don't aspirate after inserting needle. • Implant comes in preloaded syringe. If pkg damaged, don't use syringe. Make sure drug is visible. • When used for prostate cancer, may initially cause worsening of symptoms.

granisetron hydrochloride

Kytril

Selective 5-hydroxytryptamine (5-HT₃) receptor antagonist

Antiemetic and antinauseant

Preg. Risk Category: B

Prevention of nausea and vomiting associated with emetogenic cancer chemotherapy — **Adults and children 2 to 16 yr:** 10 mcg/kg IV infused over 5 min. Begin infusion within 30 min before chemotherapy administration. Alternatively, 1 mg PO up to 1 hr before chemotherapy, and repeated 12 hr later.

- **IV use:** Dilute with 0.9% NaCl or D₅W to volume of 20 to 50 ml.
- Don't mix with other drugs.
- Stress importance of taking second dose of oral drug 12 hr later for maximum effectiveness.
- Instruct to report adverse reactions immediately.

griseofulvin microsize

Fulcin‡, Fulvicin-U/F, Grifulvin V, Grisactin, Grisovin‡, Grisovin 500‡, Grisovin-FP

griseofulvin ultramicrosize

Fulvicin P/G, Grisactin Ultra, Griseostatin‡, Gris-PEG

Penicillium antibiotic

Antifungal

Preg. Risk Category: C

Ringworm infections of skin, hair, nails — **Adults:** 500 mg microsize PO qd in single or divided doses. Severe infections may require up to 1 g qd. Or, 330 to 375 mg ultramicrosize PO qd in single or divided doses. **Children > 2 yr:** 3.3 mg/lb microsize PO qd or 125 to 250 mg microsize PO qd for child 13.1 to 22.7 kg; or 250 to 500 mg microsize PO qd for child > 22.7 kg.

Tinea pedis and tinea unguium — **Adults:** 0.75 to 1 g microsize PO daily. Or, 660 to 750 mg ultramicrosize PO qd in divided doses. **Children > age 2:** 3.3 mg/lb ultramicrosize PO qd or 125 to 250 mg microsize PO qd for child 13.1 to 22.7 kg; or 250 to 500 mg microsize PO qd for child > 22.7 kg.

- Advise to take drug after high-fat meal.
- Inform that prolonged treatment may be needed to control infection and prevent relapse, even if symptoms abate in first few days.
- Instruct to keep skin clean and dry and to maintain good hygiene.
- Caution to avoid intense sunlight.
- Advise to avoid alcoholic beverages.

DRUG/CLASS/CATEGORY	INDICATIONS/DOSAGES	KEY NURSING CONSIDERATIONS
guaifenesin (glyceryl guaiacolate) Anti-Tuss, Glytuss, Halotussin, Humibid L.A., Neo-Spect, Robitussin *Propanediol derivative* *Expectorant* Preg. Risk Category: C	*Expectorant* — **Adults and children ≥ 12 yr:** 100 to 400 mg PO q 4 hr, max 2.4 g/day; or 600 to 1,200 mg ext-release caps q 12 hr. Max 2,400 mg daily. **Children 6 to 12 yr:** 100 to 200 mg PO q 4 hr, max 1,200 mg daily. For ext-release caps, 600 mg q 12 hr, not to exceed 1,200 mg in 24 hr. **Children 2 to 6 yr:** 50 to 100 mg PO q 4 hr. Max 600 mg daily. For ext-release cap, 300 mg q 12 hr, not to exceed 600 mg in 24 hr.	- Explain that persistent cough may signal serious condition; instruct to contact doctor if cough lasts > 1 wk, recurs frequently, or is associated with high fever, rash, or severe headache. - Advise to take each dose with glass of water. - Encourage deep-breathing exercises.
h		
haloperidol Apo-Haloperidol†, Haldol, Novo-Peridol†, Peridol†, Serenace‡ **haloperidol decanoate** Haldol Decanoate, Haldol LA† **haloperidol lactate** Haldol *Butyrophenone* *Antipsychotic* Preg. Risk Category: C	*Psychotic disorders* — **Adults and children ≥ 12 yr:** dosage varies. Initial range 0.5 to 5 mg PO bid or tid; or 2 to 5 mg IM q 4 to 8 hr. Max 100 mg PO qd. **Children 3 to 12 yr:** 0.05 mg/kg to 0.15 mg/kg PO qd. *Chronic psychotic patients who require prolonged therapy* — **Adults:** 50 to 100 mg IM haloperidol decanoate q 4 wk. *Nonpsychotic behavior disorders* — **Children 3 to 12 yr:** 0.05 mg/kg PO qd. Max 6 mg qd.	- Don't give decanoate form IV - Monitor for tardive dyskinesia, which may follow prolonged use. - Warn to avoid activities that require alertness and good psychomotor coordination until CNS effects known. - Tell to avoid alcohol. - Instruct to relieve dry mouth with sugarless gum or hard candy.

heparin calcium
Calcilean‡, Calciparine, Caprin‡

heparin sodium
Hepalean‡, Liquaemin Sodium, Uniparin‡
Anticoagulant
Anticoagulant
Preg. Risk Category: C

Dosage highly individualized, depending on disease state, age, and renal and hepatic status.
Full-dose continuous IV infusion therapy for DVT, MI, pulmonary embolism — **Adults:** initially, 5,000 units by IV bolus, followed by 750 to 1,500 units/hr by IV infusion with pump. Adjust hourly rate 8 hr after bolus dose and according to PTT. **Children:** initially, 50 units/kg IV followed by 25 units/kg/hr or 20,000 units/m² daily by IV infusion pump. Adjust dosage according to PTT.
Full-dose SC therapy for DVT, MI, pulmonary embolism — **Adults:** initially, 5,000 units IV bolus and 10,000 to 20,000 units in conc sol SC, followed by 8,000 to 10,000 units SC q 8 hr or 15,000 to 20,000 units in conc sol q 12 hr.
Fixed low-dose therapy for venous thrombosis, pulmonary embolism, atrial fibrillation with embolism, postop DVT, and embolism prevention — **Adults:** 5,000 units SC q 12 hr. In surgical patients, give 1st dose 2 hr before procedure, then 5,000 units SC q 8 to 12 hr for 5 to 7 days or until patient can walk.
Consumptive coagulopathy (such as DIC) — **Adults:** 50 to 100 units/kg by IV bolus or continuous IV infusion q 4 hr. **Children:** 25 to 50 units/kg by IV bolus or continuous IV infusion q 4 hr. If no improvement within 4 to 8 hr, discontinue.

- Give low-dose injections sequentially between iliac crests in lower abdomen deep into SC fat. Inject slowly into fat pad. Leave needle in place for 10 sec after injection; then withdraw. Don't massage after SC injection. Watch for signs of bleeding at injection site. Alternate sites q 12 hr (right for morning, left for evening).
- ***IV use:*** Administer IV using infusion pump. Check constant IV infusions regularly.
- During intermittent IV therapy, always draw blood ½ hr before next scheduled dose to avoid falsely elevated PTT. May draw blood for PTT any time after 8 hr of initiation of continuous IV therapy. Never draw blood for PTT from IV tubing of infusion or from infused vein (falsely elevated PTT will result). Always draw blood from opposite arm.
- Never piggyback other drugs into infusion line while infusion running. Never mix with another drug in same syringe when giving bolus.
- Measure PTT carefully and regularly. Anticoagulation present when PTT values 1.5 to 2 times control values. Monitor platelet count regularly.
- To treat severe overdose, use protamine sulfate, as ordered.

151

HEPARIN SODIUM

DRUG / CLASS / CATEGORY	INDICATIONS / DOSAGES	KEY NURSING CONSIDERATIONS
hydralazine hydrochloride Alphapress‡, Apresoline, Novo-Hylazin†, Supres‡ *Peripheral vasodilator* *Antihypertensive* Preg. Risk Category: C	*Essential hypertension (orally); severe essential hypertension (parenterally) —* **Adults:** *Oral:* 10 mg PO qid; increase gradually to 50 mg qid prn. Max dosage 200 mg qd, but some patients may require 300 to 400 mg qd. *IV:* 10 to 20 mg repeated prn; switch to PO as soon as possible. *IM:* 10 to 50 mg, repeated prn; switch to PO form as soon as possible. **Children:** *Oral:* 0.75 mg/kg/day PO divided into 4 doses; increase gradually over 3 to 4 wk to max 7.5 mg/kg or 200 mg qd. *IV or IM:* 1.7 to 3.5 mg/kg or 50 to 100 mg/m² qd in 4 to 6 divided doses. Initial parenteral dose shouldn't exceed 20 mg.	• **IV use:** Give slowly and repeat as necessary, generally every 4 to 6 hr. Undergoes color changes in most infusion solutions; changes don't indicate potency loss. Check with pharmacist for compatibility information. • Monitor BP, pulse, and weight frequently. • Elderly patients may be more sensitive to hypotensive effects. • Watch closely for lupuslike syndrome — call doctor immediately if these symptoms develop. • Instruct to take oral form with meals to increase absorption. • Advise rising slowly and avoiding sudden position changes to minimize orthostatic hypotension.
hydrochloro-thiazide Apo-Hydro†, Aquazide-H, Diaqua, Dichlotride‡, HydroDIURIL *Thiazide diuretic* *Diuretic/antihypertensive* Preg. Risk Category: B	*Edema —* **Adults:** 25 to 100 mg PO daily or intermittently. **Children 2 to 12 yr:** 37.5 to 100 mg PO daily in 2 divided doses. **Children 6 mo to 2 yr:** 12.5 to 37.5 mg PO daily in 2 divided doses. **Infants < 6 mo:** up to 3 mg/kg PO daily in 2 divided doses. Maximum dosage may range from 12.5 to 37.5 mg qd. *Hypertension —* **Adults:** 25 to 50 mg PO daily as single dose or divided bid. Increase	• Monitor I&O, weight, BP, and serum electrolytes. • Monitor serum creatinine, BUN, and serum uric acid regularly. Cumulative drug effects may occur with impaired renal function. • Monitor elderly patients, who are especially susceptible to excessive diuresis.

	or decrease daily dosage according to BP. Doses > 50 mg/day not required when combined with other antihypertensives.	• Monitor blood glucose, especially in diabetics. • In hypertension, therapeutic response may be delayed several weeks.
hydrocortisone Cortef, Hydrocortone **hydrocortisone acetate** Cortifoam, Hydrocortone Acetate **hydrocortisone sodium phosphate** Hydrocortone Phosphate **hydrocortisone sodium succinate** A-hydroCort, Solu-Cortef *Glucocorticoid/mineralocorticoid* *Adrenocortical replacement* Preg. Risk Category: C	*Severe inflammation, adrenal insufficiency* — **Adults:** 5 to 30 mg PO bid, tid, or qid (up to 80 mg qid in acute situations); or initially, 100 to 500 mg succinate IM or IV, and then 50 to 100 mg IM, as indicated; or 15 to 240 mg phosphate IM or IV daily in divided doses q 12 hr; or 5 to 75 mg acetate into joints or soft tissue. Dosage varies with size of joint. Local anesthetics often injected with dose. *Shock* — **Adults:** initially, 50 mg/kg succinate IV, repeated in 4 hr. Repeat q 24 hr as needed. Alternatively, 100 to 500 mg to 2 g q 2 to 6 hr; continue until patient stabilized (usually not longer than 48 to 72 hr). **Children:** phosphate (IM) or succinate (IM or IV) 0.16 to 1 mg/kg or 6 to 30 mg/m² qd or bid.	• May mask or exacerbate infections. • Watch for depression or psychotic episodes. • Diabetics may need increased insulin; monitor blood glucose. • Instruct to take oral form with milk or food. • Warn patient on long-term therapy about cushingoid symptoms. • Teach about symptoms of early adrenal insufficiency: fatigue, muscular weakness, joint pain, fever, anorexia, nausea, dyspnea, dizziness, and fainting. • Instruct to carry card identifying need for supplemental systemic glucocorticoids during stress. • Warn about easy bruising.

DRUG/CLASS/CATEGORY	INDICATIONS/DOSAGES	KEY NURSING CONSIDERATIONS
hydrocortisone Acticort, CaldeCort, Cortef, Cortizone 5, Squibb-HC‡ **hydrocortisone acetate** CortaGel, Cortaid, Cortamed†, Dermacort‡, Hydrocortisone Acetate **hydrocortisone butyrate** Locoid **hydrocortisone valerate** Westcort Cream *Glucocorticoid* *Topical adrenocorticoid* Preg. Risk Category: C	*Inflammation associated with corticosteroid-responsive dermatoses; adjunctive topical management of seborrheic dermatitis of scalp* — **Adults and children:** clean area; apply cream, gel, lotion, oint, or topical sol sparingly daily to qid. Spray aerosol onto affected area daily to qid until acute phase controlled; then reduce dosage to 1 to 3 times weekly as needed. *Inflammation associated with proctitis* — **Adults:** 1 applicatorful of rectal foam PR daily or bid for 2 to 3 wk, then qod as necessary.	• Gently wash skin before applying. To prevent skin damage, rub in gently, leaving thin coat. When treating hairy sites, part hair and apply directly to lesions. Don't apply near eyes, mucous membranes, or in ear canal; may be safely used on face, groin, armpits, and under breasts. • Stop drug and tell doctor if skin infection, striae, atrophy, or fever develops. • When using aerosol around face, cover patient's eyes and warn against inhaling spray. Don't spray for > 3 sec or closer than 6″ (15 cm). Apply to dry scalp after shampooing. No need to massage medication into scalp after spraying. • Systemic absorption likely with use of occlusive dressings, prolonged treatment, or extensive body-surface treatment. Watch for symptoms. • Continue treatment for several days after lesions clear, as ordered.
hydromorphone hydrochloride (dihydromorphinone hydrochloride)	*Moderate to severe pain* — **Adults:** 2 to 10 mg PO q 3 to 6 hr, prn or around the clock; or 2 to 4 mg IM, SC, or IV (slowly over at least 3 to 5 min) q 4 to 6 hr prn or around the clock; or 3 mg rectal supp hs, prn or	• Respiratory depression and hypotension possible with IV use. Give very slowly and monitor constantly. Keep resuscitation equipment available. • Keep narcotic antagonist available.

Dilaudid, Dilaudid-HP
Opioid
Analgesic/Antitussive
Preg. Risk Category: C
Controlled Sub. Sched.: II

around the clock. (Give 1 to 14 mg Dilaudid-HP SC or IM q 4 to 6 hr.)
Cough — Adults and children > 12 yr: 1 mg PO q 3 to 4 hr prn. **Children 6 to 12 yr:** 0.5 mg PO q 3 to 4 hr, prn.

- Dilaudid-HP highly concentrated.
- Instruct to request or to take drug before pain becomes intense.
- Warn outpatient to avoid hazardous activities that require mental alertness until CNS effects known.
- Tell to take drug with food if GI upset occurs.

---

hydroxyzine embonate‡
Atarax
hydroxyzine hydrochloride
Apo-Hydroxyzine†, Atarax, Hyzine-50, Multipaxt, Vistaquel, Vistaril, Vistazine 50
hydroxyzine pamoate
Hy-Pam, Vamate, Vistaril
Antihistamine (piperazine derivative)
Antianxiety agent/sedative/antipruritic/antiemetic/antispasmodic
Preg. Risk Category: C

Anxiety, tension, hyperkinesia — **Adults:** 50 to 100 mg PO qid. **Children ≥ 6 yr:** 50 to 100 mg PO daily in divided doses. **Children < 6 yr:** 50 mg PO daily in divided doses.
Preop and postop adjunctive sedation, to control vomiting (excluding pregnancy), or as adjunct to asthma treatment — **Adults:** 25 to 100 mg IM q 4 to 6 hr. **Children:** 1.1 mg/kg IM q 4 to 6 hr.
Pruritus due to allergies — **Adults:** 25 mg PO tid or qid. **Children < 6 yr:** 50 mg PO daily in divided doses. **Children ≥ 6 yr:** 50 to 100 mg PO daily in divided doses.

- Parenteral form (hydroxyzine hydrochloride) for IM use only; never administer IV. Z-track method preferred.
- Aspirate IM injection carefully to prevent inadvertent intravascular injection. Inject deeply into large muscle mass.
- If patient receiving other CNS drugs, observe for oversedation. Warn to avoid hazardous activities that require alertness and good psychomotor coordination until CNS effects known.
- Tell to avoid alcohol.
- To relieve dry mouth, suggest sugarless hard candy or gum.

DRUG/CLASS/ CATEGORY	INDICATIONS/ DOSAGES	KEY NURSING CONSIDERATIONS
hyoscyamine *Cystospaz* **hyoscyamine sulfate** Anaspaz, Bellaspaz, Levsin, Levsin S/L, Neoquess *Belladonna alkaloid Anticholinergic* Preg. Risk Category: C	*GI tract disorders caused by spasm; to di-minish secretions and block cardiac vagal reflexes preop; adjunctive therapy for peptic ulcerations* — **Adults and children ≥ 12 yr:** 0.125 to 0.25 mg PO or SL tid or qid before meals and hs; 0.375 mg to 0.75 mg PO (ext-release form) PO q 12 hr; or 0.25 to 0.5 mg (1 or 2 ml) IM, IV, or SC q 4 hr bid to qid. Max 1.5 mg daily. **Children < 12 yr:** dosage individualized according to weight.	• Give 30 min to 1 hr before meals and hs. Bedtime dose can be larger; give at least 2 hr after last meal of day. • Monitor vital signs and urine output care-fully. • Injection may cause allergic reaction in certain patients. • Advise to avoid hazardous activities if ad-verse CNS effects occur; to drink plenty of fluids and to report rash or other skin eruption.
ibuprofen Aches-N-Pain, ACT-3‡, Advil, Children's Advil, Chil-dren's Motrin, Motrin, Motrin IB Caplets, Motrin IB Tablets, Nuprin Caplets, Nuprin Tablets, PediaProfen *Nonsteroidal anti-inflamma-tory* *Nonnarcotic analgesic/an-tipyretic/anti-inflammatory* Preg. Risk Category: B	*Rheumatoid arthritis, osteoarthritis, arthri-tis* — **Adults:** 300 to 800 mg PO tid or qid, not to exceed 3.2 g/day. *Mild to moderate pain, dysmenorrhea* — **Adults:** 400 mg PO q 4 to 6 hr, prn. *Fever* — **Adults:** 200 to 400 mg PO q 4 to 6 hr. Don't exceed 1.2 g daily or give > 3 days. **6 mo to 12 yr:** If fever < 102.5° F (39.2° C), 5 mg/kg PO q 6 to 8 hr. Treat higher fevers with 10 mg/kg PO q 6 to 8 hr. Max 40 mg/kg qd. *Juvenile arthritis* — **Children:** 30 to 70 mg/kg/day in 3 or 4 divided doses.	• Check renal and hepatic function periodi-cally with long-term therapy. • Changes in vision may occur. • Instruct not to give to children < 12 years, and not to self-medicate for extended peri-ods without consulting doctor. • Caution that using with aspirin, alcohol, or corticosteroids may increase risk of ad-verse GI reactions. • Teach about signs and symptoms of GI bleeding, and tell to contact doctor imme-diately if these occur.

ibutilide fumarate
Corvert
Ibutilide derivative
Supraventricular antiar-rhythmic
Preg. Risk Category: C

Rapid conversion of fibrillation or atrial flut-ter of recent onset to sinus rhythm —

Adults > 60 kg (132 lb): 1 mg IV over 10 min. **Adults < 60 kg:** 0.01 mg/kg IV over 10 min. Stop infusion if arrhythmia ends or if ventricular tachycardia or marked prolonga-tion of QT or QTc occurs. If arrhythmia doesn't end 10 min after infusion ends, may give second 10-min infusion of equal strength.

- Should be given only by skilled personnel.
- Before therapy, correct hypokalemia and hypomagnesemia.
- Patients with atrial fibrillation of > 2 to 3 days' duration must be adequately antico-agulated, generally for at least 2 wk.
- Monitor ECG continuously during and at least 4 hr after administration or until QTc returns to baseline.
- *IV use:* May give undiluted or diluted in 50 ml diluent.

idarubicin hydrochloride
Idamycin
Antibiotic/antineoplastic
Antineoplastic
Preg. Risk Category: D

Dosage and indications vary. Check treat-ment protocol with doctor.
Acute myeloid leukemia, including FAB (French-American-British) classifications M1 through M7, in combination with other approved antileukemic agents — **Adults:** 12 mg/m²/day for 3 days by slow IV injec-tion (over 10 to 15 min) in combination with 100 mg/m²/day of cytarabine by continuous IV infusion; or as 25 mg/m² bo-lus (cytarabine), followed by 200 mg/m²/day (cytarabine) for 5 days by continuous infusion. Second course may be given prn. If patient experiences severe mucositis, de-lay until recovery complete, and reduce dosage by 25%. Also reduce dosage in he-patic or renal impairment. Don't give if bilirubin > 5 mg/dl.

- Cardiotoxicity is dose-limiting toxicity.
- Take preventive steps, such as adequate hydration, before treatment starts. Hyper-uricemia may result from rapid lysis of leukemic cells; allopurinol may be or-dered.
- Give over 10 to 15 min into free-flowing IV infusion of 0.9% NaCl or 5% dextrose so-lution running into large vein.
- Vesicant; tissue necrosis may result. If ex-travasation occurs, discontinue infusion immediately and notify doctor. Apply in-termittent ice packs — for ½ hr immedi-ately, and then for ½ hr qid for 4 days.
- Monitor hepatic and renal function tests and CBC frequently, as ordered.
- Notify doctor if signs or symptoms of heart failure occur.

IDARUBICIN HYDROCHLORIDE   157

†Canadian ‡Australian

DRUG / CLASS / CATEGORY	INDICATIONS / DOSAGES	KEY NURSING CONSIDERATIONS
idoxuridine (IDU) Herplex *Halogenated pyrimidine* *Antiviral agent* Preg. Risk Category: C	*Herpes simplex keratitis* — **Adults and children:** 1 drop sol instilled into conjunctival sac q hr during day and q 2 hr at night. Continue until definite improvement occurs, usually ≤ 7 days.	• Don't mix with other topical eye drugs. • Apply light finger pressure on lacrimal sac for 1 min after instilling drops. • Don't use for > 21 days. • Keep solution in tightly closed, light-resistant container at room temp.
ifosfamide IFEX *Alkylating agent (cell cycle–phase nonspecific)* *Antineoplastic* Preg. Risk Category: D	*Testicular cancer* — **Adults:** 1.2 g/m²/day IV for 5 consecutive days. Infuse each dose over ≥ 30 min. Repeat treatment q 3 wk or after patient recovers from hematologic toxicity. Administer with protecting agent (mesna) to prevent hemorrhagic cystitis.	• Adequate fluid intake (2 L/day) essential before and for 72 hr after therapy. • Assess for mental status changes. • Don't give at bedtime. If cystitis develops, discontinue and notify doctor. • Monitor CBC and renal and liver function tests, as ordered.
imipenem/cilastatin sodium Primaxin IM, Primaxin IV *Carbapenem (thienamycin class) beta-lactam antibiotic* *Antibiotic* Preg. Risk Category: C	*Serious lower respiratory, urinary tract, intra-abdominal, gyn, bone and joint, and skin and soft-tissue infections; bacterial septicemia and endocarditis* — **Adults and children > 40 kg:** 250 mg to 1 g by IV infusion q 6 to 8 hr. Max 50 mg/kg/day or 4 g/day, whichever is less. Alternatively, 500 to 750 mg IM q 12 hr. Max 1,500 mg/day. **Children < 40 kg:** 60 mg/kg IV daily in divided doses. **Premature infants < 36 wk gestational age:** 20 mg/kg IV q 12 hr.	• Obtain culture and sensitivity tests before first dose. • **IV use:** Give each 250- or 500-mg dose by IV infusion over 20 to 30 min. Infuse each 1-g dose over 40 to 60 min. If nausea occurs, infusion may be slowed. • Adjust dosage for creatinine clearance < 70 ml/min. • If seizures develop and persist, notify doctor. Drug should be discontinued. • Monitor for superinfections and resistant infections.

imipramine hydrochloride

Apo-Imipramine†, Imipril†, Janimine‡, Melipramine†, Norfranil, Tipramine, Tofranil

imipramine pamoate

Tofranil-PM

Dibenzazepine tricyclic antidepressant

Antidepressant

Preg. Risk Category: B

Depression — **Adults:** 75 to 100 mg PO or IM daily in divided doses, increased in 25- to 50-mg increments. Max for outpatients 200 mg daily; 300 mg daily may be used for hospital patients. Entire dosage may be given hs. **Elderly and adolescent patients:** initially, 30 to 40 mg daily; usually not necessary to exceed 100 mg daily.

Childhood enuresis — **Children ≥ 6 yr:** 25 mg PO 1 hr before bedtime. If no response within 1 wk, increase to 50 mg if child < 12 yr; 75 mg for children ≥ 12 yr. In either case, max 2.5 mg/kg/day.

- Reduce dosage in elderly or debilitated persons and adolescents or in patient with aggravated psychotic symptoms.
- Don't withdraw abruptly.
- Should discontinue gradually several days before surgery.
- Warn to avoid hazardous activities until CNS effects known.
- If signs of psychosis occur or increase, reduce dosage. Monitor for suicidal tendencies, and allow only minimum drug supply.

---

indapamide

Lozide†, Lozol, Natrilix‡

Thiazide-like diuretic

Diuretic/antihypertensive

Preg. Risk Category: B

Edema — **Adults:** initially, 2.5 mg PO daily in morning. Increase to 5 mg daily after 1 wk, if needed.

Hypertension — **Adults:** initially, 1.25 mg PO daily in morning. Increase to 2.5 mg daily after 4 wk, if needed. Increase to 5 mg daily after 4 more wk, if needed.

- Monitor I&O, weight, BP, serum electrolytes, BUN, creatinine, uric acid, and glucose.
- Watch for signs of hypokalemia.
- May be used with potassium-sparing diuretic to prevent potassium loss.
- Monitor elderly patients closely.

---

indinavir sulfate

Crixivan

Human immunodeficiency virus (HIV) protease inhibitor

Antiviral agent

Preg. Risk Category: C

Treatment of HIV infection when antiretroviral therapy warranted — **Adults:** 800 mg PO q 8 hr. Reduce to 600 mg PO q 8 hr in mild to moderate hepatic insufficiency due to cirrhosis.

- Maintain adequate hydration (≥ 48 oz [1½ L] fluids q 24 hr while on indinavir).
- Inform that drug won't cure HIV infection and may not prevent complications of HIV. Has not been shown to reduce risk of HIV transmission.
- Advise females to avoid breast-feeding.

†Canadian ‡Australian

INDINAVIR SULFATE   159

DRUG/CLASS/CATEGORY

indomethacin
Apo-Indomethacin‡, Indochron E-R, Indocid SR‡, Indocin, Indocin SR, Novomethacin‡, Rheumacin‡

indomethacin sodium trihydrate
Apo-Indomethacin‡, Indocid PDA‡, Indocin IV, Novomethacin‡

Nonsteroidal anti-inflammatory

Nonnarcotic analgesic/antipyretic/anti-inflammatory
Preg. Risk Category: NR

INDICATIONS/DOSAGES

Moderate to severe rheumatoid arthritis or osteoarthritis, ankylosing spondylitis —
Adults: 25 mg PO or PR bid or tid with food or antacids; increase daily dosage 25 or 50 mg q 7 days, up to 200 mg daily. Or, SR cap (75 mg): 75 mg PO to start, in morning or hs, followed, if necessary, by 75 mg bid.

Acute gouty arthritis — **Adults:** 50 mg PO tid. Reduce as soon as possible; then stop.

Acute painful shoulders (bursitis or tendinitis) — **Adults:** 75 to 150 mg PO daily in divided doses tid or qid for 7 to 14 days.

To close hemodynamically significant PDA in premature infants (IV form only) —
Neonates < 48 hr: 0.2 mg/kg IV followed by 2 doses of 0.1 mg/kg at 12- to 24-hr intervals. **Neonates 2 to 7 days:** 0.2 mg/kg IV followed by 2 doses of 0.2 mg/kg at 12- to 24-hr intervals. **Neonates > 7 days:** 0.2 mg/kg IV followed by 2 doses of 0.25 mg/kg at 12- to 24-hr intervals.

KEY NURSING CONSIDERATIONS

- Monitor carefully for bleeding and for reduced urine output with IV use. Don't give second or third scheduled IV dose if anuria or marked oliguria evident; instead, notify doctor. Monitor for bleeding in coagulation defects, in patients receiving anticoagulants, and in neonates.
- If ductus arteriosus reopens, second course of 1 to 3 doses may be given. If still ineffective, surgery may be necessary.
- May lead to reversible renal impairment; monitor patient closely.
- Causes sodium retention. Monitor for weight gain and increased BP.
- May mask signs and symptoms of infection.
- Give oral dosage with food, milk, or antacid if GI upset occurs.

insulin inj (regular insulin, crystalline zinc insulin)
Humulin R, Novolin R, Regular (Conc.) Iletin II

insulin zinc susp, prompt (semilente)
Semilente MC‡

isophane insulin susp (NPH)
Humulin N, Humulin NPH‡, Novolin N, NPH Insulin

isophane insulin susp with insulin inj
Humulin 50/50, Humulin 70/30, Novolin 70/30

insulin zinc susp (lente)
Humulin L, Lente Insulin, Lente MC‡, Novolin L

protamine zinc susp (PZI)
Protamine Zinc Insulin MC‡

insulin zinc susp, ext (ultralente)
Humulin U, Ultralente Insulin
Pancreatic hormone
Antidiabetic agent
Preg. Risk Category: NR

Diabetic ketoacidosis (use reg insulin only) — **Adults:** 0.33 units/kg as IV bolus, followed by 0.1 units/kg/hr by continuous infusion. Continue infusion until blood glucose drops to 250 mg/dl; then begin SC insulin with dosage and intervals adjusted according to blood glucose level. Or, 50 to 100 units IV and 50 to 100 units SC stat; then additional doses q 2 to 6 hr based on blood glucose levels. To prepare infusion, add 100 units reg insulin and 1 g albumin to 100 ml 0.9% NaCl. Insulin concentration will be 1 unit/ml. **Children:** 0.1 unit/kg as IV bolus, then 0.1 unit/kg/hr by continuous infusion until blood glucose drops to 250 mg/dl; then start SC insulin. Alternatively, 1 to 2 units/kg in 2 divided doses, one IV and other SC, followed by 0.5 to 1 unit/kg IV q 1 to 2 hr based on blood glucose levels.
Type 1 diabetes, adjunct to type 2 diabetes: **Adults and children:** therapeutic regimen adjusted according to blood glucose levels.

- Reg insulin used in circulatory collapse, diabetic ketoacidosis, or hyperkalemia. Don't use reg insulin (Concentrated), 500 units/ml, IV. Don't use intermediate or long-acting insulins for emergencies requiring rapid drug action.
- *IV use:* Give reg insulin only IV. Inject directly, at ordered rate, into vein through intermittent infusion device or into port close to IV access site. Intermittent infusion not recommended.
- Dosage expressed in USP units. Use syringes calibrated for specific insulin concentration.
- U-500 insulin available for patients requiring large doses.
- Monitor pregnant patients closely.
- When mixing reg insulin with intermediate or long-acting insulins, always draw up reg insulin into syringe first.
- Rotate injection sites, and chart to avoid overusing one area.
- Store in cool area.

‡Canadian †Australian

DRUG/CLASS/ CATEGORY	INDICATIONS/ DOSAGES	KEY NURSING CONSIDERATIONS
interferon alfa-2a, recombinant (rIFN-A) Roferon-A *Biological response modifier* *Antineoplastic* Preg. Risk Category: C	*Hairy-cell leukemia* — **Adults:** for induction, 3 million IU SC or IM daily for 16 to 24 wk. For maintenance, 3 million IU SC or IM 3 times weekly. *AIDS-related kaposi's sarcoma* — **Adults:** for induction, 36 million IU SC or IM daily for 10 to 12 wk. For maintenance, 36 million IU SC or IM 3 times/wk. *Philadelphia chromosome-positive chronic myelogenous leukemia* — **Adults:** initially, 3 million IU daily for 3 days; then 6 million IU for 3 days, then 9 million IU for duration of treatment.	• Obtain allergy history. Contains phenol as preservative and serum albumin as stabilizer. • Give by SC route if platelet count <50,000/mm³. • Administer hs to minimize daytime drowsiness. • Keep patient well hydrated, especially during initial treatment stage. • Monitor for CNS adverse reactions, such as decreased mental status and dizziness. • Different brands may not be equivalent and may require different dosage. • Neurotoxicity and cardiotoxicity more common in elderly patients, especially those with underlying CNS or cardiac impairment.
interferon alfa-2b, recombinant (IFN-alpha 2) Intron A *Biological response modifier* *Antineoplastic* Preg. Risk Category: C	*Hairy-cell leukemia* — **Adults:** 2 million IU/m² IM or SC, 3 times/wk. *AIDS-related Kaposi's sarcoma* — **Adults:** 30 million IU/m² SC or IM 3 times/wk. *Chronic hepatitis B* — **Adults:** 30 to 35 million IU weekly IM or SC, given either as 5 million IU daily or 10 million IU 3 times/wk for 16 wk.	• Give by SC route if platelet count <50,000/mm³. • Administer hs to minimize daytime drowsiness. • Keep patient well hydrated. • Monitor for adverse CNS reactions. • May increase bone marrow suppressant effects when used with blood dyscrasia-causing therapies.

interferon alfa-n3

Alferon N
Biological response modifier
Antineoplastic
Preg. Risk Category: C

Condylomata acuminata (genital or venereal warts) — **Adults:** 0.05 ml (250,000 units) for each wart by intralesional injection. Treatment usually continues twice weekly for up to 8 wk. Dosage shouldn't exceed 0.5 ml (2.5 million units) per session.

- Be prepared to treat acute hypersensitivity reactions.
- Inject each lesion at base of wart, using 30G needle.
- Administer acetaminophen for flulike symptoms.

interferon beta-1a

Avonex
Biological response modifier
Antiviral immunoregulator
Preg. Risk Category: C

Treatment of relapsing forms of multiple sclerosis to slow accumulation of physical disability and decrease frequency of clinical exacerbation — **Adults:** 30 mcg IM q wk.

- Monitor closely for depression and suicidal ideation.
- Monitor WBC counts, platelet counts, and blood chemistries, including liver function tests.
- To reconstitute, inject 1.1 ml supplied diluent (sterile water for injection) into vial and gently swirl to dissolve drug. Don't shake.

interferon beta-1b, recombinant

Betaseron
Biological response modifier
Antiviral immunoregulator
Preg.Risk Category: C

To reduce frequency of exacerbations in relapsing-remitting multiple sclerosis — **Adults:** 8 million IU (0.25 mg) SC qod

- To reconstitute, inject 1.2 ml supplied diluent (0.54% NaCl injection) into vial and gently swirl to dissolve drug. Don't shake.
- Discard vials containing particulates or discolored solution.
- Inject immediately after preparation.
- Rotate injection sites to minimize local reactions.
- Monitor for mental depression.

DRUG/CLASS/CATEGORY	INDICATIONS/DOSAGES	KEY NURSING CONSIDERATIONS
interferon gamma-1b Actimmune *Biological response modifier* *Antineoplastic* Preg. Risk Category: C	*Chronic granulomatous disease* — **Adults with BSA > 0.5 m²**: 50 mcg/m² (1.5 million units/m²) SC 3 times weekly, preferably at hs. Preferred injection site deltoid or anterior or thigh muscle. **Adults with BSA ≤ 0.5 m²**: 1.5 mcg/kg 3 times weekly.	• Premedicate with acetaminophen to minimize symptoms at start of therapy. Flulike symptoms tend to diminish with continued therapy. • Discard unused portion. • Refrigerate immediately. Store vials at 36° to 46° F (2° to 8° C); don't freeze. Don't shake vial; avoid excessive agitation. Discard vials left at room temp for > 12 hr.
ipratropium bromide Atrovent *Anticholinergic* *Bronchodilator* Preg. Risk Category: B	*Bronchospasm associated with COPD* — **Adults**: 1 to 2 inhalations qid. More may be needed. Total inhalations shouldn't exceed 12 in 24 hr, or use inhalation sol. Give 500 mcg dissolved in 0.9% NaCl and administer by nebulizer q 6 to 8 hrs. **Children 5 to 12 yr**: 125 to 250 mcg nebulizer sol dissolved in 0.9% NaCl and administer by nebulizer q 6 to 8 hr. *Perennial rhinitis* — **Adults and children > 12 yr**: 2 sprays (42 mcg) of 0.03% nasal spray per nostril 2 to 3 times qd. *Common cold-induced rhinorrhea* — **Adults and children > 12 yr**: 2 sprays (84 mcg) of 0.06% nasal spray per nostril 3 or 4 times qd.	• If using face mask for nebulizer, avoid leakage around mask. • Warn that drug is ineffective for treating acute episodes of bronchospasm. • Teach to perform oral inhalation correctly: Clear nasal passages and throat. Breathe out as much as possible. Place mouthpiece well into mouth as dose is released, and then inhale deeply. Hold breath for several seconds, and then exhale slowly. If > 1 exhalation ordered, wait at least 2 min before repeating. • If patient also uses steroid inhaler, tell to use ipratropium first, then wait 5 min before using steroid.

ipecac syrup

ipecac syrup
Alkaloid emetic
Emetic
Preg. Risk Category: C

To induce vomiting in poisoning — Adults and children > 12 yr: 15 to 30 ml PO, followed by 3 to 4 glasses of water. *Children 1 to 12 yr:* 15 ml PO, followed by 240 to 480 ml water. *Children 6 mo to 1 yr:* 5 to 10 ml PO, followed by 120 to 240 ml water. May repeat dose in patients > 1 yr if vomiting doesn't occur within 20 min. If no vomiting occurs within 30 to 35 min after 2nd dose, gastric lavage should be performed.

- Usually induces vomiting within 20 to 30 min.
- If 2 doses don't induce vomiting, be prepared for gastric lavage.
- No systemic toxicity with doses of ≤ 30 ml (1 oz) or less.
- In antiemetic toxicity, usually effective if < 1 hr has passed since antiemetic ingested.

irinotecan hydrochloride

Camptosar
Topoisomerase inhibitor
Antineoplastic agent
Preg. Risk Category: D

Treatment of metastatic carcinoma of colon or rectum that has recurred or progressed after fluorouracil (5-FU) therapy — Adults: initially, 125 mg/m² IV infusion over 90 min. Recommended treatment 125 mg/m² IV q wk for 4 wk followed by 2-wk rest period. Thereafter, may repeat additional treatment course q 6 wk (4 wk on therapy, followed by 2 wk off). May adjust subsequent doses to low of 50 mg/m² or to max 150 mg/m² in 25- to 50-mg/m² increments, depending on tolerance. Treatment with additional courses may continue indefinitely if patient responds favorably or if disease remains stable, unless intolerable toxicity occurs.

- Don't add other drugs to infusion.
- Avoid extravasation. If it occurs, flush site with sterile water and apply ice. Notify doctor.
- Can induce severe diarrhea. Diarrhea occurring ≤ 24 hr of use may be relieved by atropine IV, unless contraindicated. Late diarrhea (occurring after 24 hr) may be prolonged and life-threatening. Treat late diarrhea with loperamide, as ordered. Monitor fluid status and serum electrolytes.
- Monitor WBC count with differential, Hgb, and platelet count before each dose. If low, dosages may need to be reduced or held.

†Canadian ‡Australian

DRUG / CLASS / CATEGORY

isoniazid (isonicotinic acid hydride, INH)
Isotamine†, Laniazid, Nydrazid, PMS Isoniazid†
Isonicotinic acid hydrazine
Antitubercular agent
Preg. Risk Category: C

isoproterenol (isoprenaline)
Dey-Dose Isoproterenol, Isuprel, Vapo-Iso
isoproterenol hydrochloride
Isuprel, Norisodrine Aerotrol
isoproterenol sulfate

INDICATIONS / DOSAGES

Actively growing tubercle bacilli — **Adults:** 5 mg/kg PO or IM daily in single dose, up to 300 mg/day for 9 mo to 2 yr. **Infants and children:** 10 mg/kg PO or IM daily in single dose, up to 300 mg/day, for 18 mo to 2 yr. Give with one other antitubercular.
Prevention of tubercle bacilli in those exposed to TB or those with tests consistent with nonprogressive TB — **Adults:** 300 mg PO daily in single dose, continued for 6 mo to 1 yr. **Infants and children:** 10 mg/kg PO daily in single dose, up to 300 mg/day, continued for 6 mo to 1 yr.

Shock — **Adults and children:** (hydrochloride) 0.5 to 5 mcg/min by continuous IV infusion titrated to response. Usual concentration 1 mg (5 ml) in 500 ml D_5W.
Bronchodilation — **Adults:** 10 to 15 mg hydrochloride SL tid or qid. Max daily SL, 60 mg. **Children:** 5 to 10 mg hydrochloride SL tid. Max daily SL dosage 30 mg.
Bronchospasm during mild acute asthma attacks— **Adults:** 1 inhalation of sulfate form initially; repeat if needed after 2 to 5 min, with max 6 inhalations daily.

KEY NURSING CONSIDERATIONS

- Should always be given with other antituberculars to prevent development of resistant organisms.
- Monitor hepatic function closely for changes.
- Advise to avoid alcoholic beverages, fish, and tyramine-containing products such as aged cheese, beer, and chocolate.
- Give pyridoxine, as ordered, to prevent peripheral neuropathy, especially in malnourished patients.

- Correct volume deficit and hypotension before administering vasopressors.
- If HR > 110 with IV infusion, notify doctor. Doses sufficient to increase HR > 130 may induce ventricular arrhythmias.
- When giving IV to treat shock, monitor BP, CVP, ECG, ABGs, and urine output. Adjust infusion rate according to results.
- May aggravate ventilation-perfusion abnormalities.
- May cause slight rise in systolic BP and slight to marked drop in diastolic BP.

Medihaler-Iso
Adrenergic
Bronchodilator/cardiac
stimulant
Preg. Risk Category: C

Bronchospasm in COPD — **Adults and children:** (hydrochloride) by hand-held nebulizer; 5 to 15 deep inhalations of 0.5% sol. In adults requiring stronger sol, 3 to 7 deep inhalations of 1% sol no more frequently than q 3 to 4 hr.

Heart block and ventricular arrhythmias — **Adults:** (hydrochloride) 0.02 to 0.06 mg IV. Subsequent doses 0.01 to 0.2 mg IV or 5 mcg/min IV titrated to response; or 0.2 mg IM, then 0.02 to 1 mg IM prn. **Children:** (hydrochloride): IV infusion of 2.5 mcg/min to 0.1 mcg/kg/min. Dosage based on response.

- **IV use:** Give by direct injection or infusion. For infusion, don't use with sodium bicarbonate injection.
- Don't use injection or inhalation solution if discolored or contains precipitate.
- If administering via inhalation with oxygen, make sure O_2 conc won't suppress respiratory drive.
- Signs of overdose include exaggeration of common adverse reactions.
- Monitor for rebound bronchospasms when drug effects end.

isosorbide
Ismotic
Osmotic diuretic
Antiglaucoma agent
Preg. Risk Category: B

Short-term reduction of IOP caused by glaucoma — **Adults:** initially, 1.5 g/kg PO. Usual dosage range 1 to 3 g/kg bid to qid, as indicated.

- To improve palatability, pour over cracked ice and instruct to sip.
- Monitor patient closely for adverse effects for 5 to 10 min after administration.
- Especially useful in reducing IOP rapidly. May be used to interrupt acute glaucoma attack before laser surgery.
- In diseases associated with sodium retention, carefully monitor fluid and electrolyte balance.

DRUG/CLASS/ CATEGORY	INDICATIONS/ DOSAGES	KEY NURSING CONSIDERATIONS
isosorbide dinitrate Apo-ISDN†, Dilatrate-SR, Isonate, Isorbid, Isordil, Isordil Tembids, Isotrate, Sorbitrate **isosorbide mononitrate** Imdur, ISMO, Monoket *Nitrate* *Antianginal agent/vasodilator* Preg. Risk Category: C	*Acute anginal attacks (SL and chew tab of isosorbide dinitrate only), prophylaxis in situations likely to cause anginal attacks —* **Adults:** *SL form —* 2.5 to 5 mg under tongue, repeated q 5 to 10 min (max 3 doses for each 30-min period). For prophylaxis, 2.5 to 10 mg q 2 to 3 hr. *Chewable form —* 5 to 10 mg prn for acute attack or q 2 to 3 hr for prophylaxis, but only after initial test dose of 5 mg. *Oral form (dinitrate) —* 5 to 30 mg PO tid or qid for prophylaxis (use smallest effective dose); 20 to 40 mg PO (SR form) q 6 to 12 hr. *Oral form (mononitrate, using Imdur) —* 30 to 60 mg PO qd on arising; increased to 120 mg qd after several days, prn. *Oral form (mononitrate, using ISMO or Monoket) —* 20 mg PO bid with 2 doses given 7 hr apart.	■ Monitor BP and intensity and duration of drug response. ■ May cause headaches, especially when therapy begins. Dosage may be reduced temporarily, but tolerance usually develops. Give aspirin or acetaminophen for headache as ordered. ■ Inform that abrupt discontinuation may cause coronary vasospasm with increased anginal symptoms and potential risk of MI. ■ Tell to take SL tab at first sign of attack. Warn not to confuse SL with oral form. ■ To prevent development of tolerance, nitrate-free interval of 8 to 12 hr per day recommended.
isotretinoin Accutane, Roaccutane‡ *Retinoic acid derivative* *Antiacne agent/keratinization stabilizer* Preg. Risk Category: X	*Severe recalcitrant nodular acne unresponsive to conventional therapy —* **Adults and adolescents:** 0.5 to 2 mg/kg PO daily in 2 divided doses for 15 to 20 wk.	■ Monitor serum lipids, glucose, and CK levels, and liver function tests before and during therapy. ■ Most adverse reactions occur at daily dosages > 1 mg/kg.

- Screen patients who experience headache, nausea and vomiting, or visual disturbances for papilledema. Signs and symptoms of pseudotumor cerebri require immediate drug stoppage and prompt neurologic intervention.
- Anticipate 2nd course of therapy, if needed, not to start for ≥ 8 wk after completion of 1st course.

---

isradipine
DynaCirc
Calcium channel blocker
Antihypertensive
Preg. Risk Category: C

Hypertension — **Adults:** initially, 2.5 mg PO bid, alone or with thiazide diuretic. If response inadequate after first 2 to 4 wk, make dosage adjustments of 5 mg daily at 2- to 4-wk intervals to max 20 mg daily.

- May cause symptomatic hypotension; monitor for adverse reactions. Most adverse reactions mild, transient, and related to vasodilation (dizziness, edema, flushing, palpitations, and tachycardia).
- Monitor BP closely.
- Advise to avoid hazardous tasks if adverse CNS reactions occur.
- Before surgery, inform anesthesiologist that patient receiving calcium channel blocker.

---

itraconazole
Sporanox
Synthetic triazole
Antifungal
Preg. Risk Category: C

Pulmonary and extrapulmonary blastomycosis; nonmeningeal histoplasmosis — **Adults:** 200 mg PO daily. Increase dosage as needed and tolerated in 100-mg increments to max 400 mg daily. Give dosages > 200 mg daily in 2 divided doses.
Aspergillosis — **Adults:** 200 to 400 mg PO daily.

- Perform baseline liver function tests, as ordered, and monitor periodically.
- Teach to recognize and report signs and symptoms of liver disease (anorexia, dark urine, pale stools, unusual fatigue, or jaundice).
- Tell to take with food to ensure maximal absorption.

ITRACONAZOLE 169

---

†Canadian ‡Australian

K

DRUG/CLASS/ CATEGORY	INDICATIONS/ DOSAGES	KEY NURSING CONSIDERATIONS
ketoconazole Nizoral *Imidazole derivative* *Antifungal* Preg. Risk Category: C	*Fungal infections caused by susceptible organisms* — **Adults:** 200 mg PO qd in single dose. Max 400 mg qd. **Children ≥ 2 yr:** 3.3 to 6.6 mg/kg PO qd as single dose. *Topical treatment of tinea infestations* — **Adults and children:** Apply qd or bid for about 2 wk; for tinea pedis, apply for 4 wk.	▪ To minimize nausea, divide daily dosage into 2 doses or give with meals. ▪ Monitor for elevated liver enzymes, nausea that doesn't subside, unusual fatigue, jaundice, dark urine, or pale stools.
ketoconazole Nizoral *Imidazole derivative* *Antifungal* Preg. Risk Category: C	*Tinea corporis, tinea cruris, tinea pedis, and tinea versicolor caused by susceptible organisms; seborrheic dermatitis; cutaneous candidiasis* — **Adults:** cover affected and surrounding area with 2% cream qd for ≥ 2 wk; for seborrheic dermatitis, apply bid for 4 wk, with ≥ 3 days between shampoos prn.	▪ Most patients show improvement soon after treatment begins. ▪ Treatment of tinea cruris or tinea corporis should continue for ≥ 2 wk. ▪ If condition worsens, may have to be discontinued and diagnosis redetermined. ▪ For shampoo, wet hair, lather, and massage for 1 min. Rinse and repeat, but leave drug on scalp for 3 min before rinsing.
ketoprofen Actron, Orudis *Nonsteroidal anti- inflammatory* *Nonnarcotic analgesic/an- tipyretic/anti-inflammatory* Preg. Risk Category: B	*Rheumatoid arthritis and osteoarthritis* — **Adults:** 75 mg tid or 50 mg qid or 200 mg as ext-release pm. Max 300 mg/day. *Mild to moderate pain; dysmenorrhea* — **Adults:** 25 to 50 mg PO q 6 to 8 hrs, pm. *Minor aches and pain or fever* — **Adults:** 12.5 mg q 4 to 6 hr. Don't exceed 75 mg in 24 hr.	▪ May lead to reversible renal impairment. Check renal and hepatic function every 6 mo or pm. ▪ May mask signs of infection. ▪ Full effect may be delayed for 2 to 4 wk. ▪ Warn to avoid hazardous activities until CNS effects known.

**ketorolac
tromethamine**
Acular
*Nonsteroidal anti-inflamma-
tory*
Ophthalmic anti-inflammatory
Preg. Risk Category: C

**ketorolac
tromethamine**
Toradol
*Nonsteroidal anti-inflamma-
tory*
Analgesic
Preg. Risk Category: C

*Relief of ocular itching caused by seasonal
allergic conjunctivitis* — **Adults:** 1 drop instilled into conjunctival sac of each eye qid.

Short-term management of pain — **Adults
< 65 yr:** 60 mg IM or 30 mg IV as single
dose, or multiple doses of 30 mg IM or IV q
6 hr; max 120 mg daily. **Adults 65 yr or older, renally impaired patients, or patients <
50 kg:** 30 mg IM or 15 mg IV as single
dose, or multiple doses of 15 mg IM or IV q
6 hr; max 60 mg daily.
*Short-term management of moderately se-
vere, acute pain when switching from parenteral to oral therapy* — **Adults < 65 yr:** 20
mg PO as a single dose, then 10 mg PO q 4
to 6 hr, not to exceed 40 mg/day. Adults ≥
65 yr, renally impaired patients, or patients
< 50 kg: 10 mg PO as single dose followed
by 10 mg PO q 4 to 6 hr, not to exceed
40 mg/day.

- Apply light finger pressure on lacrimal sac
for 1 min after instillation.
- Store away from heat in dark, tightly
closed container and protect from freezing.

- Limit duration of therapy to 5 days.
- IM administration may cause pain at injection site. Apply pressure over site after injection.
- Don't mix with morphine sulfate, meperi-
dine hydrochloride, promethazine hydrochloride, or hydroxyzine hydrochloride.
- Inhibits platelet aggregation and can prolong bleeding time; carefully observe patients with coagulopathies and those taking anticoagulants. Won't alter platelet
count, PTT, or PT.
- May mask signs and symptoms of infection.

DRUG / CLASS / CATEGORY	INDICATIONS / DOSAGES	KEY NURSING CONSIDERATIONS
labetalol hydrochloride Normodyne, Presolol‡, Trandate *Alpha- and beta-adrenergic blocking agent Antihypertensive* Preg. Risk Category: C	*Hypertension* — **Adults:** 100 mg PO bid with or without diuretic. May increase by 100 mg bid daily q 2 or 4 days until optimum response reached. Usual maint. 200 to 400 mg bid; max 2,400 mg daily. *Hypertensive emergencies* — **Adults:** infuse 2 mg/min and titrate; usual cumulative dose 50 to 200 mg. Or, by repeated IV injection: initially, 20 mg IV slowly over 2 min. Then repeat injections of 40 to 80 mg q 10 min to max 300 mg.	▪ When given IV for hypertensive emergencies, produces rapid, predictable BP drop within 5 to 10 min. ▪ *IV use:* Give injection with infusion control device. Monitor BP q 5 min for 30 min, q 30 min for 2 hr, then hourly for 6 hr. Keep patient supine for 3 hr. ▪ Masks common signs of shock. ▪ IV form incompatible with sodium bicarbonate injection. ▪ May mask signs of hypoglycemia.
lactulose Chronulac, Constulose, Enulose, Lactulax†, Lactulose, Portalac *Disaccharide Laxative* Preg. Risk Category: B	*Constipation* — **Adults:** 10 to 20 g (15 to 30 ml) PO daily, increased to 60 ml/day, if needed. *Hepatic encephalopathy* — **Adults:** 20 to 30 g PO tid or qid, until q 2 or 3 soft stools qd. Or, 300 ml diluted with 700 ml water or saline solution PR and retained for 40 to 60 min q 4 to 6 hr, prn.	▪ To minimize sweet taste, dilute with water or fruit juice or give with food. ▪ Monitor serum sodium for possible hypernatremia, especially when giving to treat hepatic encephalopathy. ▪ Be prepared to replace fluid loss.
lamivudine Epivir *Synthetic nucleoside analogue Antiviral* Preg. Risk Category: C	*Treatment of HIV infection concomitantly with zidovudine* — **Adults ≥ 50 kg and children ≥ 12 yr:** 150 mg PO bid. **Adults < 50 kg:** 2 mg/kg PO bid. **Children 3 mo to 12 yr:** 4 mg/kg PO bid. Max 150 mg bid.	▪ Monitor CBC, platelet count, and liver function studies, as ordered. ▪ Stop treatment immediately and notify doctor if clinical signs, symptoms, or lab results suggest pancreatitis.

lamotrigine
Lamictal
Phenyltriazine
Anticonvulsant
Preg. Risk Category: C

Adjunct therapy in treatment of partial seizures caused by epilepsy — **Adults:** 50 mg PO qd for 2 wk, then 100 mg qd in 2 divided doses for 2 wk. Usual maintenance dosage 300 to 500 mg PO qd in 2 divided doses. For patients also taking valproic acid, 25 mg PO qod for 2 wk, then 25 mg PO qd for 2 wk. Max 150 mg PO qd in 2 divided doses.

- Don't discontinue abruptly. Instead, taper over at least 2 weeks. Check adjunct anticonvulsant serum levels, as ordered.
- Use reduced maintenance dosage in severe renal impairment.
- Warn not to engage in hazardous activities until CNS effects known.

lansoprazole
Prevacid
Acid (proton) pump inhibitor
Antiulcer agent
Preg. Risk Category: B

Short-term treatment of active duodenal ulcer — **Adults:** 15 mg PO qd before meals for 4 wk.
Short-term treatment of erosive esophagitis — **Adults:** 30 mg PO qd before meals for up to 8 wk. If healing doesn't occur, may give for 8 more wk.
Long-term treatment of pathologic hypersecretory conditions, including Zollinger-Ellison syndrome — **Adults:** initially, 60 mg PO qd. Increase dosage prn. Give daily dosages of >120 mg in divided doses.

- Instruct to take before eating.
- May open capsules and sprinkle contents over applesauce.
- Breast-feeding may need to be discontinued during therapy.
- Don't use as maintenance therapy for treatment of duodenal ulcer or erosive esophagitis.
- Monitor closely if patient also receiving ampicillin esters, digoxin, iron salts, or ketoconazole. May inhibit lansoprazole absorption.

latanoprost
Xalatan
Prostaglandin analogue
Antiglaucoma/ocular antihypertensive agent
Preg. Risk Category: C

Treatment of increased IOP in patients with ocular hypertension or open-angle glaucoma who can't tolerate or who respond insufficiently to other IOP-lowering medications — **Adults:** 1 drop in conjunctival sac of affected eye qd in evening.

- Don't administer while patient wears contact lenses.
- More frequent administration than recommended may decrease IOP-lowering effects.
- May gradually change eye color, increasing amount of brown pigment in iris.

LATANOPROST 173

†Canadian ‡Australian

DRUG / CLASS / CATEGORY	INDICATIONS / DOSAGES	KEY NURSING CONSIDERATIONS
leucovorin calcium (citrovorum factor, folinic acid) Wellcovorin *Formyl derivative (active reduced form of folic acid)* Vitamin/antidote Preg. Risk Category: C	*Overdose of folic acid antagonist* — **Adults and children:** IM or IV dose equiv to weight of antagonist given. *Leucovorin rescue after high methotrexate dose* — **Adults and children:** 10 mg/m² PO, IM, or IV q 6 hr until methotrexate levels < 5 ×10⁻⁸ M. *Megaloblastic anemia caused by congenital enzyme deficiency* — **Adults and children:** 3 to 6 mg IM daily. *Folate-deficient megaloblastic anemia* — **Adults and children:** up to 1 mg IM daily.	▪ *IV use:* When using powder for injection, reconstitute 50-mg vial with 5 ml, 100-mg vial with 10 ml, or 350-mg vial with 17 ml sterile or bacteriostatic water for injection. With doses > 10 mg/m², don't use diluents containing benzyl alcohol. ▪ Don't exceed 160 mg/min when giving by direct injection. ▪ Don't confuse folinic acid with folic acid. ▪ Don't administer simultaneously with systemic methotrexate.
levobunolol hydrochloride Betagan *Beta-adrenergic blocker* Antiglaucoma agent Preg. Risk Category: C	*Chronic open-angle glaucoma and ocular hypertension* — **Adults:** 1 to 2 drop qd (0.5%) or bid (0.25%).	▪ Apply light pressure on lacrimal sac for 1 min after instilling. ▪ Avoid letting dropper touch eye or surrounding tissue.
levocabastine hydrochloride Livostin *Cyclohexyl/piperidine derivative* Antihistamine/antiallergic Preg. Risk Category: C	*Temporary relief of seasonal allergic conjunctivitis* — **Adults and children ≥ 12 yr:** 1 drop qid for up to 2 wk.	▪ For ophthalmic use only. Never inject.

levodopa

Dopar, Larodopa

Dopamine precursor

Antiparkinsonism agent

Preg. Risk Category: C

Parkinsonism — **Adults:** initially, 0.5 to 1 g PO daily, bid, tid, or qid with food; increase by no more than 0.75 g daily q 3 to 7 days as tolerated; usual optimal dose 3 to 6 g daily divided into 3 doses. Don't exceed 8 g/day except for exceptional patients. Significant therapeutic response may not occur for 6 mo.

- Report muscle twitching.
- With long-term therapy, test regularly for diabetes and acromegaly; periodically monitor renal, liver, and hematopoietic function.
- Multivitamins, fortified cereals, and OTC medications may block drug effects.

levofloxacin

Levaquin

Fluoroquinolone antibiotic

Antibiotic

Preg. Risk Category: C

Acute maxillary sinusitis caused by susceptible organisms — **Adults:** 500 mg PO or IV qd for 10 to 14 days.

Acute exacerbation of chronic bronchitis caused by susceptible organisms — **Adults:** 500 mg PO or IV qd for 7 days.

Community-acquired pneumonia caused by susceptible organisms — **Adults:** 500 mg PO or IV qd for 7 to 14 days.

Mild to moderate skin and skin structure infections caused by susceptible organisms — **Adults:** 500 mg PO or IV qd for 7 to 10 days.

UTIs caused by susceptible organisms — **Adults:** 250 mg PO or IV qd for 10 days.

Acute pyelonephritis caused by E. coli — **Adults:** 250 mg PO or IV qd for 10 days.

- Discontinue and notify doctor if symptoms of excessive CNS stimulation occur. Institute seizure precautions. Use cautiously in renal impairment.
- Notify doctor if diarrhea occurs.
- Obtain specimen for C+S before therapy and to detect bacterial resistance.
- Monitor blood glucose and renal, hepatic, and hematopoietic blood studies.
- *IV use:* Give injection only by IV infusion. Dilute drug in single-use vials according to manufacturer's instructions. Reconstituted solution should be clear and slightly yellow. Reconstituted drug stable for 72 hr at room temp, for 14 days when refrigerated in plastic containers, and for 6 mo when frozen. Thaw at room temp or in refrigerator for IV use only. Don't mix with other medications. Infuse over 60 min.

DRUG/CLASS/ CATEGORY	INDICATIONS/ DOSAGES	KEY NURSING CONSIDERATIONS
levonorgestrel Norplant System *Progestin* *Contraceptive* Preg. Risk Category: X	*Prevention of pregnancy* — **Women:** 6 caps implanted subdermally in midportion of upper arm, about 8 cm above elbow crease, during first 7 days of onset of menses. Caps placed in fanlike position, 15° apart (total of 75°). Contraceptive efficacy lasts for 5 yr.	• Irregular bleeding may mask symptoms of cervical or endometrial cancer. • Expect implant to be removed if patient develops active thrombophlebitis, thromboembolic disease, will be immobilized for significant time, or if jaundice develops.
levothyroxine sodium (T₄ or L-thyroxine sodium) Eltroxin, Levo-T, Levothroid, Levoxine, Levoxyl, Synthroid *Thyroid hormone* *Thyroid hormone replacement therapy* Preg. Risk Category: A	*Myxedema coma* — **Adults:** 200 to 500 mcg IV; if no response in 24 hrs, give 100 to 300 mcg IV. Maintenance dose 50 to 200 mcg IV qd. *Thyroid hormone replacement* — **Adults:** initially, 50 mcg PO qd, increased by 25 to 50 mcg PO daily q 2 to 4 wk. May give IV or IM. **Adults > 65 yr:** 12.5 to 50 mcg PO qd. Increase by 12.5 to 25 mcg at 2- to 8-wk prn. **Children > 12 yr:** over 150 mcg or 2 to 3 mcg/kg/day. **Children 6 to 12 yr:** 100 to 150 mcg/kg/day or 4 to 5 mcg/kg/day. **Children 1 to 5 yr:** 75 to 100 mcg or 5 to 6 mcg/kg/day. **Children 6 to 12 mo:** 50 to 75 mcg or 6 to 8 mcg/kg/day. **Children < 6 mo:** 25 to 50 mcg or 8 to 10 mcg/kg/day.	• Rapid replacement in arteriosclerotic patients may trigger angina, coronary occlusion, or CVA; use cautiously. • **IV use:** Prepare IV dose immediately before injection. Don't mix with other solutions. Inject into vein over 1 to 2 min. • Monitor BP and HR closely. Normal serum T₄ levels should occur within 24 hr, followed by threefold increase in serum T₃ in 3 days. • When switching *to* liothyronine (T₃), stop levothyroxine and begin liothyronine. Increase dosage of levothyroxine after residual effects of levothyroxine disappear. When switching *from* liothyronine, start levothyroxine several days before withdrawing liothyronine. • Must be discontinued 4 wk before radioactive iodine uptake studies.

lidocaine hydrochloride (lignocaine hydrochloride)

LidoPen Auto-Injector, Xylocaine

Amide derivative
Ventricular antiarrhythmic/local anesthetic

Preg. Risk Category: B

Ventricular arrhythmias resulting from MI, cardiac manipulation, or cardiac glycosides — **Adults:** 50 to 100 mg (1 to 1.5 mg/kg) by IV bolus at 25 to 50 mg/min. Give half this amount to elderly patients or patients < 50 kg and to those with heart failure or hepatic disease. Repeat bolus dose q 3 to 5 min until arrhythmias subside or adverse reactions develop. Don't exceed 300-mg total bolus over 1-hr period. Simultaneously, begin constant infusion of 20 to 50 mcg/kg/min (1 to 4 mg/min). **Children:** 0.5 to 1 mg/kg by IV bolus, followed by infusion of 10 to 50 mcg/kg/min.

- **IV use:** Patient must be on cardiac monitor. Use infusion control device. Don't exceed rate of 4 mg/min. Seizures may be first clinical sign of toxicity. Therapeutic levels 2 to 5 mcg/ml.
- If signs of toxicity occur, stop drug at once and notify doctor. Keep O_2 and CPR equipment available.
- Discontinue infusion and notify doctor if arrhythmias worsen or ECG changes appear.
- Give IM injections in deltoid muscle only.
- Monitor patient response, especially BP, electrolytes, BUN, and creatinine levels.

lindane

gBHt, G-Well, Kwell, Kwelladat, Scabene

Chlorinated hydrocarbon insecticide
Scabicide/pediculicide

Preg. Risk Category: B

Parasitic infestation (scabies, pediculosis) — **Adults and children:** CDC recommends avoiding bathing before skin application. If patient bathes, let skin dry and cool thoroughly before using. Apply thin layer of cream or lotion over entire skin surface (with special attention to folds, creases, interdigital spaces, and genital area) for scabies, or to hairy areas for pediculosis. After 8 to 12 hr, wash off drug. Repeat in 1 wk if mites appear or new lesions develop. Apply shampoo undiluted to affected area and work into lather for 4 to 5 min.

- Apply topical corticosteroids or administer oral antihistamines for pruritus.
- Place hospitalized patient in isolation, with special linen-handling precautions.
- Modest amounts (6% to 13%) absorbed through intact skin.
- Wash off skin and notify doctor immediately if skin irritation or hypersensitivity develops.
- In case of accidental contact with eyes, flush with water and notify doctor.

DRUG / CLASS / CATEGORY	INDICATIONS / DOSAGES	KEY NURSING CONSIDERATIONS
liothyronine sodium (T₃) Cyronine, Cytomel, Tertroxin‡, Triostat *Thyroid hormone* *Thyroid hormone replacement agent* Preg. Risk Category: A	*Cretinism* — **Children:** 5 mcg PO daily with 5-mcg increase q 3 to 4 days prn. *Myxedema* — **Adults:** initially, 5 mcg PO daily, increased by 5 to 10 mcg q 1 or 2 wk. Maintenance dosage 50 to 100 mcg daily. *Myxedema coma, premyxedema coma* — **Adults:** initially, 10-20 mcg IV for known or suspected CV disease; 25 to 50 mcg IV for patients without known CV disease. *Nontoxic goiter* — **Adults:** initially, 5 mcg PO daily; increase by 12.5 to 25 mcg daily q 1 to 2 wk. Maintenance dose 75 mcg qd. *Thyroid hormone replacement* — **Adults:** initially, 25 mcg PO daily, increased by 12.5 to 25 mcg q 1 to 2 wk prn. Maintenance dose 25 to 75 mcg qd. **Geriatric patients:** 5 mcg daily, increased in 5-mcg daily increments.	• Rapid replacement in patients with arteriosclerosis may trigger angina, coronary occlusion, or CVA; use cautiously. In CAD patients, observe carefully for possible coronary insufficiency. • Alters thyroid function tests. Monitor PT; decreased anticoagulant dosage usually required. • When switching *from* levothyroxine, stop that drug and start liothyronine at low dosage. Increase dosage in small increments after residual effects of levothyroxine disappear. When switching *to* levothyroxine, start levothyroxine several days before withdrawing liothyronine. • Must be discontinued 7 to 10 days before radioactive iodine uptake studies.
lisinopril Prinivil, Zestril *ACE inhibitor* *Antihypertensive* Preg. Risk Category: C (1st trimester), D (2nd and 3rd trimesters)	*Hypertension* — **Adults:** initially, 10 mg PO daily. Most patients well controlled on 20 to 40 mg daily as single dose. *Treatment adjunct in heart failure (with diuretics and cardiac glycosides)* — **Adults:** initially, 5 mg PO daily. Most patients well controlled on 5 to 20 mg daily as single dose. *Acute MI* — **Adults:** initially 5 mg PO, followed by 5 mg in 24 hr, 10 mg in 48 hr, and	• Monitor BP often. If drug doesn't adequately control BP, diuretics may be added. • Monitor WBC with differential before therapy, every 2 wk for first 3 months of therapy, and periodically thereafter. • When used in acute MI, patient should receive standard recommended treatment as appropriate (such as thrombolytics, aspirin, and beta blockers).

then 10 mg daily for 6 wk. In patients with low systolic BP ≤ (120) when treatment starts or during first 3 days after MI, reduce to 2.5 mg PO. If systolic BP ≤ 100, may reduce daily maintenance dose of 5 mg to 2.5 mg.

- Angioedema (including laryngeal edema) may occur, especially after first dose. Advise to report swelling of face, eyes, lips, or tongue or breathing difficulty.
- Light-headedness may occur, especially during first few days. Tell to rise slowly and report symptoms. Advise to stop drug and call doctor immediately if fainting occurs.

lithium carbonate
Carbolith‡, Eskalith CR, Lithane, Lithizine‡, Lithobid, Lithonate, Lithotabs

lithium citrate
Cibalith-S

Alkali metal
Antimanic/antipsychotic
Preg. Risk Category: D

Prevention or control of mania — **Adults:** 300 to 600 mg PO up to qid or 900 mg PO q 12 hr of CR tab; increase on basis of blood levels to achieve optimal dosage.

- Blood drug level measurements crucial to safe use. Monitor weekly to monthly during maintenance therapy.
- Monitor baseline ECG, thyroid, and renal studies, and electrolyte levels, as ordered.
- May alter glucose tolerance in diabetics.
- Check fluid I&O. Weigh daily; check for edema or sudden weight gain. Normally, daily fluid intake should be 2,500 to 3,000 ml and patient should eat balanced diet with adequate salt intake.
- Warn to watch for toxicity signs and to expect transient nausea, polyuria, thirst, and discomfort in first few days. Tell to withhold one dose and call doctor if toxicity signs appear, but not stop drug abruptly.
- Warn ambulatory patient to avoid hazardous activities until CNS effects known.

DRUG/CLASS/ CATEGORY	INDICATIONS/ DOSAGES	KEY NURSING CONSIDERATIONS
lodoxamide tromethamine Alomide *Cromolyn-like mast cell stabilizer* *Antiallergic ophthalmic* Preg. Risk Category: B	*Vernal conjunctivitis, vernal keratoconjunctivitis; vernal keratitis* — **Adults and children ≥2 yr:** 1 to 2 drop in affected eye qid for up to 3 mo.	• For ophth use only; never inject. • Check expiration date before using.
lomefloxacin hydrochloride Maxaquin *Fluoroquinolone* *Broad-spectrum antibiotic* Preg. Risk Category: C	*Acute bacterial exacerbations of chronic bronchitis caused by susceptible organisms* — **Adults:** 400 mg PO daily for 10 days. *Uncomplicated UTI (cystitis) caused by susceptible organisms* — **Adults:** 400 mg PO daily for 10 days. *Complicated UTI caused by susceptible organisms* — **Adults:** 400 mg PO daily for 14 days. *Prophylaxis of UTI after transrectal prostate biopsy* — **Adults:** 400 mg PO as single dose 1 to 6 hr before procedure.	• Obtain culture and sensitivity tests before first dose. Begin therapy pending results. • Photosensitization and phototoxicity may be common. • Prolonged use may result in overgrowth of resistant organisms. • Warn to avoid hazardous tasks until CNS effects known. • Drug interactions may occur when using with antacids, sucralfate, cimetidine, probenecid, warfarin, or cyclosporine. Give no less than 4 hr before or 2 hr after lomefloxacin dose.
lomustine (CCNU) CeeNU *Alkylating agent/nitrosourea* *(cell cycle–phase nonspecific)*	*Brain tumor, Hodgkin's disease* — **Adults and children:** 100 to 130 mg/m² PO as single dose q 6 wk. Reduce dosage according to degree of bone marrow suppression.	• Give 2 to 4 hr after meals for more complete absorption. • Monitor CBC weekly. Usually not given more often than q 6 wk; bone marrow tox-

Antineoplastic
Preg. Risk Category: D

Don't repeat doses until WBC count > 4,000/mm³ and platelet count > 100,000/mm³.

- icity cumulative and delayed, usually occurring 4 to 6 wk after administration.
- Periodically monitor liver function tests.
- Therapeutic effects often accompanied by toxicity.

---

loperamide
Imodium, Kaopectate II Caplets
Piperadine derivative
Antidiarrheal
Preg. Risk Category: B

Acute, nonspecific diarrhea — **Adults and children > age 12:** initially, 4 mg PO, then 2 mg after each unformed stool. Max 16 mg daily **Children 9 to 11 yr:** 2 mg tid on first day. **Children 6 to 8 yr:** 2 mg bid on first day. **Children 2 to 5 yr:** 1 mg tid on first day. Maintenance dose 1/3 to 1/2 of initial dose.

- In acute diarrhea, tell to discontinue and seek medical attention if no improvement within 48 hr; in chronic diarrhea, tell to notify doctor and discontinue if no improvement after taking 16 mg daily for at least 10 days.
- Advise patient with acute colitis to stop drug immediately.

---

loracarbef
Lorabid
Synthetic beta-lactam antibiotic of carbacephem class
Antibiotic
Preg. Risk Category: B

Secondary bacterial infections of acute bronchitis — **Adults:** 200 to 400 mg PO q 12 hr for 7 days.
Acute bacterial exacerbations of chronic bronchitis — **Adults:** 400 mg PO q 12 hr for 7 days.
Pneumonia — **Adults:** 400 mg PO q 12 hr for 14 days.
Pharyngitis, sinusitis, or tonsillitis — **Adults:** 200 mg PO q 12 hr for 10 days. **Children:** 15 mg/kg PO daily in divided doses q 12 hr for 10 days.
Acute otitis media — **Children:** 30 mg/kg (oral susp) PO daily in divided doses q 12 hr for 10 days.

- Obtain specimen for culture and sensitivity tests before first dose.
- Monitor for superinfection.
- To reconstitute powder for oral suspension, add 30 ml water in 2 portions to 50-ml bottle or 60 ml water in 2 portions to 100-ml bottle; shake after each addition. After reconstitution, store oral suspension for 14 days at room temp (59° to 86° F [15° to 30° C]).
- Monitor for seizures. If seizures occur, discontinue and notify doctor. Give anticonvulsants as ordered.

LORACARBEF   181

---

†Canadian ‡Australian

DRUG / CLASS / CATEGORY	INDICATIONS / DOSAGES	KEY NURSING CONSIDERATIONS
loratadine Claratyne†, Claritin *Tricyclic antihistamine* Antihistaminic agent Preg. Risk Category: B	*Symptomatic treatment of seasonal allergic rhinitis* — **Adults and children 12 ≥ yr:** 10 mg PO daily.	▪ May affect allergy skin tests results. ▪ Advise to stop drug 7 days before allergy skin tests to preserve test accuracy.
lorazepam Alzapam, Apo-Lorazepam†, Ativan, Lorazepam Intensol, Novo-Lorazem†, Nu-Loraz† *Benzodiazepine* Antianxiety agent/sedative-hypnotic Preg. Risk Category: D Controlled Sub. Sched.: IV	*Anxiety, agitation, irritability* — **Adults:** 2 to 6 mg PO daily in divided doses. Max 10 mg daily. Or, 0.05 mg/kg up to 4 mg IM daily in divided doses or 0.044 to 0.05 mg/kg up to 4 mg IV daily in divided doses. *Insomnia due to anxiety* — **Adults:** 2 to 4 mg PO hs. *Preop sedation* — **Adults:** 0.05 mg/kg IM 2 hr before procedure. Max 4 mg. Or, 0.044 mg/kg (max total dose 2 mg) IV, 15 to 20 min before surgery. In adults < 50 yr, may give 0.05 mg/kg (max 4 mg) if increased lack of recall of preop events desired.	▪ Monitor respirations q 5 to 15 minutes and before each repeated IV dose. Have emergency resuscitation equipment and O₂ available. ▪ *IV use:* Give slowly, at rate not > 2 mg/min. Dilute with equal volume of sterile water for injection, 0.9% NaCl for injection, or dextrose 5% injection. ▪ Reduce dosage in elderly or debilitated patients. ▪ Inject IM doses deeply into muscle mass. ▪ With repeated or prolonged therapy, monitor liver, renal, and hematopoietic function studies periodically, as ordered. ▪ Possibility of abuse and addiction exists. Don't withdraw abruptly after long-term use; withdrawal symptoms may occur.

losartan potassium

Cozaar

Angiotensin II receptor antagonist

Antihypertensive

Preg. Risk Category: C (1st trimester), D (2nd and 3rd trimesters)

Hypertension — **Adults:** initially, 25 to 50 mg PO daily, given qd or bid.

- If pregnancy suspected, notify doctor.
- Monitor BP closely to evaluate effectiveness.
- Closely monitor patient with severe heart failure; acute renal failure possible.
- Tell to avoid sodium substitutes.
- Regularly assess renal function, as ordered.

lovastatin (mevinolin)

Mevacor

Lactone‡

Cholesterol-lowering agent

Preg. Risk Category: X

Reduction of LDL and total cholesterol levels in primary hypercholesterolemia (types IIa and IIb) — **Adults:** initially, 20 mg PO qd with evening meal. For patients with severely elevated cholesterol (for example, > 300 mg/dl), initial dose 40 mg. Recommended daily dosage range 20 to 80 mg in single or divided doses.

- Initiate only after diet and other nonpharmacologic therapies prove ineffective. Patient should be on low-cholesterol diet.
- Liver function tests should be done at start of therapy and periodically thereafter.
- Inform female that drug contraindicated during pregnancy.
- Advise to have periodic eye exams.

loxapine hydrochloride

Loxapac‡, Loxitane C, Loxitane IM

loxapine succinate

Loxapac‡, Loxitane

Dibenzoxazepine

Antipsychotic

Preg. Risk Category: NR

Psychotic disorders — **Adults:** 10 mg PO bid to qid, rapidly increasing to 60 to 100 mg PO daily for most patients; dosage varies among individuals. If patient can't take oral dose, 12.5 to 50 mg IM q 4 to 6 hr or longer, both dose and interval depending on patient response. Dosages > 250 mg/day not recommended.

- Monitor for tardive dyskinesia. Acute dystonic reactions may be treated with diphenhydramine.
- Monitor for neuroleptic malignant syndrome.
- Warn to avoid hazardous activities until CNS effects known.
- Obtain baseline BP before therapy and monitor regularly.
- Dilute liquid concentrate with orange or grapefruit juice just before giving.

LOXAPINE SUCCINATE 183

DRUG/CLASS/ CATEGORY	INDICATIONS/ DOSAGES	KEY NURSING CONSIDERATIONS
magaldrate (aluminum-magnesium complex) Antiflux, Iosopan, Lowsium, Riopan *Aluminum magnesium salt* *Antacid* Preg. Risk Category: C	*Antacid* — **Adults:** 480 to 960 mg PO (or 5 to 10 ml of susp) with water between meals and hs; or 1 to 2 chew tab (chewed before swallowing) between meals and hs.	• Monitor serum magnesium in mild kidney impairment. Symptomatic hypermagnesemia usually occurs only in severe renal failure. • Not typically used in renal failure to help control hypophosphatemia. • Very low sodium content; good choice for patients on restricted sodium intake.
magnesium citrate (citrate of magnesia) Citroma, Citro-Mag†, Citro-Nesia, Evac-Q-Mag **magnesium hydroxide (milk of magnesia)** Milk of Magnesia, Phillips' Milk of Magnesia **magnesium sulfate (epsom salts)** *Magnesium salts* *Antacid/antiulcer agent/laxative* Preg. Risk Category: NR	*Constipation; to evacuate bowel before surgery* — **Adults and children ≥ 12 yr:** 11 to 25 g magnesium citrate PO daily; 2.4 to 4.8 g (30 to 60 ml) magnesium hydroxide PO daily; 10 to 30 g magnesium sulfate PO daily. **Children 6 to 12 yr:** 5.5 to 12.5 g magnesium citrate PO daily; 1.2 to 2.4 g (15 to 30 ml) magnesium hydroxide PO daily; 5 to 10 g magnesium sulfate PO daily. **Children 2 to 6 yr:** 2.7 to 6.25 g magnesium citrate PO daily; 0.4 to 1.2 g (5 to 15 ml) magnesium hydroxide PO daily; 2.5 to 5 g magnesium sulfate PO daily. **Note:** All doses may be single or divided. *Antacid* — **Adults:** 5 to 15 ml milk of magnesia PO tid or qid.	• Produces watery stools in 3 to 6 hr. Time doses so drug won't interfere with scheduled activities or sleep. • Before giving for constipation, determine if patient has adequate fluid intake, exercise, and diet. • Chill magnesium citrate before use to make more palatable. • Shake suspension well; give with large amount of water when used as laxative. • May accumulate in renal insufficiency. Monitor serum electrolytes as ordered during prolonged use.

magnesium oxide
Mag-Ox 400, Maox-420,
Uro-Mag
Magnesium salt
Antacid/laxative
Preg. Risk Category: NR

Antacid — **Adults:** 140 mg PO with water or milk after meals and hs.
Laxative — **Adults:** 4 g PO with water or milk, usually hs.
Oral replacement therapy in mild hypomagnesemia — **Adults:** 400 to 840 mg PO daily.

- Monitor serum magnesium. With prolonged use and renal impairment, watch for symptoms of hypermagnesemia (hypotension, nausea, vomiting, depressed reflexes, respiratory depression, and coma).
- If diarrhea occurs, use another drug.

magnesium salicylate
Doan's, Mobidin, Bayer Select Maximum Strength Backache Pain Relief Formula
Salicylate
Nonnarcotic analgesic/antipyretic/anti-inflammatory
Preg. Risk Category: NR

Arthritis — **Adults:** 545 mg to 1.2 g PO tid or qid.
Mild pain or fever — **Adults and children >11 yr:** 300 to 600 mg PO q 4 hr, not to exceed 3.5 g/day.

- Don't give to children or teenagers with chickenpox or flulike illness.
- Febrile, dehydrated children can develop toxicity rapidly.
- Therapeutic level in arthritis 10 to 30 mg/100 ml. With chronic therapy, mild toxicity may occur at 20 mg/100 ml.
- Monitor Hgb and PT in long-term, high-dose treatment.

magnesium sulfate
Mineral/electrolyte
Anticonvulsant
Preg. Risk Category: A

Prevention or control of seizures in preeclampsia or eclampsia — **Adults:** 4 g IV in 250 ml D_5W and 4 to 5 g deep IM alternate buttock; then 4 g deep IM alternate buttock q 4 hr, prn. Or, 4 g IV loading dose, then 1 to 2 g hourly as IV infusion. Max 40 g daily.
Hypomagnesemia; seizures — **Adults:** 1 to 2 g (as 10% sol) IV over 15 min, then 1 g IM q 4 to 6 hr per response and drug levels.
Seizures, hypomagnesemia associated with acute nephritis in children — **Children:** 0.2 ml/kg of 50% sol IM q 4 to 6 hr, prn, or

- **IV use:** If necessary, dilute to max concentration of 20%. Infuse no faster than 150 mg/min (1.5 ml/min of 10% solution or 0.75 ml/min of 20% solution). Compatible with D_5W.
- Monitor vital signs q 15 min when giving IV. Watch for respiratory depression and signs of heart block.
- Keep IV calcium gluconate at hand to reverse magnesium intoxication; however,

(continued)

DRUG / CLASS / CATEGORY	INDICATIONS / DOSAGES	KEY NURSING CONSIDERATIONS
magnesium sulfate *(continued)*	100 to 200 mg/kg of 1% to 3% solution IV slowly. Titrate dosage according to blood magnesium levels and seizure response. *Management of paroxysmal atrial tachycardia* — **Adults:** 3 to 4 g IV over 30 seconds. *Management of life-threatening ventricular arrhythmias, such as sustained ventricular tachycardia or torsades de pointes* — **Adults:** 2 to 6 g IV over several min, then IV infusion of 3 to 20 mg/min for 5 to 48 hr. Dosage and duration of therapy based on response and serum magnesium levels.	use cautiously in patients undergoing digitalization. ■ Check blood magnesium levels after repeated doses. Disappearance of knee-jerk and patellar reflexes signals impending toxicity. ■ Observe neonates for signs of magnesium toxicity, including neuromuscular or respiratory depression, when giving IV form to toxemic mothers within 24 hours before delivery.
magnesium chloride Slow-Mag **magnesium sulfate** *Mineral/electrolyte* *Anticonvulsant* Preg. Risk Category: NR	*Mild hypomagnesemia* — **Adults:** 1 g IV by piggyback or IM q 6 hr for 4 doses, depending on serum magnesium level. Or, 3 g PO q 6 hr for 4 doses. *Severe hypomagnesemia (serum magnesium 0.8 mEq/L or less, with symptoms)* — **Adults:** 2 to 5 g IV in 1 L sol over 3 hr. Subsequent doses depend on serum magnesium levels. *Magnesium supplementation* — **Adults:** 64 mg (1 tab) PO tid.	■ **IV use:** Inject IV bolus dose slowly, using infusion pump for continuous infusion. Max infusion rate 150 mg/min. ■ When giving IV for severe hypomagnesemia, watch for respiratory depression and signs of heart block. Respirations should be > 16 before dose given. ■ Monitor I&O. ■ Test knee-jerk and patellar reflexes before each additional dose. If absent, notify doctor and withhold drug until reflexes return. ■ Incompatible with alkalis.

mannitol

Osmitrol

Osmotic diuretic

Diuretic/prevention and management of acute renal failure or oliguria/reduction of ICP or IOP/treatment of drug intoxication

Preg. Risk Category: B

Test dose for marked oliguria or suspected inadequate renal function — **Adults and children > 12 yr:** 200 mg/kg or 12.5 g as 25% IV sol over 3 to 5 min. Response adequate if 30 to 50 ml urine/hr excreted over 2 to 3 hr; if response inadequate, give 2nd test dose. If still no response, discontinue. *Oliguria* — **Adults and children > 12 yr:** 50 to 100 g IV as 5% to 25% sol over 1 ½ hr to several hr.

- To redissolve crystallized solution, warm bottle in hot water bath and shake vigorously. Cool to body temp before giving.
- *IV use:* Give as intermittent or continuous infusion, using in-line filter. Direct injection not recommended.
- Monitor vital signs, including CVP, and I&O hourly. Check weight, renal function, and serum sodium and urine sodium and potassium qd.

measles, mumps, and rubella virus vaccine, live

M-M-R II

Vaccine

Viral vaccine

Preg. Risk Category: C

Routine immunization — **Adults:** 1 vial SC. Persons born after 1957 should receive 2 doses ≥ 1 mo apart. **Children:** 1 vial SC. 2-dose schedule recommended, with 1st dose given at 15 mo (12 mo in high-risk areas) and 2nd given either at 4 to 6 yr or at 11 or 12 yr.

- Obtain history of allergies, anaphylactic reactions to antibiotics, or immunization.
- Keep epinephrine 1:1,000 available to treat anaphylaxis.
- Use only diluent supplied. Discard 8 hr after reconstituting. Refrigerate.
- Protect from light. Solution may be red, pink, or yellow, but must be clear.
- Review immunization sched. with parents.

measles and rubella virus vaccine, live attenuated

M-R-Vax II

Vaccine

Viral vaccine

Preg. Risk Category: C

Immunization — **Adults and children ≥ 15 mo:** 0.5 ml (1,000 units) SC. Inject into outer upper arm. Don't inject IV.

- Obtain history of allergies, especially anaphylactic reactions to antibiotics.
- Keep epinephrine 1:1,000 available to treat anaphylaxis.
- Use only diluent supplied. Discard 8 hr after reconstituting.
- Refrigerate and protect from light. Solution may be red, pink, or yellow, but must be clear.

†Canadian ‡Australian

DRUG/CLASS/CATEGORY	INDICATIONS/DOSAGES	KEY NURSING CONSIDERATIONS
measles virus vaccine, live attenuated Attenuvax *Vaccine* *Viral vaccine* Preg. Risk Category: C	*Immunization* — **Adults and children ≥ 15 mo:** 0.5 ml (1,000 units) SC. Two-dose schedule recommended, with 1st dose given at age 15 mo and 2nd at age 4 to 6 yr or age 11 to 12 yr. *Measles outbreak control* — **Adults:** School personnel or those in a medical facility born in or after 1957 who lack proof of measles immunity should be revaccinated. **Children:** if cases occur in children < 1 yr, children should be vaccinated as young as 6 mo. All students and siblings without documentation of measles immunity should be revaccinated.	• Obtain history of allergies, especially anaphylactic reactions to antibiotics, or reaction to immunization. Defer immunization in patients with acute illness or after blood or plasma administration. • Keep epinephrine 1:1,000 available to treat anaphylaxis. • Use only diluent supplied. Discard 8 hr after reconstituting. • Don't give IV. • Refrigerate and protect from light. Reconstituted solution is clear yellow with no precipitation. Don't use if discolored.
mebendazole Vermox *Benzimidazole* *Anthelmintic* Preg. Risk Category: C	*Pinworm* — **Adults and children > 2 yr:** 100 mg PO as single dose; repeated if infection persists 2 to 3 wk later. *Roundworm, whipworm, hookworm* — **Adults and children > 2 yr:** 100 mg PO bid for 3 days; repeated if infection persists 3 wk later.	• Tablets may be chewed, swallowed whole, or crushed and mixed with food. • Administer to all family members, as prescribed, to decrease risk of spreading infection.
mechlorethamine hydrochloride (nitrogen mustard)	*Chronic lymphocytic leukemia, Hodgkin's disease, bronchogenic cancer* — **Adults:** 0.4 mg/kg IV as single dose or in divided doses of 0.1 to 0.2 mg/kg/day. Give through run-	• Prepare immediately before infusion. Very unstable solution. Inspect before using; use within 15 min. Discard unused solution.

ning IV infusion. Give subsequent courses when patient recovers hematologically from previous course (usually 3 to 6 wk).

- If extravasation occurs, apply cold compresses and infiltrate area with isotonic sodium thiosulfate.
- Neurotoxicity increases with dose and patient age.
- Watch for signs of infection and bleeding.

Mustargen
Alkylating agent (cell cycle-phase nonspecific)
Antineoplastic
Preg. Risk Category: D

---

meclizine hydrochloride
Antivert, Bonamine†, D-Vert, Meni-D, Vergon
Piperazine-derivative antihistamine
Antiemetic/antivertigo agent
Preg. Risk Category: B

Vertigo — **Adults:** 25 to 100 mg PO in divided doses. Dosage varies with response.
Motion sickness — **Adults:** 25 to 50 mg PO 1 hr before travel, then daily for duration of trip.

- May mask symptoms of ototoxicity, brain tumor, or intestinal obstruction.
- Advise to avoid hazardous activities that require alertness until CNS effects known.

---

medroxyprogesterone acetate
Amen, Curretab, Cycrin, Depo-Provera, Provera
Progestin
Progestin/antineoplastic
Preg. Risk Category: X

Abnormal uterine bleeding caused by hormonal imbalance — **Adults:** 5 to 10 mg PO daily for 5 to 10 days starting on 16th day of menstrual cycle. If patient also has received estrogen, 10 mg PO daily for 10 days starting on 16th day of cycle.
Secondary amenorrhea — **Adults:** 5 to 10 mg PO daily for 5 to 10 days.
Endometrial or renal cancer — **Adults:** 400 to 1,000 mg IM weekly.
Contraception in women — **Adults:** 150 mg IM q 3 mo; give first injection during first 5 days of menstrual cycle.

- Shouldn't be used as test for pregnancy; may cause birth defects and masculinization of female fetus.
- IM injection may be painful. Monitor sites for sterile abscess. Rotate injection sites.
- Tell to report unusual symptoms immediately and to stop drug and call doctor if visual disturbances or migraines occur.
- FDA regulations require that patient read package insert before first dose for information on possible side effects. Also give verbal information.

MEDROXYPROGESTERONE ACETATE 189

---

†Canadian ‡Australian

DRUG/CLASS/ CATEGORY	INDICATIONS/ DOSAGES	KEY NURSING CONSIDERATIONS
medrysone HMS Liquifilm Ophthalmic *Corticosteroid* *Ophth anti-inflammatory* Preg. Risk Category: C	*Allergic conjunctivitis, vernal conjunctivitis, episcleritis, ophth epinephrine sensitivity reaction* — **Adults and children:** 1 drop instilled into conjunctival sac q 4 hr.	• Don't touch dropper tip to eye or surrounding tissue. • Apply light finger pressure on lacrimal sac for 1 min after instillation. • Tell not to share medication, washcloths, or towels with family members and to notify doctor if anyone in household develops eye symptoms. • Do not use leftover drug for new eye inflammation.
mefloquine hydrochloride Lariam *Quinine derivative* *Antimalarial* Preg. Risk Category: C	*Acute malaria infections caused by mefloquine-sensitive strains of* P. falciparum *or* P. vivax — **Adults:** 1,250 mg PO (5 tab) as single dose. *Malaria prophylaxis* — **Adults:** 250 mg PO q wk. Initiate 1 wk before entering endemic area and continue 4 wk after returning.	• Therapy shouldn't begin sooner than 12 hr after last dose of quinine or quinidine. • Patients with P. vivax infections at high risk for relapse. Follow-up therapy with primaquine advisable. • Monitor liver function tests periodically as ordered.
megestrol acetate Megace, Megostat‡ *Progestin* *Antineoplastic* Preg. Risk Category: D	*Breast cancer* — **Adults:** 40 mg PO qid. *Endometrial cancer* — **Adults:** 40 to 320 mg PO daily in divided doses. *Treatment of unexplained significant weight loss* — **Adults:** 800 mg PO (oral susp) daily.	• Advise to discontinue breast-feeding during therapy; possible infant toxicity. • Advise women of childbearing age to use effective contraception during therapy. • Inform that therapeutic response isn't immediate.

melphalan (l-phenylalanine mustard)

Alkeran

Alkylating agent (cell cycle-phase nonspecific

Antineoplastic

Preg. Risk Category: D

Multiple myeloma — Adults: initially, 6 mg PO qd for 2 to 3 wk; then drug stopped for up to 4 wk, or until WBC and platelet counts stop decreasing and begin to rise again; then maintenance dosage of 2 mg daily. Or, 16 mg/m² by IV infusion over 15 to 20 min at 2-wk intervals for 4 doses. After recovery from toxicity, give at 4-wk intervals. May reduce dose up to 50% in renal insufficiency.

Nonresectable advanced ovarian cancer —
Adults: 0.2 mg/kg PO daily for 5 days. Repeat q 4 to 5 wk.

- **IV use:** Reconstitute immediately before administering, with 10 ml of sterile diluent supplied by manufacturer. Shake vigorously until solution clear.
- Promptly dilute and administer; reconstituted product begins to degrade within 30 min. Don't refrigerate reconstituted product.
- Give oral form on empty stomach.
- Monitor serum uric acid and CBC, as ordered.
- To prevent bleeding, avoid all IM injections when platelet count < 100,000/mm³.

---

meningococcal polysaccharide vaccine

Menomune-A/C/YW-135 Vaccine

Bacterial vaccine

Preg. Risk Category: C

Meningococcal meningitis prophylaxis —
Adults and children ≥ 2 yr: 0.5 ml SC.

- Obtain history of allergies and reaction to immunization.
- Keep epinephrine 1:1,000 available to treat anaphylaxis.
- Stress importance of avoiding pregnancy for 3 mo after vaccination. Offer contraception information.

---

menotropins

Pergonal

Gonadotropin

Ovulation stimulant/spermatogenesis stimulant

Preg. Risk Category: X

Production of follicular maturation —
Women: 75 IU each of FSH and LH IM qd for 7 to 12 days, then 5,000 to 10,000 USP human chorionic gonadotropin (HCG) IM 1 day after last dose of menotropins; repeat for 2 more menstrual cycles. May increase to 150 IU each of FSH and LH IM qd for 7 to 12 days, then 5,000 to 10,000 USP units

- Monitor closely to ensure adequate ovarian stimulation without hyperstimulation.
- Reconstitute with 1 to 2 ml sterile 0.9% NaCl for injection. Use immediately.
- Rotate injection sites.

(continued)

MENOTROPINS 191

†Canadian ‡Australian

DRUG / CLASS / CATEGORY	INDICATIONS / DOSAGES	KEY NURSING CONSIDERATIONS
menotropins *(continued)*	HCG IM 1 day after last dose of menotropins; repeat for 2 menstrual cycles. *Stimulation of spermatogenesis* — **Adults:** 75 IU IM 3 times weekly (with 2,000 USP units HCG twice weekly) for 4 mo. After 4 mo, may continue with 75 IU FSH/LH 3 times weekly or 150 IU FSH/LH 3 times weekly prn.	• Advise that multiple births possible. • Initiate treatment for stimulation of spermatogenesis after 4 to 6 mo of treatment with HCG.
meperidine hydrochloride (pethidine hydrochloride) Demerol *Opioid* *Analgesic/adjunct to anesthesia* Preg. Risk Category: C Controlled Sub. Sched.: II	*Moderate to severe pain* — **Adults:** 50 to 150 mg PO, IM, IV or SC q 3 to 4 hr. **Children:** 0.5 to 0.8 mg/lb PO, IM, IV, or SC q 3 to 4 hr or 175 mg/m² daily in 6 divided doses. Max single dose not to exceed 100 mg. *Preoperatively* — **Adults:** 50 to 100 mg IM, IV, or SC 30 to 90 min before surgery. **Children:** 0.5 to 1 mg/lb IM, IV or SC up to adult dose 30 to 90 min before surgery. Don't exceed adult dosage.	• Monitor respiratory and CV status. Don't give if respirations < 12, if respiratory rate or depth decreases, or if pupil change occurs. • *IV use:* Give slowly by direct IV injection. May also give by slow infusion. • Keep narcotic antagonist (naloxone) available when giving IV. • Watch for withdrawal symptoms if drug stopped abruptly after long-term use.
mercaptopurine (6-mercaptopurine, 6-MP) Purinethol *Antimetabolite (cell cycle–phase specific, S phase)* *Antineoplastic* Preg. Risk Category: D	*Acute myeloblastic leukemia, chronic myelocytic leukemia* — **Adults:** 80 to 100 mg/ m² PO daily as single dose up to 5 mg/kg/ day. **Children:** 70 mg/m² PO daily. *Acute lymphoblastic leukemia* — **Children:** 70 mg/m² PO daily. **Usual maintenance for adults and children:** 1.5 to 2.5 mg/kg/day.	• Watch for hepatic dysfunction, reversible on discontinuation. If hepatic tenderness occurs, stop drug and notify doctor. • Watch for signs of bleeding or infection. • To prevent bleeding, avoid all IM injections when platelet count < 100,000/mm³.

meropenem
Merrem IV
Carbapenem derivative
Antibiotic
Preg. Risk Category: B

Complicated appendicitis and peritonitis caused by susceptible organisms; bacterial meningitis (pediatric patients only) caused by susceptible organisms — **Adults:** 1 g IV q 8 hr over 15 to 30 min as IV infusion or over about 3 to 5 min as IV bolus injection (5 to 20 ml). **Children ≥ 3 mo:** 20 to 40 mg/kg q 8 hr over 15 to 30 min as IV infusion or over about 3 to 5 min as IV bolus injection (5 to 20 ml). Max 2 g IV q 8 hr. **Children >50 kg:** 1 to 2 g IV q 8 hr for meningitis.

- Obtain specimen for culture and sensitivity test before giving first dose.
- Monitor for superinfection.
- Serious and occasionally fatal hypersensitivity reactions reported. Determine if previous hypersensitivity reactions to antibiotics have occurred.
- If seizures occur, discontinue infusion and notify doctor.
- Periodic assessment of organ system functions recommended during prolonged therapy.

mesalamine
Asacol, Salofalk, Mesasal, Pentasa, Rowasa
Salicylate
Anti-inflammatory
Preg. Risk Category: B

Active mild to moderate distal ulcerative colitis, proctitis, or proctosigmoiditis — **Adults:** 800 mg PO (tab) tid for total dose of 2.4 g/day for 6 wk; 1 g PO (cap) qid for total dose of 4 g up to 8 wk; 500 mg PR (supp) bid, or 4 g as retention enema qd (preferably hs). Rectal dosage form should be retained overnight (for about 8 hr).

- Monitor periodic renal function studies with long-term therapy, as ordered.
- May cause hypersensitivity reactions in patients sensitive to sulfites.
- Instruct to discontinue if fever or rash occurs.
- Advise to carefully follow instructions supplied with medication.

mesna
Mesnex, Dromitexan
Thiol derivative
Uroprotectant
Preg. Risk Category: B

Prophylaxis of hemorrhagic cystitis in patients receiving ifosfamide — **Adults:** dosage varies with amount of ifosfamide administered; calculated as 20% (w/w) of ifosfamide dose at time of ifosfamide administration. Usual dosage 240 mg/m² as IV bolus with ifosfamide administration; repeat at 4 and 8 hr after ifosfamide given.

- **IV use:** Prepare solution by diluting commercially available ampules with D₅W solution, dextrose 5% and 0.9% NaCl for injection, 0.9% NaCl for injection, or lact Ringer's to obtain final solution of 20 mg mesna/ml.
- Monitor urine samples daily in patients receiving mesna for hematuria.

MESNA   193

DRUG / CLASS / CATEGORY	INDICATIONS / DOSAGES	KEY NURSING CONSIDERATIONS
mesoridazine besylate Serentil, Serentil Concentrate *Phenothiazine (piperidine derivative)* *Antipsychotic* Preg. Risk Category: NR	*Alcoholism* — **Adults and children > 12 yr:** 25 mg PO bid up to max 200 mg daily. *Behavioral problems associated with chronic organic mental syndrome* — **Adults and children > 12 yr:** 25 mg PO tid.to max 300 mg daily. *Psychoneurotic manifestations (anxiety)* — **Adults and children > 12 yr:** 10 mg PO tid to max 150 mg daily. *Schizophrenia* — **Adults and children > 12 yr:** initially, 50 mg PO tid or 25 mg IM, repeated in 30 to 60 min, prn. Max oral dosage 400 mg daily; max IM dosage 200 mg.	■ Monitor for tardive dyskinesia. Acute dystonic reactions may be treated with diphenhydramine. ■ Assess for neuroleptic malignant syndrome. ■ Withhold dose and notify doctor if patient develops jaundice, symptoms of blood dyscrasia, or persistent extrapyramidal reactions (> several hours). ■ Arrange for weekly bilirubin tests during first month; periodic blood tests (CBC and liver function); and ophthalmic tests. ■ Wear gloves when preparing solutions, and prevent contact with skin and clothing. ■ Obtain baseline BP before starting.
metaproterenol sulfate Alupent, Dey-Dose Metaproterenol, Dey-Lute Metaproterenol, Metaprel *Adrenergic* *Bronchodilator* Preg. Risk Category: C	*Acute episodes of bronchial asthma* — **Adults and children > 9 yr:** 2 to 3 inhalations. Don't repeat inhalation more often than q 3 to 4 hr. Max 12 inhalations/day. *Bronchial asthma and reversible bronchospasm* — **Adults and children > 9 yr or > 60 lbs (27 kg):** 20 mg PO q 6 to 8 hr. **Children 6 to 9 yr or < 27 kg:** 10 mg PO q 6 to 8 hr. Alternatively, via IPPB or nebulizer: **Adults and children ≥ 12 yr:** 0.2 to 0.3 ml of 5% solution diluted in approx 2.5 ml of 0.45%	■ May use tablets and aerosol together. ■ Inhalant solution can be given by IPPB with drug diluted in 0.45% or 0.9% NaCl solution or with hand nebulizer at full strength. ■ If patient also uses steroid inhaler, tell to use bronchodilator first, then wait about 5 min before using steroid. ■ Warn to discontinue immediately and notify doctor if paradoxical bronchospasm occurs.

- or 0.9% NaCl or 2.5 ml commercially available 0.4% or 0.6% solution q 4 hr prn.
Children 6 to 12 yr: 0.1 to 0.2 ml of 5% solution diluted in 0.9% NaCl to final volume of 3 ml q 4 hr prn.

- Instruct to notify doctor if drug ineffective or to request dosage adjustment.

---

metformin hydrochloride
Glucophage
Biguanide
Antidiabetic agent
Preg. Risk Category: B

Adjunct to diet to lower blood glucose in type 2 diabetes — **Adults:** initially, 500 mg PO bid with morning and evening meals, or 850 mg PO qd with morning meal. When 500-mg dose form used, increase dosage 500 mg weekly to max 2,500 mg PO daily in divided doses as needed. When 850-mg dose form used, increase dosage 850 mg every other wk to max 2,550 mg PO daily in divided doses as needed. Use conservative dose with elderly and debilitated patients.

- Monitor renal function. If renal impairment detected, expect to switch to different antidiabetic agent.
- Give with meals.
- Monitor blood glucose regularly to evaluate effectiveness.
- Monitor closely during times of increased stress. Insulin therapy may be needed then.

---

methadone hydrochloride
Dolophine, Methadose, Physeptone‡
Opioid
Analgesic/narcotic detoxification adjunct
Preg. Risk Category: C
Controlled Sub. Sched.: II

Severe pain — **Adults:** 2.5 to 10 mg PO, IM, or SC q 3 to 4 hr, prn.
Narcotic withdrawal syndrome — **Adults:** 15 to 40 mg PO daily (highly individualized). Maintenance 20 to 120 mg PO daily. Adjust dosage as needed. Daily dosages > 120 mg dosage require special state and federal approval.

- Oral liquid form legally required in maintenance programs. Completely dissolve tablets in 120 ml orange juice or powdered citrus drink.
- For parenteral use; IM injection preferred.
- Around-the-clock regimen necessary to manage severe, chronic pain.

DRUG / CLASS / CATEGORY	INDICATIONS / DOSAGES	KEY NURSING CONSIDERATIONS
methamphetamine hydrochloride Desoxyn *CNS stimulant/adjunctive anorexigenic/sympathomimetic amine* Preg. Risk Category: C Controlled Sub. Sched.: I	*Attention deficit disorder with hyperactivity* — **Children ≥ 6 yr:** 2.5 to 5 mg PO qd or bid, with 5-mg increments weekly, prn. Usual effective dosage 20 to 25 mg daily. *Short-term adjunct in exogenous obesity* — **Adults:** 2.5 to 5 mg PO bid to tid, 30 min before meals; or 10 to 15 mg long-acting tab PO daily before breakfast.	• Not recommended for first-line treatment of obesity. Use as anorexigenic agent prohibited in some states. • When used for obesity, be sure patient on weight-reduction program. • If tolerance to anorexigenic effect develops, notify doctor.
methimazole Tapazole *Thyroid hormone antagonist* *Antihyperthyroid agent* Preg. Risk Category: D	*Hyperthyroidism* — **Adults:** if mild, 15 mg PO daily; if moderately severe, 30 to 45 mg PO daily; if severe, 60 mg daily. All given in 3 equally divided doses q 8 hr. Maintenance 5 to 15 mg daily. **Children:** 0.4 mg/kg/day PO divided q 8 hr. Maintenance 0.2 mg/kg/day divided q 8 hr.	• Monitor hepatic function and CBC. • Dosages > 30 mg/day increase agranulocytosis risk. • Watch for signs of hypothyroidism. • Discontinue and notify doctor of severe rash or enlarged cervical lymph nodes. • Advise not to take OTC cough medicines.
methocarbamol Robaxin, Robaxin-7500 *Carbamate derivative of guaifenesin* *Skeletal muscle relaxant* Preg. Risk Category: NR	*Adjunct in acute, painful musculoskeletal conditions* — **Adults:** 1.5 g PO qid for 2 to 3 days. Maintenance 4 to 4.5 g PO daily in 3 to 6 divided doses. Or, 1 g IM or IV. Max 3 g daily IM or IV or 3 consecutive days. *Supportive therapy in tetanus management* — **Adults:** 1 to 2 g IV push or 1 to 3 g as infusion q 6 hr. **Children:** 15 mg/kg IV q 6 hr.	• Irritates veins; may cause fainting or phlebitis or aggravate seizures if injected rapidly. Keep patient supine during infusion. Avoid infiltration. • Give IM deeply, only into upper outer quadrant of buttock, with max 5 ml in each buttock. Don't give SC. • Warn to avoid activities that require alertness until CNS effects known.

methotrexate (amethopterin, MTX) methotrexate sodium

Folex, Folex PFS, Mexate-AQ, Rheumatrex

Antimetabolite (cell cycle-phase specific, S phase)

Antineoplastic

Preg. Risk Category: X

Trophoblastic tumors (choriocarcinoma, hydatidiform mole) — **Adults:** 15 to 30 mg PO or IM daily for 5 days. Repeat after ≥ 1 wk, according to response or toxicity.

Acute lymphocytic leukemia — **Adults and children:** 3.3 mg/m² /day PO, IM, or IV for 4 to 6 wk or until remission; then 20 to 30 mg/m² PO or IM weekly in 2 divided doses or 2.5 mg/kg IV q 14 days.

Meningeal leukemia — **Adults and children:** 12 mg/m² or less (max 15 mg) intrathecally q 2 to 5 days until CSF normal, then 1 additional dose.

- Reconstitute solutions without preservatives just before use; discard unused drug.
- Leucovorin rescue necessary with high-dose (> 100 mg) protocols; started 24 hr after methotrexate therapy begins.
- Rash, redness, or ulcerations in mouth or adverse pulmonary reactions may signal serious complications.
- Monitor pulmonary function tests periodically, as ordered.
- Monitor I&O daily. Encourage intake of 2 to 3 L daily.
- Watch for infection or bleeding.

methoxsalen (topical)

Oxsoralen

Psoralen derivative

Pigmenting antipsoriatic

Preg. Risk Category: C

To induce repigmentation in vitiligo; psoriasis — **Adults and children > 12 yr:** apply lotion to small, well-defined vitiliginous lesions. For optimum effect, apply about 1 to 2 hr before exposure to UV light.

- Treated area may be exposed to UV light for limited time.
- After exposure, wash lesions with soap and water, and protect area with sunblock. Overdosage or overexposure to light can cause serious burning or blistering.
- Inform of need for monthly blood tests.
- Protect patient's eyes and lips during light exposure treatments.

methylcellulose

Citrucel, Cologel

Adsorbent

Bulk-forming laxative

Preg. Risk Category: C

Chronic constipation — **Adults:** max 6 g daily, divided into 0.45 to 3 g/dose. **Children 6 to 12 yr:** Max 3 g daily, divided into 0.45 to 1.5 g/dose.

- Especially useful in debilitated patients and in those with postpartum constipation, irritable bowel syndrome, diverticulitis, and colostomies.

†Canadian ‡Australian

DRUG/CLASS/ CATEGORY	INDICATIONS/ DOSAGES	KEY NURSING CONSIDERATIONS
methyldopa Aldomet, Apo-Methyldopa†, Dopamet†, Novomedopa† **methyldopate hydrochloride** Aldomet, Aldomet Ester Injection‡ *Centrally acting antiadrenergic agent* *Antihypertensive* Preg. Risk Category: B	*Hypertension, hypertensive crisis* — **Adults:** *oral* — initially, 250 mg PO bid to tid in first 48 hr. Then increase as needed q 2 days. Maintenance 500 mg to 2 g daily in 2 to 4 divided doses; max recommended 3 g daily. Or, 250 to 500 mg IV q 6 hr, diluted in D₅W and given over 30 to 60 min; max dose 1 g q 6 hr. **Children:** 10 mg/kg PO qd in 2 to 4 divided doses; or 20 to 40 mg/kg IV qd in 4 divided doses. Dosage increased qd prn. Max daily dosage 65 mg/kg or 3 g.	▪ *IV use:* Observe for and report involuntary choreoathetoid movements. ▪ After dialysis, monitor for hypertension and notify doctor if necessary. ▪ Monitor Coombs' test results. ▪ Monitor CBC with differential. ▪ Caution not to stop taking suddenly but to contact doctor if unpleasant adverse reactions occur.
methylergonovine maleate Methergine *Ergot alkaloid* *Oxytocic* Preg. Risk Category: C	*Prevention and treatment of postpartum hemorrhage caused by uterine atony or subinvolution* — **Adults:** 0.2 mg IM q 2 to 4 hr; for excessive uterine bleeding or other emergencies, 0.2 mg IV over 1 min while BP and uterine contractions monitored. After initial IM or IV dose, 0.2 mg PO q 6 to 8 hr for 2 to 7 days. Decrease dosage if severe cramping occurs.	▪ *IV use:* Shouldn't be routinely given IV; risk of severe hypertension and CVA. If IV route necessary, administer slowly over 1 min with careful BP monitoring. May dilute IV dose to 5 ml with 0.9% NaCl solution. Contractions begin immediately after IV use and continue for up to 45 min. ▪ Monitor and record BP, pulse rate, and uterine response; report sudden change in vital signs, frequent periods of uterine relaxation, and character and amount of vaginal bleeding. ▪ Monitor contractions, which may last ≥ 3 hr after PO or IM administration.

methylphenidate hydrochloride

PMS-Methylphenidate‡, Ritalin, Ritalin-SR

Piperidine CNS stimulant
CNS stimulant (analeptic)
Preg. Risk Category: NR
Controlled Sub. Sched.: II

Attention deficit hyperactivity disorder (ADHD) — **Children ≥ 6 yr:** initial dose, 5 to 10 mg PO daily before breakfast and lunch, with 5- to 10-mg increments weekly prn, up to 2 mg/kg or 60 mg daily. Usual effective dose 20 to 30 mg.
Narcolepsy — **Adults:** 10 mg PO bid or tid 30 to 45 min before meals. Dosage varies with patient needs; average 40 to 60 mg/day.

- May trigger Tourette syndrome in children.
- Observe for signs of excessive stimulation. Monitor BP.
- Monitor height and weight in children on long-term therapy. May delay growth spurt, but children will attain normal height when drug stopped.
- Monitor for tolerance or psychological dependence.

methylprednisolone
Medrol

methylprednisolone acetate
depMedalone-40, Depoject-40, Depo-Medrol, Depopred-40, Depo-Predate 40, Duralone-40, Medralone-40, Rep-pred 40

methylprednisolone sodium succinate
A-methaPred, Solu-Medrol

Glucocorticoid
Anti-inflammatory/immunosuppressant
Preg. Risk Category: C

Multiple sclerosis — **Adults:** 200 mg PO daily for 1 wk, followed by 80 mg qod for 1 month.
Severe inflammation or immunosuppression — **Adults:** 2 to 60 mg PO daily in 4 divided doses; 10 to 80 mg acetate IM daily, or 10 to 250 mg succinate IM or IV up to q 4 hr; or 4 to 40 mg acetate into smaller joints or 20 to 80 mg acetate into larger joints. **Children:** succinate 0.03 to 0.2 mg/kg or 1 to 6.25 mg/m² IM qd or bid.
Shock — **Adults:** 100 to 250 mg succinate IV at 2- to 6-hr intervals; or 30 mg/kg IV initially, repeated q 4 to 6 hr, prn. Continue therapy for 2 to 3 days or until patient stable.

- Give oral dose with food when possible.
- Critically ill patients may require concomitant antacid or histamine₂-receptor antagonist.
- **IV use:** Use only methylprednisolone sodium succinate; never use acetate form for IV use. Reconstitute according to manufacturer's directions.
  Direct injection, inject over at least 1 min.
  Give massive doses over at least 10 min.
  If used for continuous infusion, change solution q 24 hr.
- May mask or exacerbate infections.
- Watch for depression or psychotic episodes.
- Diabetics may need increased insulin.

METHYLPREDNISOLONE SODIUM SUCCINATE   199

‡Canadian †Australian

DRUG/CLASS/ CATEGORY	INDICATIONS/ DOSAGES	KEY NURSING CONSIDERATIONS
methyltestosterone Android, Metandren, Testred *Androgen* Androgen replacement Preg. Risk Category: X Controlled Sub. Sched.: II	*Breast cancer in women* — **Adults:** 50 to 200 mg PO daily; or 25 to 100 mg buccally daily. *Male hypogonadism* — **Adults:** 10 to 50 mg PO daily; or 5 to 25 mg buccally daily. Semen evaluation q 3 to 4 months.	• In children, wrist bone X-rays should be taken before therapy to establish bone maturation level. • Check Hgb, HCT, cholesterol, calcium, and cardiac and liver function. • Therapy should be stopped if disease progression occurs.
methysergide maleate Deseril; Sansert *Ergot alkaloid* *Vasoconstrictor* Preg. Risk Category: X	*Prevention of frequent, severe, uncontrollable, or disabling migraine or vascular headaches* — **Adults:** 4 to 8 mg PO daily with meals.	• Monitor lab studies of cardiac and renal function, and CBC. • May be withdrawn gradually q 6 mo, then restarted after at least 3 wk.
metipranolol hydrochloride OptiPranolol *Beta-adrenergic blocker* *Antiglaucoma agent* Preg. Risk Category: C	*IOP reduction in ocular conditions, including ocular hypertension and chronic open-angle glaucoma* — **Adults:** 1 drop into affected eye bid. If IOP not at satisfactory level, may institute concomitant therapy to lower IOP.	• To administer, wash hands. Have patient tilt head back or lie down. Gently grasp lower eyelid and pull eyelid away from eye to form pouch. Place dropper directly over eye, avoiding contact with eye or any surface.
metoclopramide hydrochloride Apo-Metoclop†, Clopra, Maxolon, Octamide, Reclomide, Reglan	*Prevention or reduction of nausea and vomiting associated with cancer chemotherapy* — **Adults:** 1 to 2 mg/kg IV 30 min before cancer chemotherapy, then repeated q 2 hr for 2 doses, then q 3 hr for 3 doses.	• **IV use:** Give lower doses (≤ 10 mg) by direct injection over 1 to 2 min. Dilute doses > 10 mg in 50 ml compatible diluent; infuse over ≥ 15 min. Protection from light unnecessary if mixture given ≤ 24 hr.

Para-aminobenzoic acid
(PABA) derivative
Antiemetic/GI stimulant
Preg. Risk Category: B

Prevention of postop nausea and vomiting — **Adults:** 10 to 20 mg IM near end of procedure; then q 4 to 6 hr prn.
To facilitate small-bowel intubation and to aid in radiologic exams — **Adults and children > 14 yr:** 10 mg IV as single dose over 1 to 2 min. **Children < 6 yr:** 0.1 mg/kg IV. **Children 6 to 14 yr:** 2.5 to 5 mg IV.
Gastroesophageal reflux — **Adults:** 10 to 15 mg PO qid, prn, 30 min before meals and hs.

- Compatible with D$_5$W, 0.9% NaCl for injection, and D$_5$ in 0.45% NaCl.
- Use diphenhydramine 25 mg IV as ordered to counteract extrapyramidal adverse effects associated with high doses.
- Advise to avoid activities requiring alertness for 2 hr after each dose.
- Closely monitor BP in patient receiving IV form.

metolazone
Diulo, Mykrox, Zaroxolyn
Quinazoline derivative (thiazide-like) diuretic
Diuretic/antihypertensive
Preg. Risk Category: B

Edema in heart failure or renal disease — **Adults:** 5 to 20 mg (ext-release) PO daily.
Hypertension — **Adults:** 2.5 to 5 mg (ext-release) PO daily. Maintenance dosage based on BP. Or 0.5 mg (prompt-release) PO daily in AM, increased to 1 mg PO daily.

- To prevent nocturia, give in morning.
- Monitor I&O, weight, BP, and electrolytes.
- Watch for signs of hypokalemia, such as muscle weakness and cramps.
- Advise to avoid sudden posture changes.

metoprolol succinate
Toprol XL

metoprolol tartrate
Apo-Metoprolol†, Lopresor
Apo-Metoprolol†, Lopressor, Minax‡
SR†, Lopressor, Minax‡
Beta-adrenergic blocker
Antihypertensive/adjunctive treatment of acute MI
Preg. Risk Category: C

Hypertension — **Adults:** 100 mg PO in single or divided doses; maint. 100 to 450 mg qd in 2 or 3 divided doses. Or, 50 to 100 mg of ext-release tab qd (max 400 mg qd).
Early intervention in acute MI — **Adults:** three 5-mg (tartrate) IV boluses q 2 min. Then, 15 min after last dose, 25 to 50 mg PO q 6 hr for 48 hr. Maint. 100 mg PO bid.
Angina pectoris — **Adults:** initially, 100 mg PO daily in 2 divided doses. Maint. 100 to 400 mg qd.

- Check apical pulse before giving. If < 60, withhold dose and call doctor immediately.
- Masks common signs of hypoglycemia. Monitor blood glucose closely in diabetics.
- Masks common signs of shock. Monitor BP frequently.

METOPROLOL TARTRATE   201

DRUG / CLASS / CATEGORY	INDICATIONS / DOSAGES	KEY NURSING CONSIDERATIONS
metronidazole Apo-Metronidazole†, Flagyl, Metrozine‡, Neo-Metric†, PMS Metronidazole†, Protostat, Trikacide† **metronidazole hydrochloride** Flagyl IV RTU, Metro IV, Novonidazol† *Nitroimidazole* *Antibacterial/antiprotozoal/ amebicide* Preg. Risk Category: B	*Intestinal amebiasis* — **Adults:** 750 mg PO tid for 5 to 10 days. **Children:** 30 to 50 mg/kg daily (in 3 doses) for 10 days. *Trichomoniasis* — **Adults:** 250 mg PO tid for 7 days or 2 g PO in single dose; 4 to 6 wk should elapse between courses of therapy. **Children:** 5 mg/kg dose PO tid for 7 days. *Refractory trichomoniasis* — **Adults:** 250 or 500 mg PO bid for 10 or 7 days, respectively. *Bacterial infections caused by anaerobic microorganisms* — **Adults:** load: 15 mg/kg IV infused over 1 hr. Maint. dose 7.5 mg/kg IV or PO q 6 hr. Give 1st maint. dose 6 hr after loading dose. Max 4 g qd. *Prevention of postop infection in contaminated or potentially contaminated colorectal surgery* — **Adults:** 15 mg/kg IV infused over 30 to 60 min 1 hr before surgery. Then, 7.5 mg/kg IV infused over 30 to 60 min at 6 and 12 hr after initial dose.	▪ Infuse over ≥ 1 hr. Don't give IV push. ▪ Record number and character of stools when used to treat amebiasis. Should be used only after *T. vaginalis* confirmed by wet smear or culture or *E. histolytica* identified. Asymptomatic sexual partners of patients being treated for *T. vaginalis* should be treated simultaneously to avoid reinfection. ▪ Instruct to take oral form with food. ▪ Tell to avoid alcohol or alcohol-containing medications during therapy and for at least 48 hr afterward. ▪ Inform that metallic taste and dark or reddish-brown urine may occur. ▪ Don't refrigerate neutralized diluted solution; precipitation may occur. If Flagyl IV RTU refrigerated, crystals may form; these disappear after sol warms to room temp.
metronidazole (topical) MetroGel, MetroGel-Vaginal *Nitroimidazole* *Antiprotozoal/antibacterial* Preg. Risk Category: B	*Acne rosacea* — **Adults:** apply thin film to affected area bid, morning and evening. Frequency and duration of therapy adjusted after response evaluated. *Bacterial vaginosis* — **Adults:** 1 applicatorful bid, morning and evening, for 5 days.	▪ Avoid using topical gel around eyes. Clean area before use and wait 15 to 20 min before applying drug. Cosmetics may be used after applying drug. ▪ If local reactions occur, tell to apply less frequently or to stop and contact doctor.

mexiletine hydrochloride

Mexitil

Lidocaine analog, sodium channel antagonist

Ventricular antiarrhythmic

Preg. Risk Category: C

Refractory life-threatening ventricular arrhythmias, including ventricular tachycardia and PVCs — **Adults:** 200 mg PO q 8 hr. May increase dose in increments of 50 to 100 mg q 8 hr. Or, loading dose of 400 mg with maintenance dose of 200 mg q 8 hr. Max shouldn't exceed 1,200 mg daily.

- When switching from lidocaine, stop lidocaine infusion when first mexiletine dose given. Keep infusion line open until arrhythmia appears to be satisfactorily controlled. Monitor therapeutic levels, as ordered. Levels range from 0.5 to 2 mcg/ml.
- Monitor for toxicity. Tremor early toxicity sign; progresses to dizziness and later to ataxia and nystagmus.
- Monitor BP and heart rate and rhythm frequently.

mezlocillin sodium

Mezlin

Extended-spectrum penicillin, acylaminopenicillin

Antibiotic

Preg. Risk Category: B

Systemic infections caused by susceptible strains of gram-pos and especially gram-neg organisms — **Adults:** 200 to 300 mg/kg daily IV or IM in 4 to 6 divided doses. Usual dose 3 g q 4 hr or 4 g q 6 hr. For very serious infections, up to 24 g daily may be given. **Children ≤ 12 yr:** 200 to 300 mg/kg per day IM or IV in divided doses q 4 to 6 hr.

- Before giving, ask about previous allergic reactions to penicillin. (However, negative history doesn't preclude future reaction.) Obtain specimen for culture and sensitivity tests before first dose.
- With IM, don't give > 2 g per injection.
- May cause thrombocytopenia. Check CBC and platelet counts frequently, as ordered.
- Monitor serum potassium.

miconazole nitrate

Micatin, Monistat-Derm Cream and Lotion, Monistat 3 Vaginal Suppository, Monistat 7

Imidazole derivative

Antifungal

Preg. Risk Category: C

Tinea pedis, tinea cruris, tinea corporis — **Adults and children:** apply or spray sparingly bid for 2 to 4 wk. *Vulvovaginal candidiasis —* **Adults:** 1 applicatorful or 100 mg supp (Monistat 7) inserted intravaginally hs for 7 days; repeat course if necessary. Or, 200 mg supp (Monistat 3) intravaginally hs for 3 days.

- Concurrent use of intravag forms and certain latex products, such as vag contraceptive diaphragms, not recommended.
- Instruct to avoid sexual intercourse during vag treatment.
- Caution to discontinue if sensitivity or chemical irritation occurs.

MICONAZOLE NITRATE　　203

†Canadian ‡Australian

DRUG/CLASS/ CATEGORY	INDICATIONS/ DOSAGES	KEY NURSING CONSIDERATIONS
midazolam hydrochloride Hypnovel†; Versed *Benzodiazepine* *Preoperative sedative/agent for conscious sedation/adjunct for induction of general anesthesia/amnesic agent* Preg. Risk Category: D Controlled Sub. Sched.: IV	*Preop sedation* — **Adults:** 0.07 mg to 0.08 mg/kg IM 1 hr before surgery. *Conscious sedation before short diagnostic procedures* — **Adults:** 1 to 2 mg by slow IV injection before procedure. *Induction of general anesthesia* — **Adults:** 0.15 to 0.35 mg/kg given over 20 to 30 sec. Additional increments of 25% of initial dose may be needed. Max dose of up to 0.6 mg/kg. **Unpremedicated adults 55 yr and older:** initially, 0.3 mg/kg. For debilitated patients, initial dose 0.2 to 0.25 mg/kg.	▪ Monitor BP, heart rate and rhythm, respirations, airway integrity, and SaO₂. ▪ Have oxygen and resuscitation equipment available. ▪ May mix in same syringe with morphine sulfate, meperidine, atropine sulfate, or scopolamine. ▪ *IV use:* Administer slowly over at least 2 min, and wait at least 2 min when titrating.
midodrine hydrochloride ProAmatine *Peripheral alpha-adrenergic agonist* *Vasopressor/antihypertensive* Preg. Risk Category: C	*Treatment of symptomatic orthostatic hypotension unresponsive to standard clinical care* — **Adults:** 10 mg PO tid. Suggested dosing schedule: first dose shortly before or on arising in morning; second dose at midday; third dose in late afternoon (no later than 6 PM). Use cautiously in abnormal renal function; initially, 2.5-mg doses recommended.	▪ Monitor supine and sitting BP closely; notify doctor if supine BP increases excessively. ▪ Advise to take in daytime when patient can be upright and performing daily activities. Space doses at least 3 hr apart. Tell not to take after evening meal or within 4 hr before bedtime. ▪ Renal and hepatic tests should be done before and during therapy as ordered. ▪ Instruct to consult doctor before taking OTC medications.

milrinone lactate
Primacor

Bipyridine phosphodiesterase inhibitor

Inotropic vasodilator

Preg. Risk Category: C

Short-term treatment of heart failure —
Adults: initial loading dose 50 mcg/kg IV, given slowly over 10 min, followed by continuous IV infusion of 0.375 to 0.75 mcg/kg/min. Adjust infusion dose according to clinical and hemodynamic responses, as ordered.

- Improved cardiac output may enhance urine output. Potassium loss may predispose to digitalis toxicity.
- Monitor fluid and electrolyte status, BP, HR, and renal function. Excessive BP decrease requires discontinuing or slowing rate of infusion.

minocycline hydrochloride
Apo-Minocycline†, Dynacin, Minocin, Minomycin IV‡, Syn-Minocycline†

Tetracycline

Antibiotic

Preg. Risk Category: NR

Infections caused by susceptible gram-neg and gram-pos organisms — **Adults:** initially, 200 mg IV; then 100 mg IV q 12 hr. Not to exceed 400 mg/day. Or, 200 mg PO initially; then 100 mg PO q 12 hr. Some clinicians use 100 or 200 mg PO initially, followed by 50 mg qid. **Children > 8 yr:** initially, 4 mg/kg PO or IV, followed by 2 mg/kg q 12 hr. Given IV in 500- to 1,000-ml sol without calcium over 6 hr.

Gonorrhea in patients allergic to penicillin — **Adults:** initially, 200 mg PO; then 100 mg q 12 hr for at least 4 days.

Syphilis in patients allergic to penicillin — **Adults:** initially, 200 mg PO; then 100 mg q 12 hr for 10 to 15 days.

Meningococcal carrier state — **Adults:** 100 mg PO q 12 hr for 5 days.

Uncomplicated urethral, endocervical, or rectal infection caused by C. trachomatis — 100 mg PO bid for at least 7 days.

- Obtain specimen for culture and sensitivity tests before first dose. Therapy may begin pending test results.
- With large doses or prolonged therapy, monitor for superinfection, especially in high-risk patients.
- Check tongue for signs of candidal infection. Stress good oral hygiene.
- May cause tooth discoloration in young adults. Observe for brown pigmentation; inform doctor if present.
- Don't expose to heat or light. Keep cap tightly closed.
- Thrombophlebitis may occur with IV administration. Avoid extravasation. Switch to oral therapy as soon as possible.
- Tell to take oral form with full glass of water. May be taken with food.
- Instruct not to take within 1 hr of bedtime.

MINOCYCLINE HYDROCHLORIDE   205

DRUG/CLASS/CATEGORY	INDICATIONS/DOSAGES	KEY NURSING CONSIDERATIONS
minoxidil Loniten, Minodyl *Peripheral vasodilator* *Antihypertensive* Preg. Risk Category: C	*Severe hypertension* — **Adults:** initially, 5 mg PO as single dose. Effective dosage range usually 10 to 40 mg daily. Max 100 mg daily. **Children < 12 yr:** 0.2 mg/kg PO (max 5 mg) as single daily dose. Effective dosage range usually 0.25 to 1 mg/kg daily. Max 50 mg daily.	• Closely monitor BP and HR at start of therapy. Elderly patients may be more sensitive to hypotensive effects. • Removed by hemodialysis. Be sure to administer dose after dialysis. • Monitor fluid I&O. Check for weight gain and edema.
minoxidil (topical) Rogaine *Direct-acting vasodilator* *Hair-growth stimulant* Preg. Risk Category: C	*Androgentic alopecia* — **Adults:** 1 ml of 2% sol applied to affected area bid. Max 2 ml daily.	• Patient must have normal, healthy scalp before beginning therapy. • Hair and scalp should be thoroughly dry before application, and drug shouldn't be applied to any other body areas. Tell not to use on irritated or sunburned scalp or with any other medication on scalp. Instruct to wash hands thoroughly after application. • Warn to avoid inhaling any spray or mist from drug. Avoid spraying around eyes.
mirtazapine Remeron *Piperazinoazepine* *Tetracyclic antidepressant* Preg. Risk Category: C	*Depression* — **Adults:** initially, 15 mg PO hs. Maintenance range 15 to 45 mg daily. Dosage adjustments at intervals of at least 1 to 2 wk.	• Caution not to perform hazardous activities if somnolence occurs. • Instruct not to use alcohol or other CNS depressants. • Monitor closely for signs of dependence; not known if drug causes physical or psychological dependence.

misoprostol
Cytotec
Prostaglandin E1 analog
Antiulcer agent/gastric mucosal protectant
Preg. Risk Category: X

Prevention of NSAID-induced gastric ulcer in elderly or debilitated patients at high risk for complications from gastric ulcer and in patients with history of NSAID-induced ulcer — **Adults:** 200 mcg PO qid with food; if not tolerated, may decrease to 100 mcg PO qid. Give for duration of NSAID therapy. Give last dose hs.

- Provide oral and written warnings about dangers to fetus. Ensure that patient can comply with contraception and has negative serum pregnancy test within 2 wk of starting drug.
- Advise not to begin therapy until second or third day of next menstrual period.

mitomycin (mitomycin-C)
Mutamycin
Antineoplastic antibiotic (cell cycle-phase nonspecific)
Antineoplastic
Preg. Risk Category: NR

Dosage and indications vary. Check treatment protocol with doctor.
Disseminated adenocarcinoma of stomach or pancreas — **Adults:** 20 mg/m² as IV single dose. Cycle repeated after 6 to 8 wk when WBC and platelet counts return to normal.

- Stop infusion immediately and notify doctor if extravasation occurs.
- Monitor for dyspnea with cough.
- Watch for signs of infection and bleeding.

mitotane (o,p'-DDD)
Lysodren
Chlorophenothane (DDT) analogue
Antineoplastic/antiadrenal agent
Preg. Risk Category: C

Inoperable adrenocortical cancer — **Adults:** initially, 2 to 6 g PO daily in divided doses tid or qid; increase to 9 to 10 g PO daily, in divided doses tid or qid. Adjust dosage until max tolerated dosage achieved (varies from 2 to 16 g/day; usually 8 to 10 g/day).

- To reduce nausea, give antiemetic before.
- Assess and record behavioral and neurologic signs daily.
- Notify doctor if severe adverse GI or skin reactions occur.
- Monitor effectiveness according to reduction in pain, weakness, and anorexia.
- Obese patients may need higher dosage and may have longer-lasting adverse reactions.

DRUG/CLASS/ CATEGORY	INDICATIONS/ DOSAGES	KEY NURSING CONSIDERATIONS
moexipril hydrochloride Univasc *ACE inhibitor* *Antihypertensive* Preg. Risk Category: C (1st trimester), D (2nd and 3rd trimesters)	*Hypertension* — **Adults:** initially, 7.5 mg (3.75 mg if patient receiving diuretic) PO qd 1 hr before meal. If control inadequate, dose may be increased or divided. Recommended maintenance dosage 7.5 mg to 30 mg daily, in 1 or 2 divided doses 1 hr ac. Subsequent dosage depends on response.	▪ Monitor for excessive hypotension. Measure BP at trough (just before dose) to verify BP control. ▪ Assess renal function before and during therapy. Monitor serum potassium level. ▪ Monitor CBC with differential before therapy, especially if patient has collagen-vascular disease with impaired renal function. ▪ Angioedema can cause fatal airway obstruction. Be prepared with SC epinephrine 1:1,000 (0.3 to 0.5 ml), and equipment to ensure patent airway.
molindone hydrochloride Moban *Dihydroindolone* *Antipsychotic* Preg. Risk Category: NR	*Psychotic disorders* — **Adults:** initially, 50 to 75 mg PO daily, increased to 100 to 225 mg/day in 3 or 4 days. Maintenance dosage as follows: mild severity — 5 to 15 mg PO tid or qid; moderate severity — 10 to 25 mg PO tid or qid; extreme severity — 225 mg/day PO.	▪ Monitor for tardive dyskinesia. ▪ Assess for neuroleptic malignant syndrome. ▪ Acute dystonic reactions may be treated with diphenhydramine. ▪ Warn to avoid hazardous activities until CNS effects known. Drowsiness and dizziness usually subside after first few wk. ▪ Tell to avoid alcohol.
mometasone furoate	*Inflammation associated with corticosteroid-responsive dermatoses* — **Adults:** apply to affected areas qd.	▪ Gently wash skin before applying. To prevent skin damage, rub in gently, leaving

Elocon
Synthetic corticosteroid
Anti-inflammatory
Preg. Risk Category: C

thin coat. When treating hairy sites, part hair and apply directly to lesions.
- Tell to stop drug and report signs of systemic absorption, skin irritation or ulceration, hypersensitivity, or infection.
- Children may absorb larger amounts and be more prone to systemic toxicity. Avoid using plastic pants or tight-fitting diapers on treated areas in young children.
- Don't apply near eyes, mucous membranes, or in ear canal.
- Don't use with occlusive dressings.

---

moricizine hydrochloride
Ethmozine
Sodium channel blocker
Antiarrhythmic
Preg. Risk Category: B

Life-threatening ventricular arrhythmias —
Adults: individualized. Therapy should begin in hospital. Most patients respond to 600 to 900 mg PO daily in divided doses q 8 hr. Daily dosage increased q 3 days by 150 mg.

- Determine electrolyte status and correct imbalances before therapy as ordered.

---

morphine hydrochloride
Morphitec†, M.O.S.†
morphine sulfate
Astramorph PF, Duramorph, Epimorph†, Infumorph 200, Morphine H.P.†, MS Contin, Roxanol

Severe pain — **Adults:** 5 to 20 mg SC or IM, or 2.5 to 15 mg IV q 4 hr prn; or 10 to 30 mg PO or 10 to 20 mg pr q 4 hr, prn.
When given by cont IV, loading dose of 15 mg IV may be followed by continuous infusion of 0.8 to 10 mg/hour. May also give 15

- Keep narcotic antagonist (naloxone) and resuscitation equipment available.
- When given epidurally, monitor closely for respiratory depression up to 24 hr after injection.
- Monitor circulatory, respiratory, bowel, and bladder functions carefully. May cause transient BP decrease. May worsen or mask gallbladder pain.

MORPHINE SULFATE 209

---

†Canadian ‡Australian

DRUG / CLASS / CATEGORY	INDICATIONS / DOSAGES	KEY NURSING CONSIDERATIONS
morphine hydrochloride *(continued)* **morphine tartrate†** *Opioid* *Narcotic analgesic* Preg. Risk Category: C Controlled Sub. Sched.: II	to 30 mg contr-release tab PO q 8 to 12 hr. As epidural injection, 5 mg; then, if adequate pain relief not obtained within 1 hr, additional doses of 1 to 2 mg. Max total epidural dose shouldn't exceed 10 mg/24 hr. **Children:** 0.1 to 0.2 mg/kg SC or IM q 4 hr. Max single dose 15 mg.	• May cause respiratory depression, hypotension, urine retention, nausea, vomiting, ileus, or altered LOC regardless of route. Withhold dose and notify doctor if respirations < 12. • Tell patient not to crush, break, or chew contr-release tabs. • Constipation often severe with maintenance dosage.
mumps virus vaccine, live Mumpsvax *Vaccine* *Viral vaccine* Preg. Risk Category: C	*Immunization* — **Adults and children ≥ 1 yr:** 0.5 ml (20,000 units) SC.	• Obtain history of allergies, especially anaphylactic reactions to antibiotics, and reaction to immunization. • Keep epinephrine 1:1,000 available to treat anaphylaxis. • Use only diluent supplied. Discard 8 hr after reconstituting.
mupirocin Bactroban *Antibiotic* *Topical antibacterial* Preg. Risk Category: B	*Impetigo* — **Adults and children:** apply to affected areas tid for 1 to 2 wk.	• Wash and dry affected area thoroughly. Apply thin film, rubbing in gently. • If no improvement in 3 to 5 days, tell to notify doctor immediately. • Warn about local adverse reactions. • Prolonged use may cause overgrowth of nonsusceptible bacteria and fungi.

mycophenolate mofetil
CellCept
Mycophenolic acid derivative
Immunosuppressant agent
Preg. Risk Category: C

Prophylaxis of organ rejection in patients receiving allogenic renal transplants —
Adults: 1 g PO bid within 72 hr after transplantation, together with corticosteroids and cyclosporine.

- Potential teratogenic effects. Don't open or crush capsule. Avoid inhaling powder in capsule or letting it contact skin or mucous membranes. If contact occurs, wash with soap and water, and rinse eyes with plain water.
- Stress importance of not stopping therapy without consulting doctor.
- Monitor CBC regularly, as ordered.
- Instruct female to use contraception during therapy and for 6 wk after discontinuation. Tell her to notify doctor immediately of suspected pregnancy. Inform female that pregnancy test required 1 wk before therapy begins.

n

nabumetone
Relafen
Nonsteroidal anti-inflammatory
Antiarthritic agent
Preg. Risk Category: C

Rheumatoid arthritis or osteoarthritis —
Adults: initially, 1,000 mg PO daily as single dose or in divided doses bid. Max 2,000 mg daily.

- May lead to reversible renal impairment. Monitor closely.
- May cause serious GI toxicity. Teach about signs and symptoms of GI bleeding and tell to contact doctor immediately if they occur.
- With long-term therapy, periodically monitor for renal and liver function, CBC, and HCT as ordered; assess for GI bleeding.
- Warn against hazardous activities until CNS effects known.

NABUMETONE   211

DRUG / CLASS / CATEGORY	INDICATIONS / DOSAGES	KEY NURSING CONSIDERATIONS
nadolol Corgard *Beta-adrenergic blocker* *Antihypertensive/antiangi-nal* Preg. Risk Category: C	*Long-standing angina pectoris* — **Adults:** 40 mg PO qd. Increased in 40- to 80-mg increments until optimum response occurs. Usual maint. dosage 40 to 80 mg qd. *Hypertension* — **Adults:** 40 mg PO qd. Increased in 40- to 80-mg increments until optimum response occurs. Usual maint. dosage 40 to 80 mg qd. Doses of 320 mg may be needed.	• Check apical pulse before giving. If < 60, withhold dose and call doctor. Monitor BP frequently. If severe hypotension occurs, give vasopressor, as prescribed. • Masks signs of shock and hyperthy-roidism. • Abrupt discontinuation can exacerbate angina and trigger MI. Reduce dosage gradually over 1 to 2 wk.
nafcillin sodium Nafcil, Nallpen, Unipen *Penicillinase-resistant peni-cillin* *Antibiotic* Preg. Risk Category: B	*Systemic infections caused by penicillinase-producing staphylococci* — **Adults:** 2 to 4 g PO daily in divided doses q 6 hr; or with 2 to 12 g IM or IV daily in divided doses q 4 to 6 hr. **Children:** 25 to 50 mg/kg PO daily in divided doses q 6 hr. **Neonates:** 25 mg/kg IV bid.	• Ask about allergic reactions to penicillin. • Obtain specimen for culture and sensitivity tests before first dose. • Watch for superinfection. • Give PO 1 to 2 hr before or 2 to 3 hr after meals. • Give at least 1 hr before bacteriostatic an-tibiotics.
naftifine Naftin *Synthetic allylamine deriva-tive* *Antifungal agent* Preg. Risk Category: B	*Tinea corporis, tinea cruris, and tinea pedis* — **Adults:** apply cream to affected area qd, or apply gel bid in morning and evening.	• Keep cream away from mucous mem-branes. Not for ophth use. • Don't use occlusive dressings unless di-rected otherwise by doctor. • Discontinue and notify doctor if irritation or sensitivity develops. • Therapy should be reevaluated if no im-provement after 4 wk.

nalbuphine hydrochloride

Nubain

Narcotic agonist-antagonist/opioid partial agonist

Analgesic/adjunct to anesthesia

Preg. Risk Category: NR

Moderate to severe pain — **Adults:** For typical (70-kg) person, give 10 to 20 mg SC, IM, or IV q 3 to 6 hr, prn. Max 160 mg daily.

Adjunct to balanced anesthesia — **Adults:** 0.3 mg/kg to 3 mg/kg IV over 10 to 15 min, then maintenance doses of 0.25 to 0.50 mg/kg in single IV dose, prn.

- Causes respiratory depression, which can be reversed with naloxone. Keep resuscitation equipment available. Monitor circulatory and respiratory status and bladder and bowel function. Withhold dose and notify doctor if respirations shallow or if rate < 12.
- Acts as narcotic antagonist; may trigger withdrawal syndrome.
- *IV use:* Inject slowly over at least 2 to 3 min into vein or into IV line containing compatible, free-flowing IV solution.
- Psychological and physical dependence may occur with prolonged use.
- Warn outpatient to avoid hazardous activities until CNS effects known.

naloxone hydrochloride

Narcan

Narcotic (opioid) antagonist

Narcotic antagonist

Preg. Risk Category: B

Known or suspected narcotic-induced respiratory depression, including that caused by pentazocine and propoxyphene — **Adults:** 0.4 to 2 mg IV, SC, or IM repeated q 2 to 3 min, prn. If no response after 10 mg given, reconsider diagnosis of narcotic-induced toxicity. **Children:** 0.01 mg/kg IV, followed by 2nd dose of 0.1 mg/kg IV, if needed. If IV route not available, may give IM or SC in divided doses. **Neonates:** 0.01 mg/kg IV, IM, or SC. May repeat dose q 2 to 3 min prn.

Postop narcotic depression — **Adults:** 0.1 to 0.2 mg IV q 2 to 3 min prn. May repeat

- Abrupt reversal of opiate-induced CNS depression may result in nausea, vomiting, diaphoresis, tachycardia, CNS excitement, and increased BP.
- May induce tachypnea when given to reverse opioid-induced respiratory depression.
- Monitor respiratory depth and rate. Be prepared to provide O$_2$, ventilation, and other resuscitation measures.
- *IV use:* Be prepared to administer continuous IV infusion. If 0.02 mg/ml not available, may dilute adult conc (0.4 mg) by mixing 0.5 ml with 9.5 sterile water or

(continued)

NALOXONE HYDROCHLORIDE   213

DRUG / CLASS / CATEGORY	INDICATIONS / DOSAGES	KEY NURSING CONSIDERATIONS
naloxone hydrochloride *(continued)*	dosage within 1 to 2 hr, if needed. **Children:** 0.005 to 0.01 mg IV. Repeat q 2 to 3 min prn. **Neonates (asphyxia neonatorum):** 0.01 mg/kg IV into umbilical vein. May repeat q 2 to 3 min.	NaCl for injection to make neonatal conc (0.02 mg/ml). ▪ Narcotic duration of action may exceed that of naloxone; patient may relapse into respiratory depression.
naltrexone hydrochloride ReVia *Narcotic (opioid) antagonist* *Narcotic detoxification adjunct* Preg. Risk Category: C	*Adjunct for maintenance of opioid-free state in detoxified individuals* — **Adults:** 25 mg PO. If no withdrawal signs < 1 hr, give additional 25 mg. When patient on 50 mg q 24 hr, may use flexible maint. schedule. *Treatment of alcohol dependence* — **Adults:** 50 mg PO qd.	▪ Treatment for opioid dependency should not begin until patient receives naloxone challenge. If signs of withdrawal persist, don't give naltrexone. ▪ Patient must be completely opioid-free before taking, or severe withdrawal symptoms may occur.
nandrolone decanoate Androlone-D, Decolone, Hybolin Decanoate **nandrolone phenpropionate** Anabolin IM, Androlone, Durabolin, Nandrobolic *Anabolic steroid* *Erythropoietin/antineoplastic* Preg. Risk Category: X Controlled Sub. Sched.: III	*Anemias associated with renal insufficiency (decanoate)* — **Adults:** 100 to 200 mg IM weekly in males; 50 to 100 mg/wk in females. **Children 2 to 13 yr:** 25 to 50 mg decanoate IM q 3 to 4 wk. *Control of metastatic breast cancer* — **Adults:** 50 to 100 mg phenpropionate IM weekly.	▪ Inject IM deeply. Rotate injection sites to prevent muscle atrophy. ▪ Watch for signs of virilization. Semen evaluation performed q 3 to 4 mo. ▪ Periodically evaluate hepatic function. If results abnormal, stop therapy. ▪ Weigh regularly. ▪ Watch for hypoglycemia in diabetics. Check urine and serum calcium levels.

naphazoline hydrochloride

Allerest, Clear Eyes, Optazine‡, Vasoclear

Sympathomimetic agent

Decongestant/vasoconstrictor

Preg. Risk Category: C

Ocular congestion, irritation, itching — **Adults:** 1 drop 0.1% sol instilled q 3 to 4 hr, or 1 drop 0.012% to 0.03% sol up to qid.

- Wash hands before and after instilling. Apply light finger pressure on lacrimal sac. Don't touch dropper tip to eye or surrounding tissue.
- Notify doctor if photophobia, blurred vision, pain, or lid edema develops.
- Instruct not to use OTC preparations > 72 hr without consulting doctor.

---

naphazoline hydrochloride

Privine

Sympathomimetic agent

Decongestant/vasoconstrictor

Preg. Risk Category: NR

Nasal congestion — **Adults and children ≥ 12 yr:** 2 drops or sprays instilled in each nostril q 3 to 4 hr (drops) or 3 to 6 hr (spray). **Children 6 to 12 yr:** 1 to 2 drops or sprays instilled in each nostril q 3 to 6 hr, prn. Don't use > 3 to 5 days.

- For nasal drops, instruct to tilt head back as far as possible, instill drops, then lean head forward while inhaling, and then repeat procedure for other nostril. For nasal spray, instruct to hold spray container and head upright. Tell not to shake container.
- Tell to contact doctor if nasal congestion persists after 5 days.

---

naproxen

Inza-250‡, Naprosyn, Naprosyn SR†‡, Novo-Naprox†

naproxen sodium

Aleve, Anaprox, Apo-Napro-Na†, Naprelan, Naprogesic‡, Synflex†

Nonsteroidal anti-inflammatory

Rheumatoid arthritis, osteoarthritis, ankylosing spondylitis, pain, dysmenorrhea, tendinitis, bursitis — **Adults:** 250 to 500 mg (naproxen) bid; max 1.5 g/day. Or, 375 to 500 mg delayed-release (EC-Naprosyn) bid; or 750 to 1,000 mg contr-release (Naprelan) bid; or 275 to 550 mg naproxen sodium bid. *Juvenile arthritis —* **Children:** 10 mg/kg PO in 2 divided doses.

Acute gout — **Adults:** 750 mg (naproxen) PO, then 250 mg q 8 hr until attack subsides. Or, 825 mg naproxen sodium, then

- May lead to reversible renal impairment, especially in preexisting renal disease, liver dysfunction, or heart failure; in elderly patients; and in patients taking diuretics.
- Serious GI toxicity, including peptic ulcers and bleeding, can occur despite absence of GI symptoms. Teach about signs and symptoms of GI bleeding, and tell to contact doctor immediately if they occur.
- Caution that concomitant use with aspirin, alcohol, or corticosteroids may increase risk of adverse GI reactions. *(continued)*

NAPROXEN SODIUM

†Canadian ‡Australian

DRUG/CLASS/ CATEGORY	INDICATIONS/ DOSAGES	KEY NURSING CONSIDERATIONS
naproxen sodium (continued) Nonnarcotic analgesic/antipyretic/anti-inflammatory Preg. Risk Category: B	275 mg q 8 hr until attack subsides; or 1,000 to 1,500 mg/day cont-release (Naprelan) on first day, then 1,000 mg qd. *Mild to moderate pain* — **Adults:** 500 mg (naproxen) PO, then 250 mg q 6 to 8 hr, up to 1.25 g/day. Or, 550 mg naproxen sodium, then 275 mg q 6 to 8 hr, up to 1.375 g/day; or 1,000 mg cont-release (Naprelan) qd.	• May mask signs and symptoms of infection. • Warn against hazardous activities that require mental alertness until CNS effects known. • Advise to take with food or milk to minimize GI upset. Instruct to take each dose with full glass of water or other fluid. • If patient taking for arthritis, inform that full therapeutic effect may be delayed 2 to 4 wk.
nedocromil sodium Tilade *Pyranoquinoline* Anti-inflammatory respiratory inhalant Preg. Risk Category: B	*Maintenance in mild to moderate bronchial asthma* — **Adults and children ≥ 12 yr:** 2 inhalations qid at regular intervals.	• Slow onset. Shouldn't be used during acute bronchospasm; isn't therapeutic in aborting acute attack.
nefazodone hydrochloride Serzone *Phenylpiperazine* Antidepressant agent Preg. Risk Category: C	*Depression* — **Adults:** initially, 200 mg/day PO in 2 divided doses. Increase in increments of 100 to 200 mg/day at intervals of no less than 1 wk, prn. Usual range 300 to 600 mg/day.	• At least 1 wk should elapse between stopping nefazodone and starting MAO inhibitor. At least 14 days should elapse before starting nefazodone after MAO inhibitor therapy ends. • Monitor for suicidal tendencies, and allow only minimum drug supply. • Warn not to engage in hazardous activity until CNS effects known.

neomycin sulfate
Mycifradin, Neo-fradin, Neo-
sulft, Neo-tabs
Aminoglycoside
Antibiotic
Preg. Risk Category: NR

*Infectious diarrhea caused by enteropatho-
genic* E. coli — **Adults:** 50 mg/kg daily PO in
4 divided doses for 2 to 3 days; max 3 g daily usually adequate. **Children:** 50 to 100
mg/kg daily PO divided q 4 to 6 hr for 2 to 3
days.
*Suppression of intestinal bacteria preopera-
tively —* **Adults:** 1 g PO q 1 hr for 4 doses,
then 1 g q 4 hr for balance of 24 hr. Saline
cathartic should precede therapy. **Children:**
40 to 100 mg/kg daily PO divided q 4 to 6
hr. First dose should follow saline cathartic.

- Monitor renal function (output, specific
  gravity, urinalysis, BUN, creatinine level,
  and creatinine clearance). Notify doctor of
  signs of decreasing renal function.
- Evaluate hearing before and during prolonged therapy. Notify doctor if tinnitus,
  vertigo, or hearing loss occurs. Deafness
  may begin several weeks after drug
  stopped.
- Watch for superinfection.
- For preoperative disinfection, provide low-
  residue diet and cathartic immediately before oral administration, as ordered.

neomycin sulfate
Mycifradin†, Myciguent,
Neo-Rx
Aminoglycoside
Antibiotic
Preg. Risk Category: C

*Prevention or treatment of superficial bacte-
rial infections —* **Adults and children:** rub
into affected area qd to tid.

- In combination products containing corticosteroids, use of occlusive dressings increases corticosteroid absorption and like-
  lihood of systemic effects.
- Enhanced systemic absorption occurs on
  denuded or abraded areas.
- Watch for signs of hypersensitivity and
  contact dermatitis.
- Watch for signs of ototoxicity with prolonged or extended use.
- If no improvement occurs or if condition
  worsens, tell to stop using and notify doctor.

NEOMYCIN SULFATE   217

DRUG / CLASS / CATEGORY	INDICATIONS / DOSAGES	KEY NURSING CONSIDERATIONS
neostigmine methylsulfate Prostigmin *Cholinesterase inhibitor* *Muscle stimulant* Preg. Risk Category: C	*Symptomatic control of myasthenia gravis* — **Adults:** 0.5 mg SC or IM. Oral dose ranges from 15 to 375 mg/day. Subsequent dosages must be individualized. **Children:** 7.5 to 15 mg PO tid to qid. *Diagnosis of myasthenia gravis* — **Adults:** 0.022 mg/kg IM 30 min after 0.011 mg/kg atropine sulfate IM. **Children:** 0.025 to 0.04 mg/kg IM after 0.011 mg/kg atropine sulfate SC. *Postop abdominal distention and bladder atony* — **Adults:** 0.25 to 0.5 mg IM or SC q 4 to 6 hr for 2 to 3 days. *Antidote for nondepolarizing neuromuscular blocking agents* — **Adults:** 0.5 to 2 mg IV slowly. Repeat prn to total of 5 mg. Before antidote dose, give 0.6 to 1.2 mg atropine sulfate IV. **Neonates and infants:** 0.04 mg/kg IV with 0.02 mg/kg of atropine sulfate.	• In myasthenia gravis, schedule doses before periods of fatigue. For example, if patient has dysphagia, schedule dose 30 min before each meal. • *IV use:* Give at slow, controlled rate, not exceeding 1 mg/min in adults and 0.5 mg/min in children. • Monitor vital signs frequently, especially respirations. Have atropine injection available; provide respiratory support, as needed. • Monitor and document response after each dose. Optimum dosage hard to judge. Observe closely for improvement in strength, vision, and ptosis 45 to 60 min after each dose. • Resistance to drug may occur.
nevirapine Viramune *Non-nucleoside reverse transcriptase inhibitor* *Antiviral agent* Preg. Risk Category: C	*Adjunctive treatment in patients with HIV-1 infection who have experienced clinical or immunologic deterioration* — **Adults:** 200 mg PO daily for first 14 days, then 200 mg PO bid. Used in combination with nucleoside analogue antiretroviral agents.	• Monitor liver function tests before and during therapy. • If therapy interrupted for > 7 days, restart as if administering for first time. • Advise women of childbearing age not to use hormonal birth control methods.

niacin (vitamin B₃,
nicotinic acid)
Niac, Niacor, Nico-400,
Nicobid, Nicolar

niacinamide
(nicotinamide)
B-complex vitamin
Vitamin B₃/antilipemic/peripheral vasodilator
Preg. Risk Category: C

Pellagra — **Adults:** 300 to 500 mg PO, SC, IM, or IV daily in divided doses, depending on severity of deficiency. **Children:** up to 300 mg PO daily in divided doses, depending on severity of niacin deficiency.

Hyperlipidemias, especially with hypercholesterolemia (niacin only) — **Adults:** 1 to 2 g PO tid with or after meals, increased at intervals to 6 g daily.

- **IV use:** Give slow IV (no faster than 2 mg/min).
- Administer aspirin to possibly reduce flushing response.
- Stress that niacin is potent medication, not just vitamin, and may cause serious adverse effects. Explain importance of adhering to therapeutic regimen.
- Monitor hepatic function and blood glucose early in therapy, as ordered.
- Give with meals to minimize adverse GI effects.

---

nicardipine
Cardene, Cardene IV, Cardene SR
Calcium channel blocking agent
Antianginal/antihypertensive
Preg. Risk Category: C

Chronic stable angina, hypertension — **Adults:** initially, 20 mg PO tid (immediate-release only). Titrate according to patient response q 3 days. Usual range 20 to 40 mg tid.

Short-term management of hypertension — **Adults:** if unable to take oral nicardipine, give 5 mg/hr IV infusion, titrated to 2.5 mg/hr q 15 min to max 15 mg/hr.

- **IV use:** When switching to oral therapy other than nicardipine, initiate therapy when infusion discontinued. If oral nicardipine to be used, give first dose of tid regimen 1 hr before infusion discontinued.
- Measure BP frequently during initial therapy.
- Check for orthostatic hypotension. Adjust infusion rate if hypotension or tachycardia occurs, as ordered.
- Advise to report chest pain immediately.

DRUG / CLASS / CATEGORY	INDICATIONS / DOSAGES	KEY NURSING CONSIDERATIONS
nicotine polacrilex (nicotine-polacrilin resin complex) Nicorette, Nicorette DS *Nicotinic agonist* *Smoking cessation aid* Preg. Risk Category: X	*Relief of nicotine withdrawal symptoms in patients undergoing smoking cessation* — **Adults:** initially, one 2-mg square; highly dependent patients should start with 4-mg squares. Patients should chew 1 piece of gum slowly and intermittently for 30 min whenever urge to smoke occurs. Most patients require 9 to 12 pieces of gum daily during first month. For patients using 4-mg squares, max 20 pieces daily. For patients using 2-mg squares, max 30 pieces daily.	• Instruct to chew gum slowly and intermittently (chew several times; then place between cheek and gum) for about 30 min. Fast chewing tends to produce more adverse reactions. • Most likely to benefit smokers with high physical nicotine dependence.
nicotine transdermal system Habitrol, Nicoderm, Nicotrol, ProStep *Nicotinic cholinergic agonist* *Smoking cessation aid* Preg. Risk Category: D	*Relief of nicotine withdrawal symptoms in patients undergoing smoking cessation* — **Adults:** initially, 1 transdermal system, delivering largest available nicotine dosage in its dosage series, applied qd to nonhairy body part. For Habitrol, Nicoderm, and ProStep, patch should be kept on for 24 hr, then removed and new system applied to alternate skin site. For Nicotrol, patch should be applied on awakening and removed at bedtime. After 4 to 12 wk, dosage tapered to next lowest available nicotine dosage in its dosage series, followed in 2 to 4 wk by lowest nicotine dosage system in series being	• To reduce exposure to nicotine, avoid unnecessary contact with system. Wash hands with water alone; soap may enhance absorption. • Teach proper disposal to prevent accidental poisoning of children or pets. • Warn not to smoke. • Advise to apply patch promptly. Patch should not be altered in any way (folded or cut) before application.

nifedipine
Adalat, Adalat CC, Anpine†, Apo-Nifed†, Procardia XL, Nu-Nifed†, Procardia
Calcium channel blocker
Antianginal
Preg. Risk Category: C

Prinzmetal's (variant) angina — **Adults:** starting dose 10 mg PO tid. Usual effective range 10 to 20 mg tid. Max 180 mg daily. *Hypertension* — **Adults:** 30 or 60 mg PO qd. Titrate over 7 to 14 days. Doses > 90 mg (for Adalat CC) and 120 mg (for Procardia XL) are not recommended.

- When rapid response to drug desired, have patient bite and swallow capsule. Continuous BP and ECG monitoring recommended.
- Patient may briefly develop anginal exacerbation.

nilutamide
Nilandron
Hormone
Antiandrogen
Preg. Risk Category: C

Adjunct therapy with surgical castration for treatment of metastatic prostate cancer — **Adults:** 6 tab (50 mg each) PO qd for total of 300 mg/day for 30 days; then 3 tablets qd for total of 150 mg/day thereafter.

- Used in combination with surgical castration; should begin on same day or day after surgery for maximum benefit.
- Tell to report dyspnea or aggravation of preexisting dyspnea immediately.
- Inform of possibility of developing hepatitis and to report symptoms of nausea, vomiting, abdominal pain, or jaundice to doctor. Tell to avoid alcohol.
- Visual disturbances, such as delay in adapting to darkness, may affect driving at night or through tunnels.
- Explain purpose of drug, how given, and importance of not stopping treatment without consulting doctor.

nisoldipine
Sular
Calcium channel blocker
Antihypertensive
Preg. Risk Category: C

Hypertension — **Adults:** initially, 20 mg (10 mg if patient ≥ 65 or has liver dysfunction) PO qd; increased by 10 mg/wk or at longer intervals, as needed. Usual maintenance dosage 20 to 40 mg/day. Dosages > 60 mg/day not recommended.

- Monitor carefully. Some patients experience increased frequency, duration, or severity of angina or even acute MI after starting drug or when dosage increased.
- Monitor BP regularly, especially during initial administration and titration.

NISOLDIPINE   221

†Canadian ‡Australian

DRUG/CLASS/ CATEGORY	INDICATIONS/ DOSAGES	KEY NURSING CONSIDERATIONS
nitrofurantoin macrocrystals Macrobid, Macrodantin **nitrofurantoin microcrystals** Furadantin, Macrodantin, Nephronex† Nitrofuran, *Urinary tract anti-infective* Preg. Risk Category: B	*UTIs caused by susceptible organisms* — **Adults and children > 12 yr:** 50 to 100 mg PO qid with meals and hs. **Children 1 mo to 12 yr:** 5 to 7 mg/kg PO daily divided qid. *Long-term suppression therapy* — **Adults:** 50 to 100 mg PO daily hs. **Children:** 1 mg/kg PO daily in single dose hs or divided into 2 doses.	• Obtain urine specimen for culture and sensitivity tests before therapy. • May cause growth of nonsusceptible organisms. • Give with food or milk to minimize GI distress and improve absorption. • Monitor fluid I&O carefully. May turn urine brown or darker.
nitrofurazone Furacin *Synthetic antibacterial nitrofuran derivative* *Topical antibacterial* Preg. Risk Category: C	*Adjunctive treatment of 2nd- and 3rd-degree burns; prevention of skin allograft rejection* — **Adults and children:** apply directly to lesion daily or q few days, depending on burn severity. May also apply to dressings used to cover affected area.	• Clean wound, as indicated by doctor, before reapplying dressings. • When using wet dressing, protect skin around wound with zinc oxide ointment. • Report irritation, sensitization, or infection.
nitroglycerin (glyceryl trinitrate) Anginine‡, Coro-Nitra, Nitro-Bid, Nitrocine, Nitrodisc, Nitro-Dur, Nitrogard, Nitroglyn, Nitrol, Nitrolingual, Nitrostat, Transderm-Nitro, Transiderm-Nitro‡, Tridil	*Prophylaxis against chronic anginal attacks* — **Adults:** 2.5 mg or 2.6 mg sustained-release capsule q 8 to 12 hr. Or, use 2% ointment topically ½" to 5". Or, transderm disc or pad 0.2 to 0.4 mg/hr qd. *Acute angina pectoris, prophylaxis to prevent or minimize anginal attacks before stressful events* — **Adults:** 1 SL tab. Repeat q 5 min. if needed, for 15 min. Or, using Ni-	• Advise that abrupt drug discontinuation can cause coronary vasospasms. • Closely monitor vital signs during infusion. Excessive hypotension may worsen MI. • Measure prescribed amount on application paper; then place on nonhairy area. Don't rub in. Cover with plastic film. If using Tape-Surrounded Appli-Ruler (TSAR)

Nitrate
Antianginal/vasodilator
Preg. Risk Category: C

trolingual spray, 1 or 2 sprays into mouth. Repeat q 3 to 5 min, prn, to max 3 doses in 15-min period. Or, 1 to 3 mg transmucosally q 3 to 5 hr during waking hours.

Hypertension, heart failure, acute angina pectoris, to produce controlled hypotension during surgery (by IV infusion) — **Adults:** 5 mcg/min, increased prn by 5 mcg/min q 3 to 5 min until response.

system, keep TSAR on skin to protect clothing.
- Remove transderm patch before defibrillation.

---

nitroprusside
sodium
Nitropress
Vasodilator
Antihypertensive
Preg. Risk Category: C

Hypertensive emergencies — **Adults and children:** 50-mg vial diluted with 2 to 3 ml of D_5W and then added to 250, 500, or 1,000 ml of D_5W; infuse at 0.3 to 10 mcg/kg/min titrated to BP. Max infusion rate 10 mcg/kg/min.

Acute heart failure — **Adults and children:** IV infusion titrated to cardiac output and systemic BP. Same dosage range as for hypertensive emergencies.

- Obtain baseline vital signs and parameters before giving. Check BP every 5 min at start of infusion and every 15 min thereafter. If severe hypotension occurs, discontinue infusion and notify doctor. Check serum thiocyanate levels every 72 hr. Levels > 100 mcg/ml associated with toxicity.
- Sensitive to light; wrap IV solution in foil. Fresh solution should have faint brownish tint.

---

nizatidine
Axid, Tazac‡
Histamine₂-receptor antagonist
Antiulcer agent
Preg. Risk Category: C

Active duodenal ulcer — **Adults:** 300 mg PO daily hs. Or, 150 mg PO bid.

Maintenance therapy for duodenal ulcer — **Adults:** 150 mg PO daily hs.

Benign gastric ulcer — **Adults:** 150 mg PO bid or 300 mg PO daily hs for 8 wk.

Gastroesophageal reflux disease — **Adults:** 150 mg PO bid.

- Tell patient who has trouble swallowing capsules that contents may be mixed with apple juice but not with tomato-based mixed vegetable juices.
- Encourage to avoid cigarette smoking; may increase gastric acid secretion and worsen disease.
- Increases serum salicylate levels when used with high doses of aspirin.

NIZATIDINE   223

DRUG/CLASS/ CATEGORY	INDICATIONS/ DOSAGES	KEY NURSING CONSIDERATIONS
norepinephrine bitartrate Levophed *Adrenergic* *Vasopressor* Preg. Risk Category: C	*To maintain BP in acute hypotensive states* — **Adults:** initially, 8 to 12 mcg/min IV infusion, then adjust to maintain normal BP. Avg maintenance dosage 2 to 4 mcg/min. **Children:** 2 mcg/m²/min IV infusion. Adjust dose per response.	• **IV use:** Check BP q 2 min until stabilized; then check q 5 min. During infusion, frequently monitor ECG, cardiac output, CVP, PCWP, pulse rate, urine output, and color and temperature of extremities. • When discontinuing, gradually slow infusion rate, as ordered.
norethindrone Micronor, Norlutin, Nor-Q.D. **norethindrone acetate** Aygestin, Norlutate *Progestin* *Contraceptive* Preg. Risk Category: X	*Amenorrhea, abnormal uterine bleeding* — **Adults:** 2.5 to 20 mg PO daily on days 5 to 25 of menstrual cycle. *Endometriosis* — **Adults:** 5 to 10 mg PO daily for 14 days; then increase by 2.5 to 5 mg daily q 2 wk up to 15 to 30 mg daily. *Contraception in women* — **Adults:** initially, 0.35 mg norethindrone PO on first day of menstruation; then 0.35 mg daily.	• Norethindrone acetate twice as potent as norethindrone. Acetate shouldn't be used for contraception. • Watch carefully for signs of edema. • Tell to report unusual symptoms immediately and to stop drug and call doctor if visual disturbances or migraine occurs.
norfloxacin Noroxin *Fluoroquinolone* *Broad-spectrum antibiotic* Preg. Risk Category: C	*UTIs caused by susceptible strains of E. faecalis, E. coli, and K. pneumoniae* — **Adults:** 400 mg PO q 12 hr for uncomplicated infections, 400 mg PO q 12 hr for 7 to 10 days. For complicated infections, 400 mg PO q 12 hr for 10 to 21 days. *Acute, uncomplicated urethral and cervical gonorrhea* — **Adults:** 800 mg PO as single dose, followed by doxycycline to treat any coexisting chlamydial infection.	• Advise to take 1 hr before or 2 hr after meals. • Tell to drink several glasses of water throughout day. • Caution to avoid hazardous tasks that require alertness until CNS effects known.

norgestrel Ovrette *Progestin* *Contraceptive* Preg. Risk Category: X	*Contraception in women* — **Adults:** 0.075 mg PO daily.	• Instruct to take every day at same time, even if menstruating.
nortriptyline **hydrochloride** Allegron‡, Aventyl‡, Nortab‡, Pamelor *Tricyclic antidepressant* *Antidepressant* Preg. Risk Category: NR	*Depression* — **Adults:** 25 mg PO tid or qid, gradually increased to max 150 mg daily. Entire dosage may be given hs. Monitor plasma levels when giving doses > 100 mg/day.	• Discontinue gradually several days before surgery. • Adverse anticholinergic effects can occur rapidly. • Warn to avoid activities that require alertness until CNS effects known. • Tell to consult doctor before taking other prescription or OTC drugs.
nystatin Mycostatin, Nadostine†, Nilstat, Nystat-Rx, Nystex *Polyene macrolide* *Antifungal* Preg. Risk Category: NR	*Intestinal candidiasis* — **Adults:** 500,000 to 1 million units as oral tab tid. *Oral infections* — **Adults and children:** 400,000 to 600,000 units oral susp qid. **Infants:** 200,000 units oral susp qid. **Neonates and premature infants:** 100,000 units oral susp qid. *Vaginal infections* — **Adults:** 100,000 units as vaginal tablets high into vagina, daily for 14 days.	• Not effective against systemic infections. • Pregnant patients can use vag tablets up to 6 wk before term. • For treatment of oral candidiasis (thrush): After mouth cleaned of food debris, instruct to hold suspension in mouth for several minutes before swallowing. When treating infants, swab medication on oral mucosa.

o

DRUG/CLASS/ CATEGORY	INDICATIONS/ DOSAGES	KEY NURSING CONSIDERATIONS
octreotide acetate Sandostatin *Synthetic octapeptide* *Somatostatin* *Somatotropic hormone* Preg. Risk Category: B	*Flushing and diarrhea associated with carcinoid tumors* — **Adults:** 100 to 600 mcg daily SC in 2 to 4 divided doses for first 2 wk of therapy, then dosage per response. *Watery diarrhea associated with vasoactive intestinal polypeptide secreting tumors* — **Adults:** 200 to 300 mcg daily SC in 2 to 4 divided doses for first 2 wk of therapy. *Acromegaly* — **Adults:** initially, 50 mcg SC tid, then adjusted according to somatomedin C levels q 2 wk.	▪ Monitor somatomedin C levels q 2 wk as ordered. ▪ Monitor thyroid function tests, urine 5-HIAA, plasma serotonin, and substance P. ▪ May be linked to development of cholelithiasis. ▪ Monitor closely for symptoms of glucose imbalance.
ofloxacin Floxin, Floxin IV *Fluoroquinolone* *Antibiotic* Preg. Risk Category: C	*Lower resp tract infections* — **Adults:** 400 mg IV or PO q 12 hr for 10 days. *Cervicitis or urethritis* — **Adults:** 300 mg IV or PO q 12 hr for 7 days. *Acute, uncomplicated gonorrhea* — **Adults:** 400 mg IV or PO as single dose with doxycycline. *Mild to moderate skin infections* — **Adults:** 400 mg IV or PO q 12 hr for 10 days. *Cystitis, UTI* — **Adults:** 200 mg IV or PO q 12 hr for 3 to 7 days. *Prostatitis* — **Adults:** 300 mg IV or PO q 12 hr for 6 wk. *Pelvic inflammatory disease (outpatient)* — **Adults:** 400 mg PO q 12 hr for 14 days.	▪ Use cautiously with dosage adjustment in renal failure, as prescribed. ▪ Patient treated for gonorrhea should have serologic test for syphilis. Drug not effective against syphilis; gonorrhea treatment may mask or delay symptoms of syphilis. ▪ Advise to take with plenty of fluids but not with meals. ▪ Instruct to stop drug and notify doctor if rash or other hypersensitivity signs occur. ▪ Advise to use sunscreen and wear protective clothing.

olanzapine
Zyprexa
Cholinergic
Antipsychotic
Preg. Risk Category: C

Psychotic disorders — **Adults:** initially, 5 to 10 mg PO qd. Dosage adjustments should occur at intervals of not less than 1 wk. Most patients respond to 10 mg/day. Don't exceed 20 mg/day.

- Monitor for signs of neuroleptic malignant syndrome. Stop drug immediately.
- Monitor for tardive dyskinesia.
- Obtain baseline and periodic liver function tests, as ordered.
- May impair body's ability to reduce core temperature. Warn against exposure to extreme heat.

olsalazine sodium
Dipentum
Salicylate
Anti-inflammatory
Preg. Risk Category: C

Maintenance of remission of ulcerative colitis in patients intolerant of sulfasalazine — **Adults:** 500 mg PO bid with meals.

- Regularly monitor BUN, creatinine, and urinalysis in preexisting renal disease.
- Administer in divided doses and with food to minimize adverse GI reactions.

omeprazole
Losec†, Prilosec
Substituted benzimidazole
Gastric acid suppressant
Preg. Risk Category: C

Severe erosive esophagitis; poorly responsive GERD — **Adults:** 20 mg PO daily for 4 to 8 wk.

Pathologic hypersecretory conditions — **Adults:** initially, 60 mg PO daily; titrate according to patient response. If daily dosage > 80 mg, give in divided doses.

Duodenal ulcer (short-term treatment) — **Adults:** 20 mg PO daily for 4 to 8 wk.

Short-term treatment of active benign gastric ulcer — **Adults:** 40 mg PO qd for 4 to 8 wk.

- Increases its own bioavailability with repeated dosages. Labile in gastric acid; less drug lost to hydrolysis because drug increases gastric pH.
- Caution not to perform hazardous activities if dizziness occurs.
- Instruct to swallow tablets whole.
- Advise to report signs and symptoms of overdose: confusion, drowsiness, blurred vision, tachycardia, nausea and vomiting, diaphoresis, dry mouth, and headache.

DRUG/CLASS/ CATEGORY	INDICATIONS/ DOSAGES	KEY NURSING CONSIDERATIONS
ondansetron hydrochloride Zofran *Serotonin (5-HT₃) receptor antagonist* *Antiemetic* Preg. Risk Category: B	*Prevention of nausea and vomiting associated with chemotherapy* — **Adults and children ≥ 12 yr:** 8 mg PO 30 min before chemotherapy. Then 8 mg PO 8 hr after first dose, then 8 mg q 12 hr for 1 to 2 days. Or, single dose of 32 mg by IV infusion over 15 min, given 30 min before chemotherapy; or 3 divided doses of 0.15 mg/kg IV given over 15 min, 4 and 8 hr after first dose (30 min before chemotherapy). **Children 4 to 12 yr:** 4 mg PO 30 min before chemotherapy. Follow with 4 mg q 8 hr for 1 to 2 days. Or, 3 doses of 0.15 mg/kg IV, given as for adults. *Prevention of nausea and vomiting associated with radiotherapy* — **Adults:** 8 mg PO tid.	■ Instruct to alert nurse immediately if difficulty breathing occurs after dose taken. ■ Tell patient receiving IV form to report discomfort at insert site promptly. ■ Generally well tolerated. Common adverse reactions include headache, malaise, dizziness, sedation, diarrhea or constipation, and musculoskeletal pain.
opium tincture opium tincture, camphorated (paregoric) *Opiate* *Antidiarrheal* Preg. Risk Category: NR Controlled Sub. Sched.: II (tincture) or III (camphorated)	*Acute diarrhea* — *tincture* — **Adults:** 0.6 ml (range 0.3 to 1 ml) PO qid. Max 6 ml daily. *camphorated tincture* — **Adults:** 5 to 10 ml PO qd, bid, tid, or qid until diarrhea subsides. **Children:** 0.25 to 0.5 ml/kg camphorated tincture PO qd, bid, tid, or qid until diarrhea subsides.	■ Mix with sufficient water to ensure passage to stomach. ■ For overdose, use narcotic antagonist naloxone, to reverse respiratory depression. ■ Opium content of tincture 25 times greater than that of camphorated tincture. Do not confuse the two. ■ Risk of physical dependence; don't use > 2 days.

oxacillin sodium
Bactocill, Prostaphlin

Penicillinase-resistant penicillin
Antibiotic
Preg. Risk Category: B

Infections caused by penicillinase-producing staphylococci — **Adults and children > 40 kg:** 500 mg to 1 g PO q 4 to 6 hr; or 2 to 12 g IM or IV. qd in divided doses q 4 to 6 hr. **Children ≤ 40 kg:** 50 to 100 mg/kg PO qd in divided doses q 6 hr; or 50 to 200 mg/kg IM or IV qd in divided doses q 4 to 6 hr.

- Obtain specimen for culture and sensitivity tests before first dose.
- Watch for superinfection.
- When given orally, give 1 to 2 hr before or 2 to 3 hr after meals.
- Give at least 1 hr before bacteriostatic antibiotics.

oxaprozin
Daypro

Nonsteroidal anti-inflammatory
Anti-inflammatory
Preg. Risk Category: C

Osteoarthritis or rheumatoid arthritis — **Adults:** initially, 600–1,200 mg PO daily. Then individualized to smallest effective dose. Max 1,800 mg or 26 mg/kg.

- May cause renal toxicity in susceptible patients. Closely monitor renal function.
- Elevated liver function tests can occur after chronic use.
- May mask signs of infection.

oxazepam
Alepam†, Serax, Zapex†

Benzodiazepine
Antianxiety agent/sedative-hypnotic
Preg. Risk Category: NR
Controlled Sub. Sched.: IV

Alcohol withdrawal, severe anxiety — **Adults:** 15 to 30 mg PO tid or qid. *Mild to moderate anxiety —* **Adults:** 10 to 15 mg PO tid or qid. **Geriatric patients:** initially 10 mg tid or qid, increased to 15 mg tid or qid prn.

- Use cautiously in elderly patients or in history of drug abuse.
- Monitor liver, renal, and hematopoietic function studies periodically.
- Possibility of abuse and addiction exists. Don't stop drug abruptly; withdrawal symptoms may occur.

oxiconazole nitrate
Oxistat

Ergosterol synthesis inhibitor
Antifungal agent
Preg. Risk Category: B

Tinea pedis, cruris, and tinea corporis caused by T. rubrum, T. mentagrophytes — **Adults:** apply to affected area qd or bid. Treat tinea cruris and tinea corporis for 2 wk and tinea pedis for 1 mo to minimize risk of recurrence.

- Not for ophth or vag administration.
- For external use only.
- Drug shouldn't touch eyes or vagina.
- Tell to stop drug and call doctor if local irritation occurs.

OXICONAZOLE NITRATE 229

†Canadian ‡Australian

DRUG/CLASS/CATEGORY	INDICATIONS/DOSAGES	KEY NURSING CONSIDERATIONS
oxycodone hydrochloride Endonet‡, Roxicodone, Roxicodone Intensol, Supeudol† **oxycodone pectinate** Proladone‡ *Opioid* *Analgesic* Preg. Risk Category: C Controlled Sub. Sched.: II	*Moderate to severe pain* — **Adults:** 5 mg PO q 6 hr, prn. Or, 1 to 3 supp rectally daily, prn.	▪ For full analgesic effect, administer before intense pain occurs. ▪ To minimize GI upset, give pc or with milk. ▪ Single-agent solution or tablets especially good for patients who shouldn't take aspirin or acetaminophen. ▪ Monitor circulatory and respiratory status. Withhold dose and notify doctor if respirations are shallow or if rate < 12. ▪ Monitor bladder and bowel patterns.
oxymetazoline hydrochloride Afrin, Allerest 12-Hr Nasal, Drixine Nasal‡, Neo-Synephrine 12 Hr *Sympathomimetic agent* *Decongestant/vasoconstrictor* Preg. Risk Category: NR	*Nasal congestion* — **Adults and children ≥ 6 yr:** 2 to 3 drops or sprays of 0.05% sol in each nostril bid. **Children 2 to 6 yr:** 2 to 3 drops of 0.025% sol in each nostril bid. Don't use > 3 to 5 days.	▪ Tell to hold head upright to minimize swallowing of drug, and then sniff spray briskly. ▪ Caution not to exceed recommended dosage and to use only when needed. ▪ Excessive use may cause bradycardia, hypotension, dizziness, and weakness. ▪ Should be used by only 1 person to prevent spread of infection.
oxymetazoline hydrochloride OcuClear, Visine L.R. *Sympathomimetic agent*	*Relief of eye redness due to minor eye irritations* — **Adults and children ≥ 6 yr:** 1 to 2 drops in conjunctival sac 2 to 4 times daily (spaced ≥ 6 hr apart).	▪ Don't use if solution cloudy or changes color. ▪ Wash hands before and after instilling. Don't touch dropper tip to eye or surrounding tissue.

Decongestant/vasoconstrictor
Preg. Risk Category: C

- Apply light finger pressure on lacrimal sac for 1 min after instillation.
- Advise to stop using and see doctor if eye pain occurs, vision changes, or redness or irritation continues, worsens, or lasts > 72 hr.

oxytocin, synthetic injection
Oxytocin, Pitocin, Syntocinon
Exogenous hormone
Oxytocic/lactation stimulant
Preg. Risk Category: NR

Induction or stimulation of labor — **Adults:** initially, 1-ml (10 units) ampule in 1,000 ml dextrose 5% inj or 0.9% NaCl sol IV infused at 1 to 2 milliunits/min. Rate increased in increments of not > 1 to 2 milliunits/min at 15- to 30-min intervals.
Reduction of postpartum bleeding after placenta expulsion — **Adults:** 10 to 40 units added to 1,000 ml D₅W or 0.9% NaCl sol infused at rate necessary to control bleeding, usually 20 to 40 milliunits/min. Also, 1 ml (10 units) can be given IM after placenta delivery.
Incomplete or inevitable abortion — **Adults:** 10 units IV in 500 ml 0.9% NaCl sol or dextrose 5% in 0.9% NaCl sol. Infuse at rate of 10 to 20 milliunits (20 to 40 drops)/min.

- **IV use:** Don't give by bolus injection. Administer by infusion only; give piggyback so drug may be discontinued without interrupting IV line. Use infusion pump.
- Monitor I&O. Antidiuretic effect may lead to fluid overload, seizures, and coma.
- Monitor and record uterine contractions, HR, BP, intrauterine pressure, fetal HR, and character of blood loss q 15 min.
- If contractions occur < 2 min apart and if contractions > 50 mm Hg recorded, or if contractions last ≥ 90 sec, stop infusion, turn patient on side, and notify doctor.

oxytocin, synthetic nasal solution
Syntocinon
Exogenous hormone
Oxytocic/lactation stimulant
Preg. Risk Category: X

Promotion of initial milk ejection — **Adults:** 1 spray into one or both nostrils 2 or 3 min before breast-feeding.

- Inspect nasal cavity for signs of irritation.
- Instruct to clear nasal passages first, then hold head vertically and, holding squeeze bottle upright, eject solution into nostril.
- Inform of adverse reactions and tell to notify doctor if severe.

OXYTOCIN, SYNTHETIC NASAL SOLUTION 231

†Canadian ‡Australian

DRUG / CLASS / CATEGORY	INDICATIONS / DOSAGES	KEY NURSING CONSIDERATIONS
paclitaxel Taxol *Novel antimicrotuble Antineoplastic* Preg. Risk Category: D	*Metastatic ovarian cancer after failure of 1st-line or subsequent chemotherapy* — **Adults:** 135 or 175 mg/m² IV over 3 hr q 3 wk. *Breast cancer after failure of combination chemotherapy for metastatic disease or relapse within 6 mo of adjuvant chemotherapy* — **Adults:** 175 mg/m² IV over 3 hr q 3 wk.	• Continuously monitor patient for 30 min after initiating infusion. Continue close monitoring throughout infusion. • Monitor blood counts during therapy. • Watch for signs of infection and bleeding. • Some patients have peripheral neuropathies, which may be cumulative and dose-related. Severe symptoms may require dose reduction.
pamidronate disodium Aredia *Bisphosphonate/pyrophosphate analogue Antihypercalcemic* Preg. Risk Category: C	*Moderate to severe hypercalcemia associated with cancer (with or without bone metastases)* — Patients with moderate hypercalcemia (CCa levels 12 to 13.5 mg/dl) may receive 60 to 90 mg by IV infusion over 4 hr for 60-mg dose and over 24 hr for 90-mg dose. Patients with severe hypercalcemia (CCa levels >13.5 mg/dl) may receive 90 mg by IV infusion over 24 hr. Min of 7 days before retreatment. *Moderate to severe Paget's disease* — **Adults:** 30 mg IV as 4-hr infusion on 3 days for total dose of 90 mg. Repeat as needed. *Osteolytic bone lesions of multiple myeloma in combination with standard antineoplastic therapy* — **Adults:** 90 mg IV infusion over 4 hr q 4 wk.	• Assess hydration status before treatment. Should be used while patient hydrated. • Give only by IV infusion. • Monitor serum electrolytes, especially calcium, phosphate, and magnesium. Also monitor creatinine, CBC and differential, Hct, and Hgb. • Carefully monitor patients with preexisting anemia, leukopenia, or thrombocytopenia during 1st 2 wk of therapy. • **IV use:** Reconstitute vial with 10 ml sterile water for injection. After completely dissolved, add to 1,000 ml 0.45% or 0.9% NaCl for injection or D₅W. Don't mix with infusion solutions that contain calcium. Inspect for precipitate before administering.

paromomycin sulfate

Humatin

Aminoglycoside

Antibacterial amebicide

Preg. Risk Category: C

Intestinal amebiasis, acute and chronic — **Adults and children:** 25 to 35 mg/kg daily PO in 3 doses with meals for 5 to 10 days. *Tapeworms (fish, beef, pork, dog) —* **Adults:** 1 g PO q 15 min for 4 doses. **Children:** 11 mg/kg PO q 15 min for 4 doses.

- Criterion of cure is absence of amoeba in stools examined weekly for 6 wk after treatment and thereafter at monthly intervals for 2 yr. Examine stools of family members or suspected contacts.
- Watch for signs of superinfection.

---

paroxetine hydrochloride

Paxil

Selective serotonin reuptake inhibitor

Antidepressant

Preg. Risk Category: B

Depression — **Adults:** initially, 20 mg PO daily, in morning. If no response, may increase in 10-mg/day increments to max 50 mg daily. **Elderly or debilitated patients, patients with severe hepatic or renal disease:** initially, 10 mg PO daily, in morning. If no response, may increase in 10-mg/day increments to max 40 mg daily. *Panic disorder —* **Adults:** initially, 10 mg/ day. May increase in 10-mg/wk increments. Max dosage ≤ 60 mg/day.

- If psychosis occurs or increases, expect to reduce dosage.
- Monitor for suicidal tendencies, and allow only minimum drug supply.
- Warn to avoid hazardous activities until CNS effects known.
- Inform that orthostatic hypotension may occur. Supervise walking. Advise to get out of bed slowly.

---

pegaspargase (PEG-L-asparaginase)

Oncaspar

Modified version of enzyme L-asparaginase

Antineoplastic

Preg. Risk Category: C

Acute lymphoblastic leukemia in patients who require L-asparaginase but have developed hypersensitivity to native forms — **Adults and children with BSA ≥ 0.6 m²:** 2,500 IU/m² IM or IV q 14 days. **Children with BSA < 0.6 m²:** 82.5 IU/kg IM or IV q 14 days.

- When giving IM, limit volume administered at single injection site to 2 ml.
- When giving IV, administer over 1 to 2 hr in 100 ml 0.9% NaCl or dextrose 5% injection through infusion already running.
- Handle with care. Gloves recommended. Avoid vapor inhalation and contact with skin or mucous membranes. In case of contact, wash with water for ≥ 15 min.

PEGASPARGASE 233

DRUG/CLASS/ CATEGORY	INDICATIONS/ DOSAGES	KEY NURSING CONSIDERATIONS
pemoline Cylert, Cylert Chewable *Oxazolidinedione deriva-tive/CNS stimulant* *Analeptic* Preg. Risk Category: B Controlled Sub. Sched.: IV	*Attention deficit hyperactivity disorder (ADHD)* — **Children ≥ 6 yr:** initially, 37.5 mg PO in morning with daily dosage raised by 18.75 mg weekly, prn. Effective dosage range 56.25 to 75 mg daily; max 112.5 mg daily.	• LFTs should be done before and during therapy. Drug should be given only to pa-tients without liver dysfunction and with normal baseline LFTs. • May induce Tourette syndrome in children. • Advise to take at least 6 hr before bedtime to avoid sleep interference.
penbutolol sulfate Levatol, Lobetat *Beta-adrenergic blocker* *Antihypertensive* Preg. Risk Category: C	*Mild to moderate hypertension* — **Adults:** 20 mg PO qd. Usually given with other anti-hypertensives, such as thiazide diuretics.	• Check apical pulse before giving. If ex-treme, withhold dose and call doctor. • Monitor BP, ECG, and heart rate often. • Tell not to stop drug suddenly but to notify doctor if adverse reactions occur. • May mask hypoglycemia.
penicillin G benzathine (benzylpenicillin benzathine) Bicillin L-A, Permapen *Natural penicillin* *Antibiotic* Preg. Risk Category: B	*Congenital syphilis* — **Children < 2 yr:** 50,000 units/kg IM once. *Group A strep up-per resp infections* — **Adults:** 1.2 million units IM once. **Children > 27 kg:** 900,000 units IM once. **Children < 27 kg:** 300,000 to 600,000 units IM once. *Prophylaxis of post-streptococcal rheumatic fever* — **Adults and children:** 1.2 million units IM q mo or 600,000 units twice monthly. *Syphilis* — **Adults:** 2.4 million units IM once (< 1-yr du-ration), or q wk for 3 wk (> 1-yr duration).	• Obtain specimen for culture and sensitivity tests before first dose. • Never give IV. Inject deeply into upper out-er quadrant of buttocks in adults; in mid-lateral thigh in infants and small children. Avoid injection into or near major nerves or blood vessels. • Give at least 1 hr before bacteriostatic an-tibiotics. • With large doses and prolonged therapy, superinfection may occur.

penicillin G potassium (benzylpenicillin potassium) Megacillin†, Pfizerpen *Natural penicillin* *Antibiotic* Preg. Risk Category: B	*Moderate to severe systemic infection —* **Adults and children ≥ 12 yr:** individualized; 1.6 to 3.2 million units PO qd in divided doses q 6 hr; 1.2 to 24 million units IM or IV qd in divided doses q 4 hr. **Children < 12 yr:** 25,000 to 100,000 units/kg PO qd in divided doses q 6 hr; or 25,000 to 400,000 units/kg IM or IV qd in divided doses q 4 hr.	• Obtain specimen for culture and sensitivity tests before first dose. • Monitor renal function closely. • Give 1 to 2 hr before or 2 to 3 hr after meals. Food may interfere with absorption. • Give at least 1 hr before bacteriostatic antibiotics.
penicillin G procaine (benzylpenicillin procaine) Ayercillin†, Crysticillin 300 A.S., Wycillin *Natural penicillin* *Antibiotic* Preg. Risk Category: B	*Moderate to severe systemic infection —* **Adults:** 600,000 to 1.2 million units IM qd in single dose. **Children > 1 mo:** 25,000 to 50,000 units/kg IM qd in single dose. *Uncomplicated gonorrhea —* **Adults and children > 12 yr:** 1 g probenecid PO; after 30 min, 4.8 million units IM, divided between 2 sites. *Pneumococcal pneumonia —* **Adults and children > 12 yr:** 600,000 to 1.2 million units IM qd for 7 to 10 days.	• Obtain specimen for culture and sensitivity tests before first dose. • Never give IV. • Give deep IM in upper outer quadrant of buttocks in adults; in midlateral thigh in small children. Don't give SC. Don't massage injection site. Avoid injection near major nerves or blood vessels.
penicillin G sodium (benzylpenicillin sodium) Crystapen† *Natural penicillin* *Antibiotic* Preg. Risk Category: B	*Moderate to severe systemic infection —* **Adults and children ≥ 12 yr:** 1.2 to 24 million units daily IM or IV in divided doses q 4 to 6 hr. **Children < 12 yr:** 25,000 to 400,000 units/kg daily IM or IV in divided doses q 6 hr.	• Obtain specimen for culture and sensitivity tests before first dose. • For patients receiving ≥ 10 million units daily, dilute in 1 to 2 L of compatible solution and give over 24 hr. Otherwise, give by intermittent IV infusion: Dilute drug in 50 to 100 ml, and give over 1 to 2 hr. • Give at least 1 hr before bacteriostatic antibiotics.

235

PENICILLIN G SODIUM

†Canadian ‡Australian

DRUG/CLASS/ CATEGORY	INDICATIONS/ DOSAGES	KEY NURSING CONSIDERATIONS
penicillin V (phenoxyethylpenicillin) **penicillin V potassium (phenoxyethylpenicillin potassium)** Abbocillin, VK, Pen Vee K *Natural penicillin* *Antibiotic* Preg. Risk Category: B	*Mild to moderate systemic infections* — **Adults and children ≥ 12 yr:** 250 to 500 mg (400,000 to 800,000 U) PO q 6 hr. **Children < 12 yr:** 15 to 62.5 mg/kg (25,000 to 100,000 U/kg) PO qd, in divided doses q 6 to 8 hr. *Endocarditis prophylaxis for dental surgery* — **Adults:** 2 g PO 30 to 60 min before procedure; then 1 g 6 hr after. **Children < 30 kg:** ½ adult dose.	▪ Obtain information about past allergic reactions to penicillins. ▪ Obtain specimen for culture and sensitivity tests before giving first dose. ▪ Give penicillin V at least 1 hr before bacteriostatic antibiotics. ▪ Regularly assess renal and hematopoietic function in patients on prolonged therapy. ▪ Observe for superinfection. ▪ AHA considers drug as alternative to amoxicillin for endocarditis prophylaxis.
pentamidine isethionate NebuPent, Pentacarinat *Diamidine derivative* *Antiprotozoal* Preg. Risk Category: C	*Pneumocystis carinii pneumonia* — **Adults and children:** 3 to 4 mg/kg IV or IM qd for 14 to 21 days. *Prevention of* P. carinii *pneumonia in high-risk individuals* — **Adults:** 300 mg by inhalation q 4 wk.	▪ Administer aerosol form only by Respirgard II nebulizer. ▪ Don't mix with other drugs. ▪ Monitor blood glucose, serum calcium, serum creatinine, and BUN daily.
pentazocine hydrochloride Fortral‡, Talwin† **pentazocine hydrochloride and naloxone hydrochloride** Talwin-Nx	*Moderate to severe pain* — **Adults:** 50 to 100 mg PO q 3 to 4 hr, prn. Max oral dosage 600 mg/day. Or, 30 mg IM, IV, or SC q 3 to 4 hr, prn. Max parenteral dosage 360 mg/day. Single doses > 30 mg IV or 60 mg IM or SC not recommended.	▪ Have naloxone available. ▪ May trigger withdrawal syndrome in narcotic-dependent patients. ▪ Psychological and physical dependence may occur with prolonged use.

pentazocine lactate

Fortral‡, Talwin
Narcotic agonist-antagonist/ opioid partial agonist
Analgesic/adjunct to anesthesia
Preg. Risk Category: C
Controlled Sub. Sched.: IV

Labor — **Adults:** 30 mg IM or 20 mg IV q 2 to 3 hr with regular contractions.

- Talwin-Nx contains naloxone. This prevents illicit IV use.

pentobarbital (pentobarbitone)

Nembutal

pentobarbital Na

Carbrital‡, Nembutal Sodium, Nova Rectal†
Barbiturate
Anticonvulsant/sedative-hypnotic
Preg. Risk Category: D (suppositories C)
Controlled Sub. Sched.: II (suppositories III)

Sedation — **Adults:** 20 to 40 mg PO bid, tid, or qid. **Children:** 2 to 6 mg/kg daily PO in 3 divided doses. Max 100 mg daily.
Insomnia — **Adults:** 100 to 200 mg PO hs or 150 to 200 mg deep IM: 100 mg initially IV, then additional doses up to 500 mg; 120 or 200 mg PR. **Children:** 2 to 6 mg/kg or 125 mg/m² IM. Max 100 mg. **For child 2 mo to 1 yr,** 30 mg PR; **1 yr to 4 yr,** 30 or 60 mg; **5 to 11 yr,** 60 mg; **12 to 14 yr,** 60 or 120 mg.
Preop sedation — **Adults:** 150 to 200 mg IM. **Children:** 5 mg/kg PO or IM ≥10 yr; 5 mg/kg IM or rectally if < 10 yr.

- **IV use:** May cause severe respiratory depression, laryngospasm, or hypotension. Have emergency resuscitation equipment available.
- Watch for signs of barbiturate toxicity.
- Assess mental status before starting therapy. Elderly patients more sensitive to adverse CNS effects.
- Inspect skin. Discontinue if skin reactions occur and call doctor. In some patients, high fever, stomatitis, headache, or rhinitis may precede skin reactions.

pentoxifylline

Trental
Xanthine derivative
Hemorheologic agent
Preg. Risk Category: C

Intermittent claudication caused by chronic occlusive vascular disease — **Adults:** 400 mg PO tid with meals. May decrease to 400 mg bid if adverse GI and CNS effects occur.

- Elderly patients may be more sensitive to effects.
- Instruct to swallow medication whole.

PENTOXIFYLLINE 237

†Canadian ‡Australian

DRUG/CLASS/ CATEGORY	INDICATIONS/ DOSAGES	KEY NURSING CONSIDERATIONS
pergolide mesylate Permax *Dopaminergic agonist* *Antiparkinson agent* Preg. Risk Category: B	*Adjunctive treatment with carbidopa-levodopa in management of Parkinson's disease* — **Adults:** initially, 0.05 mg PO daily for first 2 days, then increase to 0.1 to 0.15 mg every third day over 12 days. Subsequent dosage increased by 0.25 mg every third day, if needed, until optimum response seen. Usually given in divided doses tid.	• Monitor BP. Symptomatic orthostatic or sustained hypotension may occur, especially at start of therapy. • Advise of potential adverse reactions, especially hallucinations and confusion. • Warn to avoid activities that could result in injury from orthostatic hypotension and syncope.
perphenazine Apo-Perphenazine†, PMS Perphenazine†, Trilafon, Trilafon Concentrate *Phenothiazine (piperazine derivative)* *Antipsychotic/antiemetic* Preg. Risk Category: NR	*Psychosis in nonhospitalized patients* — **Adults:** initially, 4 to 8 mg PO tid, reduced as soon as possible to minimum effective dosage. **Children > 12 yr:** lowest adult dose. *Psychosis in hospitalized patients* — **Adults:** initially, 8 to 16 mg PO bid, tid, or qid, increased to 64 mg daily, prn. Or, 5 to 10 mg IM q 6 hr, prn. Max 30 mg. **Children > 12 yr:** lowest adult dose. *Severe nausea and vomiting* — **Adults:** 8 to 16 mg PO daily in divided doses to max 24 mg. Or, 5 to 10 mg IM, prn. May give IV, diluted to 0.5 mg/ml with 0.9% NaCl solution. Max 5 mg.	• Obtain baseline BP before therapy and monitor regularly. Watch for orthostatic hypotension. Keep patient supine for 1 hr after administration; tell to change positions slowly. • Monitor for tardive dyskinesia. • Assess for neuroleptic malignant syndrome. • Acute dystonic reactions may be treated with diphenhydramine. • Monitor weekly bilirubin tests during 1st month; periodic CBC, liver function, and ophthalmic tests (long-term use), as ordered. • Don't withdraw abruptly unless required by severe adverse reactions. • Keep drug away from skin and clothes. Wear gloves to prepare liquid forms.

phenazopyridine hydrochloride (phenylazo diamino pyridine hydrochloride)
Azo-Standard, Baridium, Phenazot, Pyrazodine, Pyridium
Azo dye
Urinary analgesic
Preg. Risk Category: B

Pain with urinary tract irritation or infection — **Adults:** 200 mg PO tid after meals for 2 days. **Children:** 12 mg/kg PO daily in 3 equal doses after meals for 2 days.

- Caution to stop taking drug and notify doctor if skin or sclera sclerae yellow-tinged.
- When used with antibacterial agent, therapy shouldn't last > 2 days.
  - Advise to take with meals.
- Tell diabetic that drug may after Clinistix or Tes-Tape results. Instruct to use Clinitest for accurate urine glucose results. Also inform that drug may interfere with urinary ketone tests (Acetest or Ketostix).
- Advise that drug turns urine red or orange and may stain fabrics or contact lenses.

phenobarbital (phenobarbitone)
Ancalixirt, Barbita, Solfoton
phenobarbital sodium (phenobarbitone sodium)
Luminal Sodium
Barbiturate
Anticonvulsant/sedative-hypnotic
Preg. Risk Category: D
Controlled Sub. Sched.: IV

All forms of epilepsy; febrile seizures —
Adults: 60 to 200 mg PO daily in divided doses tid or as single dose hs. **Children:** 3 to 6 mg/kg PO daily, usually divided q 12 hr. Can give qd, usually hs.
Status epilepticus — **Adults:** 200 to 600 mg IV. **Children:** 100 to 400 mg IV. Max 50 mg/min.
Sedation — **Adults:** 30 to 120 mg PO daily in 2 or 3 divided doses. **Children:** 3 to 5 mg/kg PO daily in divided doses tid.
Insomnia — **Adults:** 100 to 200 mg PO or IM hs.
Prep sedation — **Adults:** 100 to 200 mg IM 60 to 90 min before surgery. **Children:** 16 to 100 mg IM or 1 to 3 mg/kg IV, IM, or PO 60 to 90 min before surgery.

- **IV use:** IV injection for emergencies only. Give slowly under close supervision. Monitor respirations closely. Don't give > 60 mg/min. Have resuscitation equipment available.
- Watch for signs of barbiturate toxicity; overdose can be fatal.
- Don't stop abruptly; seizures may worsen. Call doctor if adverse reactions develop.
- Therapeutic blood levels 15 to 40 mcg/ml.

PHENOBARBITAL SODIUM   239

†Canadian ‡Australian

DRUG / CLASS / CATEGORY	INDICATIONS / DOSAGES	KEY NURSING CONSIDERATIONS
phentermine hydrochloride Fastin, Obe-Mar, Panshape M, Phentercot, Phentride *Amphetamine congener* *Short-term adjunctive anorexigenic agent/indirect acting sympathomimetic amine* Preg. Risk Category: X	*Short-term adjunct in exogenous obesity* — **Adults:** 8 mg PO tid ½ hr before meals. Or, 15 to 30 mg (resin complex) or 15 to 37.5 mg (hydrochloride) PO daily as single dose in morning.	• Use in conjunction with weight-reduction program. • Monitor for tolerance or dependence. • Tell to take at least 6 hr before bedtime to avoid sleep interference.
phentolamine mesylate Regitine, Rogitine† *Alpha-adrenergic blocker* *Antihypertensive agent for pheochromocytoma/cutaneous vasodilator* Preg. Risk Category: C	*To aid pheochromocytoma diagnosis; to control or prevent hypertension before or during pheochromocytomectomy* — **Adults:** IV diagnostic dose 2.5 mg. Before tumor removal, 5 mg IM or IV. During surgery, may give 5 mg IV. **Children:** IV diagnostic dose 1 mg. Before tumor removal, 1 mg IV or IM. During surgery, may give 1 mg IV. *Dermal necrosis and sloughing after IV extravasation of norepinephrine* — **Adults and children:** infiltrate with 5 to 10 mg in 10 ml 0.9% NaCl solution, or half through infiltrated IV and other half around site. Must be done within 12 hr.	• When given to diagnose pheochromocytoma, take BP first; monitor BP frequently during administration. Positive for pheochromocytoma if IV test dose causes severe hypotension. • Don't administer epinephrine to treat phentolamine-induced hypotension. Use norepinephrine instead. • Explain why and how drug is administered. • Tell to report adverse reactions.

- Use CV catheter or large vein to minimize extravasation. Use continuous infusion pump to regulate infusion flow rate.
- With prolonged IV infusions, avoid abrupt withdrawal. During infusion, frequently monitor ECG, BP, HR, cardiac output, CVP, PAWP, urine output, and color and temperature of extremities.
- To treat extravasation, infiltrate site promptly with phentolamine.

phenylephrine hydrochloride
Neo-Synephrine
Adrenergic
Vasoconstrictor
Preg. Risk Category: C

Mild to moderate hypotension — **Adults:** 2 to 5 mg SC or IM; repeated in 1 to 2 hr prn. Initial dose ≤ 5 mg. Alternatively, 0.1 to 0.5 mg by slow IV: repeat 10 to 15 min. **Children:** 0.1 mg/kg IM or SC; repeated in 1 to 2 hr prn.

Severe hypotension and shock — **Adults:** 10 mg in 250 to 500 ml D₅W or 0.9% NaCl. Start IV infusion at 100 to 180 mcg/min; decrease to maintenance infusion of 40 to 60 mcg/min when BP stabilizes.

- Wash hands before and after instilling. Apply light finger pressure on lacrimal sac for 1 min after drops instilled.
- Tell not to use brown solutions or solutions that contain precipitate.
- Monitor BP and pulse rate.
- Advise to contact doctor if condition persists > 12 hr after drug stopped.

phenylephrine hydrochloride
AK-Dilate, AK-Nefrin Ophthalmic, Isopto Frin, Mydfrin, Neo-Synephrine
Adrenergic
Vasoconstrictor
Preg. Risk Category: C

Mydriasis without cycloplegia — **Adults and children:** 1 drop of 2.5% or 10% sol instilled before use. May repeat in 1 hr.

Mydriasis and vasoconstriction — **Adults and adolescents:** 1 drop 2.5% or 10% sol. **Children:** 1 drop 2.5% sol.

Chronic mydriasis — **Adults and adolescents:** 1 drop 2.5% or 10% sol bid or tid. **Children:** 1 drop 2.5% sol bid or tid.

- Tell to hold head upright to minimize swallowing of medication, and then to sniff spray briskly. After use, rinse tip of spray with hot water and dry with clean tissue.
- Tell not to exceed recommended dosage and to use only when needed.
- Advise to contact doctor if symptoms persist beyond 3 days.

phenylephrine hydrochloride
Alconefrin, Neo-Synephrine, Sinex
Adrenergic
Vasoconstrictor
Preg. Risk Category: NR

Nasal congestion — **Adults and children ≥ 12 yr:** 1 to 2 sprays in nostril or small amount of jelly to nasal mucosa q 4 hr. Don't use > 3 to 5 days. **Children 6 to 12 yr:** 1 to 2 sprays of 0.25% sol in nostril q 4 hr. **Children < 6 yr:** 2 to 3 drops of 0.125% sol q 4 hr.

PHENYLEPHRINE HYDROCHLORIDE   241

†Canadian ‡Australian

DRUG / CLASS / CATEGORY	INDICATIONS / DOSAGES	KEY NURSING CONSIDERATIONS
phenytoin (diphenylhydan-toin) Dilantin, Dilantin Infatabs **phenytoin sodium** Dilantin, Phenytex **phenytoin sodium (extended)** Dilantin Kapseals *Hydantoin derivative* Anticonvulsant Preg. Risk Category: NR	*Control of tonic-clonic and complex partial seizures* — **Adults:** 100 mg PO tid, increased in increments of 100 mg PO q 2 to 4 wk until desired response obtained. **Children:** 5 mg/kg or 250 mg/m² PO divided bid or tid. Max 300 mg daily. *For patients requiring loading dose* — **Adults:** initially, 1 g PO daily divided into 3 doses given at 2-hr intervals. Or, 10 to 15 mg/kg IV at rate not > 50 mg/min. Start normal maintenance dosage 24 hr later. **Children:** 5 mg/kg/day PO in 2 or 3 equally divided doses with later dosage individualized to max 300 mg daily. *Status epilepticus* — **Adults:** loading dose 10 to 15 mg/kg IV at rate not > 50 mg/min, then maintenance doses of 100 mg PO or IV q 6 to 8 hr. **Children:** loading dose 15 to 20 mg/kg IV, at rate not > 1 to 3 mg/kg/min, then individualized maintenance dosages.	• Extravasation has caused severe local tissue damage. Avoid administering by IV push into veins on back of hand. Inject into larger veins or central venous catheter if available. • Check vital signs, BP, and ECG during IV administration. Monitor blood levels. Therapeutic level 10 to 20 mcg/ml. Monitor CBC and serum calcium level q 6 mo, and periodically monitor hepatic function. • Advise to avoid hazardous activities until CNS effects known. • Inform that drug may color urine pink, red, or reddish brown.
phytonadione (vitamin K₁) AquaMEPHYTON, Konakion, Mephyton	*Hypoprothrombinemia secondary to vitamin K malabsorption, drug therapy, or excessive vitamin A dosage* — **Adults:** 2.5 to 10 mg PO, SC, or IM; repeat and increase up to 50 mg. **Infants:** 2 mg PO, IM, or SC. **Children:** 5 to 10 mg PO, IM, or SC.	• *IV use:* Give IV by slow infusion over 2 to 3 hr. Rate ≤ 1 mg/min in adults. • For IM use in adults and older children, inject in upper outer quadrant of buttocks; for infants, inject in anterolateral aspect of thigh or deltoid region.

Vitamin K *Blood coagulation modifier* Preg. Risk Category: C	*Hypoprothrombinemia secondary to effect of oral anticoagulants* — **Adults:** 2.5 to 10 mg PO, SC, or IM based on PT and INR. In emergency, 10 to 50 mg slow IV, rate ≤ 1 mg/min, repeated q 4 hr, prn.	• Monitor PT and INR to determine effectiveness. • Watch for flushing, weakness, tachycardia, and hypotension. • If severe bleeding occurs, don't delay other measures such as blood products. • Protect parenteral products from light.
pilocarpine Ocusert Pilo **pilocarpine hydrochloride** Adsorbocarpine, Isopto Carpine, Miocarpine†, Pilocar, Pilopt‡ **pilocarpine nitrate** Pilagan, P.V. *Cholinergic agonist* *Miotic* Preg. Risk Category: C	*Primary open-angle glaucoma* — **Adults and children:** 1 drop instilled up to qid, or 1-cm ribbon of 4% gel (Pilopine HS) applied hs. Or, 1 Ocusert Pilo system (20 or 40 mcg/hr) applied q 7 days. *Emergency treatment of acute angle-closure glaucoma* — **Adults and children:** 1 drop of 2% sol instilled q 5 to 10 min for 3 to 6 doses, followed by 1 drop q 1 to 3 hr until pressure controlled. *Mydriasis caused by mydriatic or cycloplegic agents* — **Adults and children:** 1 drop 1% sol.	• Instruct to apply gel hs. Warn to avoid hazardous activities until temporary blurring subsides. • Apply light finger pressure on lacrimal sac for 1 min afterward. • If Ocusert Pilo system falls out of eye during sleep, tell to wash hands, rinse insert in cool tap water, and reposition in eye. • Inform that transient brow pain and myopia common at first but usually disappear within 10 to 14 days. • Patient with dark eyes may need stronger solutions.
pimozide Orap *Diphenylbutylpiperidine* *Antipsychotic* Preg. Risk Category: C	*Suppression of motor and phonic tics in Tourette syndrome refractory to first-line therapy* — **Adults and children > 12 yr:** initially, 1 to 2 mg PO daily in divided doses, then increased qod, prn. Maintenance dose < 0.2 mg/kg/day or 10 mg/day, whichever less. Max 10 mg daily.	• Perform ECG before treatment begins and periodically thereafter, as ordered. Monitor for prolonged QT interval. • Monitor for tardive dyskinesia. Acute dystonic reactions may be treated with diphenhydramine. • May lower seizure threshold.

†Canadian ‡Australian

DRUG/CLASS/CATEGORY	INDICATIONS/DOSAGES	KEY NURSING CONSIDERATIONS
pindolol Apo-Pindol†, Barbloc‡, Visken *Beta-adrenergic blocker* *Antihypertensive* Preg. Risk Category: B	*Hypertension* — **Adults:** initially, 5 mg PO bid. Increase as needed and tolerated to max 60 mg daily.	▪ Check apical pulse before giving. If extreme, withhold dose and call doctor. ▪ Monitor BP frequently. ▪ Withdraw over 1 to 2 wk after long-term therapy, as ordered. ▪ Masks certain signs of hypoglycemia.
piperacillin sodium Pipracil, Pipril† *Extended-spectrum peni-* *cillin/acylaminopenicillin* *Antibiotic* Preg. Risk Category: B	*Systemic infections caused by susceptible strains of gram-pos and especially gram-neg organisms* — **Adults and children > 12 yr:** 100 to 300 mg/kg IV or IM daily in divided doses q 4 to 6 hr, max 24 g daily. *Prophylaxis of surgical infections* — **Adults:** 2 g IV 30 to 60 min before surgery.	▪ Obtain specimen for culture and sensitivity tests before first dose. ▪ Monitor for superinfection. ▪ Give ≥ 1 hr before bacteriostatic antibiotics. ▪ Monitor serum potassium. ▪ Alter dosage as ordered in impaired renal function.
piperacillin sodium and tazobactam sodium Zosyn *Extended-spectrum peni-* *cillin/beta-lactamase in-* *hibitor* *Antibiotic* Preg. Risk Category: B	*Appendicitis, skin and skin-structure infections, postpartum endometritis or PID, moderately severe community-acquired pneumonia* — **Adults:** 3 g piperacillin and 0.375 g tazobactam IV q 6 hr. *In renal impairment* — **Adults:** if creatinine clearance 20 to 40 ml/min, 2 g piperacillin and 0.25 g tazobactam IV q 6 hr; if < 20 ml/min, 2 g piperacillin and 0.25 g tazobactam IV q 8 hr. *Moderate to severe nosocomial pneumonia* — **Adults:** initially, 3.375 g IV over 30 min q 4 hr. Give with aminoglycoside.	▪ Obtain specimen for culture and sensitivity tests before first dose. ▪ Superinfection may occur, especially in elderly, debilitated, or immunosuppressed patients. Observe closely. ▪ Infuse over ≥ 30 min. Don't mix with other drugs. Discard unused drug after 24 hr if stored at room temp; after 48 hr if refrigerated. Once diluted, drug stable for 24 hr at room temp for 1 wk if refrigerated.

pirbuterol

Maxair, Maxair Autohaler

Beta-adrenergic agonist

Bronchodilator

Preg. Risk Category: C

Prevention and reversal of bronchospasm, asthma — **Adults and children ≥ 12 yr:** 1 or 2 inhalations (0.2 to 0.4 mg) repeated q 4 to 6 hr. Max 12 inhalations daily.

- If > 1 inhalation ordered, tell to wait at least 2 min before repeating procedure.
- If patient also using steroid inhaler, instruct to use bronchodilator first, then wait 5 min before using steroid.

piroxicam

Apo-Piroxicam†, Feldene, Novo-Pirocam†

Nonsteroidal anti-inflammatory

Nonnarcotic analgesic/antipyretic/anti-inflammatory

Preg. Risk Category: NR

Osteoarthritis and rheumatoid arthritis — **Adults:** 20 mg PO daily. If desired, may divide dosage bid.

- May lead to reversible renal impairment. Monitor closely.
- Check renal, hepatic, and auditory function and CBC periodically during prolonged therapy. If abnormalities occur, discontinue and notify doctor.
- May mask infection.

plicamycin (mithramycin)

Mithracin

Antibiotic antineoplastic

(cell cycle–phase nonspecific)

Antineoplastic/hypocalcemic agent

Preg. Risk Category: X

Dosage and indications vary. Check treatment protocol with doctor.

Hypercalcemia and hypercalciuria associated with advanced malignant disease — **Adults:** 25 mcg/kg/day IV for 3 to 4 days. Repeat dosage at weekly intervals until desired response seen.

Testicular cancer — **Adults:** 25 to 30 mcg/kg/day IV for 8 to 10 days or until toxicity occurs. Course of therapy > 10 days not recommended.

- To reduce nausea, administer infusion slowly and give antiemetic before administering.
- Vesicant. If solution extravasates, stop immediately, notify doctor, and use ice packs. Restart IV line.
- Monitor platelets and PT. Discontinue and notify doctor if WBC count < 4,000/mm³, platelet count < 150,000/mm³, or PT > 4 sec longer than control.
- Facial flushing early sign of bleeding.
- Monitor for tetany, carpopedal spasm, Chvostek's sign, and muscle cramps; check serum calcium level.

DRUG/CLASS/ CATEGORY	INDICATIONS/ DOSAGES	KEY NURSING CONSIDERATIONS
pneumococcal vaccine, polyvalent Pneumovax 23 *Vaccine* *Bacterial vaccine* Preg. Risk Category: C	*Pneumococcal immunization* — **Adults and children ≥ 2 yr:** 0.5 ml IM or SC. Not recommended for children < 2 yr.	• Check immunization history to avoid revaccination within 3 yr. • Obtain history of allergies and reaction to immunization. Egg protein not used during manufacture; contains phenol. • Keep epinephrine 1:1,000 available. • Inject in deltoid or midlateral thigh.
poliovirus vaccine, live, oral, trivalent (TOPV) Orimune *Vaccine* *Viral vaccine* Preg. Risk Category: C	*Poliovirus immunization (TOPV)* — **Children and nonimmunized adults:** 0.5 ml PO, then 0.5 ml in 6 to 8 wk, then 0.5 ml 6 to 12 mo later. Give 0.5 ml before school entry. **Infants:** 0.5 ml PO at 2, 4, and 18 mo. *Poliovirus immunization (IPV)* — **Adults:** 0.5 ml SC, then 2nd dose in 4 to 8 wk. 3rd dose in 6 to 12 mo. **Children:** 0.5 ml SC at 2 mo and 4 mo. 3rd dose at 15 to 18 mo. Give dose of 0.5 ml SC before school entry.	• Obtain history of allergies and reaction to immunization. • Don't administer oral form parenterally. • Keep TOPV frozen until used. Once thawed, if unopened, may refrigerate up to 30 days; if opened, up to 7 days. Thaw before administration. • Parenteral form should be given to patients with altered immune status. • Don't administer to neonates < 6 wk.
poliovirus vaccine, inactivated (IPV) IPOL, Poliovax *Vaccine* *Viral vaccine* Preg. Risk Category: C		
polyethylene glycol and electrolyte solution Colovage, GoLYTELY *Polyethylene glycol 3350 nonabsorbable solution* *Bowel evacuant* Preg. Risk Category: C	*Bowel preparation before GI exam* — **Adults:** 240 ml PO q 10 min until 4 L consumed or until watery stool clear. Typically, give 4 hr before exam, allowing 3 hr for drinking and 1 hr for bowel evacuation.	• Use tap water to reconstitute powder. Shake vigorously. Refrigerate reconstituted solution; use within 48 hr. • Administer early in a.m. for midmorning exam. Orally administered solution induces diarrhea that rapidly cleans bowel, usually within 4 hr.

polymyxin B sulfate

Aerosporin
Polymyxin antibiotic
Antibiotic
Preg. Risk Category: B

Meningitis caused by sensitive organisms — **Adults and children > 2 yr:** 50,000 units intrathecally qd for 3 or 4 days, then 50,000 units qod for at least 2 wk after CSF tests negative and CSF glucose level normal. **Children < 2 yr:** 20,000 units intrathecally qd for 3 or 4 days, then 25,000 units qod for at least 2 wk after CSF tests negative and CSF glucose level normal.

- Obtain culture and sensitivity tests before first dose.
- Extremely nephrotoxic. Monitor renal function before and during therapy. Fluid intake should be sufficient to maintain output of 1,500 ml/day.
- May prolong neuromuscular blockade; notify anesthesiologist about preop treatment.

polymyxin B sulfate

Aerosporin
Polymyxin antibiotic
Ophthalmic antibiotic
Preg. Risk Category: C

Used alone or with other agents to treat superficial eye infections involving conjunctiva and cornea resulting from infection with Pseudomonas or other gram-neg organism — **Adults and children:** 1 to 3 drops of 0.1% to 0.25% (10,000 to 25,000 units/ml) instilled q hr. Increase interval according to response; or up to 10,000 units injected subconjunctivally daily.

- Clean eye before application. Wash hands before and after administering. Don't touch dropper tip to eye or surrounding tissue.
- Apply light pressure to lacrimal sac for 1 min after drops instilled.
- Advise to report itching lids, swelling, or constant burning.
- Tell not to share drug, washcloths, or towels with family members; notify doctor if anyone in household develops same symptoms.

potassium bicarbonate

K-Gen ET, K-Ide,
Klor-Con/EF, K-Lyte
Potassium supplement
Therapeutic agent for electrolyte balance
Preg. Risk Category: NR

Hypokalemia — **Adults:** 25 to 50 mEq dissolved in half-glass to full glass of water (120 to 240 ml) qd to qid.

- Dissolve tablets in 6 to 8 oz (180 to 240 ml) cold water.
- Monitor BUN, serum potassium and creatinine, and I&O.
- Tell to take with meals and sip slowly.
- Warn not to use salt substitutes, except with doctor's permission.

†Canadian ‡Australian

DRUG/CLASS/CATEGORY	INDICATIONS/DOSAGES	KEY NURSING CONSIDERATIONS
potassium chloride K+10, Kaochlor 10%, K-Dur, K-Lyte/Cl, K-Tab, Slow-K *Potassium supplement* *Therapeutic agent for electrolyte balance* Preg. Risk Category: C	*Hypokalemia* — **Adults:** 40 to 100 mEq PO daily in 3 or 4 divided doses or 10 to 20 mEq for prevention. **Children:** 3 mEq/kg daily. Max daily dosage 40 mEq/m². If potassium < 2 mEq/ml, max infusion rate 40 mEq/hr; max infusion conc 80 mEq/L; and max 24-hr dose 400 mEq. If potassium > 2 mEq/ml, max infusion rate 10 mEq/hr; max infusion conc 40 mEq/L; and max 24-hr dose 200 mEq.	• Never switch potassium products without doctor's order. • **IV use:** Give by infusion only. Give slowly as dilute solution. • Make sure powder is completely dissolved before administering. • Monitor ECG and serum electrolytes.
potassium gluconate Glu-K, Kaon Liquid *Potassium supplement* *Therapeutic agent for electrolyte balance* Preg. Risk Category: C	*Hypokalemia* — **Adults:** 40 to 100 mEq PO daily in 3 or 4 divided doses for treatment; 10 to 20 mEq daily for prevention. Further dosage adjustments based on serum potassium levels.	• Don't administer potassium supplements postop until urine flow established. • Instruct to take with or after meals with full glass of water or fruit juice. • Caution not to use salt substitutes.
potassium iodide Iostat, Pima, Thyro-Block **potassium iodide, saturated solution (SSKI), strong iodine solution** *Electrolyte* *Antihyperthyroid agent* Preg. Risk Category: D	*Preparation for thyroidectomy* — **Adults and children:** strong iodine sol (USP), 0.1–0.3 ml PO tid, or SSKI, 1 to 5 drops in water PO tid after meals for 10 to 14 days before surgery. *Thyrotoxic crisis* — **Adults and children:** 500 mg PO q 4 hr (SSKI) or 1 ml strong iodine sol tid. *Radiation protectant for thyroid gland* — **Adults and children ≥ 1 yr:** 130 mg PO daily	• Doctor may avoid prescribing enteric-coated tablets, which can lead to perforation, hemorrhage, or obstruction. • Dilute oral solutions in water, milk, or fruit juice; give after meals to prevent gastric irritation, hydrate patient, and mask salty taste. • Give iodides through straw to avoid tooth discoloration.

	for 7 to 14 days after radiation exposure. **Children <1 yr:** 65 mg PO daily for 7 to 14 days after exposure.	▪ Irritation and swollen eyelids are earliest signs of delayed hypersensitivity reactions to iodides.
pravastatin sodium (eptastatin) Pravachol *HMG-CoA reductase inhibitor* *Antilipemic* Preg. Risk Category: X	*Reduction of LDL and total cholesterol levels in primary hypercholesterolemia (types IIa and IIb)* — **Adults:** 10 or 20 mg PO daily hs. Adjust q 4 wk per response; max 40 mg daily hs. Most elderly patients respond to ≤20 mg qd.	▪ Initiate only after other nonpharmacologic therapies prove ineffective. ▪ Liver function should be tested at start of therapy and periodically thereafter. ▪ Instruct to take in evening.
prazosin hydrochloride Minipress *Alpha-adrenergic blocker* *Antihypertensive* Preg. Risk Category: C	*Mild to moderate hypertension* — **Adults:** PO test dose 1 mg hs. Initial dose 1 mg PO bid or tid. Increase slowly. Max 20 mg qd. Maint. 6 to 15 mg qd in 3 divided doses.	▪ Monitor BP and HR frequently. Elderly patients may be more sensitive to hypotensive effects.
prednisolone Cortalone, Delta-Cortef **prednisolone sodium phosphate** Hydeltrasol, Key-Pred-SP **prednisolone tebutate** Hydeltra-TBA, Nor-Pred TBA *Glucocorticoid* *Anti-inflammatory/immunosuppressant* Preg. Risk Category: C	*Severe inflammation or immunosuppression* — **Adults:** 2.5 to 15 mg PO bid, tid, or qid; 2 to 30 mg IM (phosphate) or IV (phosphate) q 12 hr; or 2 to 30 mg (phosphate) into joints (depending on joint size), lesions, or soft tissue; or 4 to 40 mg (tebutate) into joints (depending on joint size) and lesions prn.	▪ Give oral dose with food to reduce GI irritation. ▪ Give IM injection deeply into gluteal muscle. Rotate injection sites to prevent muscle atrophy. Avoid SC injection. ▪ Monitor weight, BP, and serum electrolytes.

(continued)

†Canadian ‡Australian

PREDNISOLONE ACETATE 250

DRUG / CLASS / CATEGORY	INDICATIONS / DOSAGES	KEY NURSING CONSIDERATIONS
prednisolone acetate (suspension) Pred-Forte **prednisolone sodium phosphate** AK-Pred, Inflamase Forte *Corticosteroid* *Ophth anti-inflammatory* Preg. Risk Category: C	*Inflammation* — **Adults and children:** 1 to 2 drops instilled into eye. In severe conditions, may use hourly, tapering to discontinuation as inflammation subsides. In mild conditions, may use bid to qid.	• Wash hands before and after applying. Don't touch dropper tip to eye or surrounding area. • Apply light pressure on lacrimal sac for 1 min after instillation. • Instruct to notify doctor if anyone in household develops same symptoms. • Shake suspension. Store in tightly covered container.
prednisone Apo-Prednisone†, Liquid Pred, Meticorten, Panasol, Prednicen-M, Prednisone Intensol, Winpred† *Adrenocorticoid* *Anti-inflammatory/immunosuppressant* Preg. Risk Category: C	*Severe inflammation or immunosuppression* — **Adults:** 5 to 60 mg PO daily in 2 to 4 divided doses. Give maintenance dosage qd or qod. Dosage individualized. **Children:** 0.14 to 2 mg/kg or 4 to 60 mg/m² daily PO in 4 divided doses.	• Monitor BP, sleep patterns, and serum potassium. Weigh patient daily; report sudden weight gain. • Watch for depression or psychotic episodes, especially with high-dose therapy. • Diabetics may need increased insulin; monitor blood glucose. • May mask or exacerbate infections, including latent amebiasis.
primaquine phosphate *8-aminoquinoline* *Antimalarial* Preg. Risk Category: C	*Radical cure of relapsing* P. vivax *malaria, eliminating symptoms and infection completely; prevention of relapse* — **Adults:** 15 mg (base) PO daily for 14 days. (26.3-mg tab provides 15 mg of base.) **Children:** 0.5 mg/kg/day (0.3 mg base/kg/day; max 15 mg base/dose) PO for 14 days.	• Give with fast-acting antimalarial to reduce risk of drug-resistant strains. • Obtain frequent blood and urine studies. • Monitor for sudden fall in Hgb, erythrocyte, or leukocyte count and for marked urine darkening. Discontinue immediately and notify doctor.

primidone

Apo-Primidone†, Mysoline,
PMS Primidone†, Sertan‡

Barbiturate analogue
Anticonvulsant
Preg. Risk Category: NR

Tonic-clonic, complex partial, and simple partial seizures — **Adults and children ≥ 8 yr:** initially, 100 to 125 mg PO hs on days 1 to 3; 100 to 125 mg PO bid on days 4 to 6; 100 to 125 mg PO tid on days 7 to 9; followed by dose of 250 mg PO tid. Dose increased to 250 mg qid, prn. Max 2 g qd in divided doses. **Children < 8 yr:** then 50 mg PO hs for 3 days, then 50 mg PO bid for days 4 to 6, 100 mg PO bid for days 7 to 9, followed by dose of 125 to 250 mg PO tid.

- Don't withdraw suddenly; seizures may worsen. Call doctor if adverse reactions develop.
- Therapeutic primidone blood level 5 to 12 mcg/ml; therapeutic phenobarbital level 15 to 40 mcg/ml.
- Monitor CBC and routine blood chemistry q 6 mo.

probenecid

Benemid, Benn, Benuryl†,
Probalan, Robenecid

Sulfonamide derivative
Uricosuric
Preg. Risk Category: NR

Gonorrhea — **Adults:** 3.5 g ampicillin PO with 1 g probenecid given together; or 1 g probenecid PO 30 min before dose of 4.8 million units of aqueous penicillin G procaine IM, injected at 2 different sites.

Hyperuricemia of gout, gouty arthritis — **Adults:** 250 mg PO bid for 1st wk, then 500 mg bid, to max 2 g daily.

- Give with milk, food, or antacids.
- Monitor periodic BUN and renal function tests with long-term therapy.
- Force fluids to maintain minimum output of 2 to 3 L/day.
- May increase frequency, severity, and length of gout attacks during 1st 6 to 12 mo.

procarbazine hydrochloride

Matulane, Natulan†

Antibiotic antineoplastic
(cell cycle–phase specific, S phase)
Antineoplastic

Adjunct treatment of Hodgkin's disease — **Adults:** 2 to 4 mg/kg PO qd for 1st wk. Then, 4 to 6 mg/kg/day until WBC count < 4,000/mm³ or platelet count < 100,000/mm³. After bone marrow recovers, resume maint. of 1 to 2 mg/kg/day. For MOPP regi-

- Monitor CBC and platelet counts.
- Be prepared to discontinue if confusion or paresthesia or other neuropathies develop. Notify doctor.
- Take hs and in divided doses.

(continued)

†Canadian ‡Australian

DRUG/CLASS/ CATEGORY	INDICATIONS/ DOSAGES	KEY NURSING CONSIDERATIONS
procarbazine hydrochloride *(continued)* Preg. Risk Category: D	men, 100 mg/m² /day PO for 14 days. **Children:** 50 mg/m² PO daily for 1st wk; then 100 mg/m² until response or toxicity occurs. Maintenance dosage 50 mg/m² PO daily after bone marrow recovery.	▪ Watch for signs of infection and bleeding. Take temp daily. ▪ Warn to avoid alcohol. Urge to stop drug and call doctor immediately if disulfiram-like reaction (chest pains, rapid or irregular heartbeat, severe headache, stiff neck).
procainamide hydrochloride Procanbid Durules‡, Procan SR, Promine, Pronestyl *Procaine derivative* *Ventricular antiarrhythmic/ supraventricular antiarrhythmic* Preg. Risk Category: C	*Life-threatening ventricular arrhythmias —* **Adults:** 100 mg slow IV push q 5 min, no faster than 25 to 50 mg/min until arrhythmias disappear, adverse reactions develop, or 1 g given. Usual effective dose 500 to 600 mg. When arrhythmias disappear, give continuous infusion of 1 to 6 mg/min. If arrhythmias recur, repeat bolus and increase infusion rate. Or, 0.5 to 1 g IM q 4 to 8 hr until oral therapy begins. Oral: 50 mg/kg qd in divided doses q 3 hr.	▪ **IV use:** Monitor BP and ECG continuously. If prolonged QT intervals and QRS complexes, heart block, or increased arrhythmias occur, withhold drug and notify doctor. ▪ To suppress ventricular arrhythmias, drug levels 4 to 8 mcg/ml; NAPA levels 10 to 30 mcg/ml. ▪ Monitor serum electrolytes.
prochlorperazine Compazine, PMS Prochlorperazine†, Prorazin†, Stemetil† **prochlorperazine edisylate**	*Preop nausea control —* **Adults:** 5 to 10 mg IM 1 to 2 hr before anesthesia; repeat once in 30 min, prn. Or, 5 to 10 mg IV 15 to 30 min before anesthesia; repeat once prn. *Severe nausea and vomiting —* **Adults:** 5 to 10 mg PO, tid or qid; 25 mg PR, bid; or 5 to 10 mg IM repeated q 3 to 4 hr, prn. Max IM dosage 40 mg daily. Or, 2.5 to 10 mg IV at	▪ Dilute oral solution with tomato or fruit juice, milk, coffee, carbonated beverage, tea, water, or soup or mix with pudding. ▪ **IV use:** 15 to 30 min before induction, add 20 mg prochlorperazine/L D₅W and 0.9% NaCl solution. Max infusion rate 5 mg/min. Max parenteral dosage 40 mg daily. Infuse slowly, never as bolus.

Compa-Z, Compazine, Cotranzine, Ultrazine-10

prochlorperazine maleate

Anti-Naus‡, Compazine, PMS Prochlorperazine†, Prorazin†, Stemetil†

Phenothiazine (piperazine derivative)

Antipsychotic/antiemetic/antianxiety agent

Preg. Risk Category: NR

max rate 5 mg/min. **Children 9 to 13 kg:** 2.5 mg PO or PR qd or bid. Max 7.5 mg daily. Or give 0.132 mg/kg by IM injection. **Children 14 to 17 kg:** 2.5 mg PO or PR, bid or tid. Max 10 mg daily. Or give 0.132 mg/kg by deep IM injection. Control usually obtained with one dose. **Children 18 to 39 kg:** 2.5 mg PO or PR, tid; or 5 mg PO or PR, bid. Max 15 mg daily. Or give 0.132 mg/kg by deep IM injection. Control usually obtained with one dose.

To manage symptoms of psychotic disorders — **Adults:** 5 to 10 mg PO, tid or qid. **Children 2 to 12 yr:** 2.5 mg PO or PR, bid or tid. Max 10 mg on day 1. Increase dosage gradually to recommended max (if necessary). In children 2 to 5 yr, max 25 mg daily. In children 6 to 10 yr, max 25 mg daily.

Nonpsychotic anxiety — **Adults:** 5 to 10 mg by deep IM injection q 3 to 4 hr, not to exceed 20 mg daily or for > 12 wk; or 5 to 10 mg PO, tid or qid. Or, 15 mg ext-release cap qd or 10 mg ext-release cap q 12 hr.

- Avoid getting concentrate or injection solution on hands or clothing.
- Watch for orthostatic hypotension, especially when giving IV.
- For IM use, inject deeply into upper outer quadrant of gluteal region.
- Don't give SC or mix in syringe with another drug.
- Used only when vomiting can't be controlled by other measures. Notify doctor if > 4 doses needed in 24 hours.
- Advise to wear protective clothing when exposed to sunlight.
- Store in light-resistant container. Slight yellowing does not affect potency; discard extremely discolored solutions.

---

progesterone

Gesterol 50, Progestilin†

Progestin

Progestin/contraceptive

Preg. Risk Category: X

Amenorrhea — **Adults:** 5 to 10 mg IM daily for 6 to 8 days, beginning 8 to 10 days before anticipated start of menstruation.

Dysfunctional uterine bleeding — **Adults:** 5 to 10 mg IM daily for 6 doses.

- Give oil solutions (peanut oil or sesame oil) via deep IM injection. Check sites frequently for irritation.
- Rotate injection sites.

PROGESTERONE 253

DRUG/CLASS/CATEGORY	INDICATIONS/DOSAGES	KEY NURSING CONSIDERATIONS
promethazine hydrochloride Anergan 25, Histantil†, Pentazine, Phenazine 25, Phencen-50, Phenergan, Phenerject-50, Phenoject-50, PMS-Promethazine†, Promethegan, Prothazine†, V-Gan-25 *Phenothiazine derivative* *Antiemetic/antivertigo agent/antihistamine (H₁-receptor antagonist)/preop, postop, or obstetric sedative and adjunct to analgesics* Preg. Risk Category: C **promethazine theoclate** Avomine‡	*Motion sickness* — **Adults:** 25 mg PO bid. **Children:** 12.5 to 25 mg PO, IM, or PR bid. *Nausea* — **Adults:** 12.5 to 25 mg PO, IM, or PR q 4 to 6 hr, prn. **Children:** 12.5 to 25 mg IM or PR q 4 to 6 hr, prn. *Rhinitis, allergy symptoms* — **Adults:** 12.5 mg PO qid; or 25 mg PO hs. **Children:** 6.25 to 12.5 mg PO tid or 25 mg PO or PR hs. *Sedation* — **Adults:** 25 to 50 mg PO or IM hs or prn. **Children:** 12.5 to 25 mg PO, IM, or PR hs. *Routine preop or postop sedation or adjunct to analgesics* — **Adults:** 25 to 50 mg IM, IV, or PO. **Children:** 12.5 to 25 mg IM, IV, or PO.	• Used as adjunct to analgesics; has no analgesic activity. • Don't administer SC. • In patients scheduled for myelogram, discontinue drug 48 hr before procedure and don't resume until 24 hr after procedure. • *IV use:* Don't give concentration > 25 mg/ml or give faster than 25 mg/min. • May cause pronounced sedation. Warn to avoid alcohol and activities requiring alertness until CNS effects known.
propafenone hydrochloride Rythmol *Sodium channel antagonist* *Antiarrhythmic (class IC)* Preg. Risk Category: C	*Suppression of life-threatening ventricular arrhythmias, such as SVT* — **Adults:** initially, 150 mg PO q 8 hr. May increase dosage at 3- to 4-day intervals to 225 mg q 8 hr; if necessary, increase to 300 mg q 8 hr. Max 900 mg daily.	• Continuous cardiac monitoring recommended during initiation and dosage adjustments. If PR interval or QRS complex increases by > 25%, expect to reduce dose. • During use with digoxin, frequently monitor ECG and serum digoxin.

propantheline bromide

Panthelin‡, Pro-Banthine
Anticholinergic
Antimuscarinic/GI antispasmodic
Preg. Risk Category: C

Adjunctive treatment of peptic ulceration — **Adults:** 15 mg PO tid ac and 30 mg hs. **Elderly patients:** 7.5 mg PO tid ac.

- Give 30 min to 1 hr before meals and hs. Bedtime doses can be larger; give at least 2 hr after last meal of day.
- Advise to avoid hazardous activities if drowsiness, dizziness, or blurred vision occurs; drink plenty of fluids; and report skin eruptions.

propoxyphene hydrochloride

Darvon, Dolene, Novopropoxyne, 642†
propoxyphene napsylate
Darvon-N, Doloxene‡
Narcotic analgesic
Opioid analgesic
Preg. Risk Category: C

Mild to moderate pain — **Adults:** 65 mg (hydrochloride) PO q 4 hr, prn. Max 390 mg/day.
Mild to moderate pain — **Adults:** 100 mg (napsylate) PO q 4 hr, prn. Max 600 mg/day.

- Mild narcotic analgesic.
- Warn not to exceed recommended dosage. Respiratory depression, hypotension, profound sedation, and coma may result if used in excessive doses or with other CNS depressants.
- Advise to avoid alcohol or other CNS-type drugs.

propranolol hydrochloride

Betachron E-R, Deralin†, Detensol†, Inderal, Inderal LA, Novopranol†
Beta-adrenergic blocker
Antihypertensive/antianginal/antiarrhythmic/adjunctive therapy of MI

Angina pectoris — **Adults:** total daily dose, 80 to 320 mg PO bid, tid, or qid; or one 80-mg ext-rel cap qd. Increase dosage at 7-to 10-day intervals.
Mortality reduction after MI — **Adults:** 180 to 240 mg PO tid or qid 5 to 21 days after MI.
Supraventricular and ventricular arrhythmias; tachyarrhythmias due to excessive catecholamine action during anesthesia, hyperthyroidism, or pheochromocytoma — **Adults:** 0.5 to 3 mg by slow IV push

- Check apical pulse before giving drug. If extremes detected, stop drug and call doctor at once.
- Double-check dose and route.
- *I.V. use:* Give by direct injection into a large vessel or into the tubing of a free-flowing, compatible IV solution; continuous IV infusion generally is not recommended. Or, dilute drug with 0.9% NaCl and give by intermittent infusion over 10

(continued)

PROPRANOLOL HYDROCHLORIDE 255

†Canadian ‡Australian

DRUG / CLASS / CATEGORY	INDICATIONS / DOSAGES	KEY NURSING CONSIDERATIONS
propranolol hydrochloride *(continued)* Preg. Risk Category: C	(≤1 mg/min). After 3 mg, give next dose in 2 min; other doses > q 4 hr. Maint. 10 to 30 mg PO tid or qid. *Hypertension* — **Adults:** 80 mg PO qd in 2 to 4 divided doses or ext-release qd. Increased at 3- to 7-day intervals to max 640 mg qd. Maint. 160 to 480 mg qd. *Essential tremor* — **Adults:** 40 mg PO bid. Maint. 120 to 320 mg PO in 3 divided doses. *Hypertrophic subaortic stenosis* — **Adults:** 20 to 40 mg PO tid or qid, or 80 to 160 mg ext-rel capsules once daily. *Adjunct therapy in pheochromocytoma* — **Adults:** 60 mg PO qd in divided doses with an alpha blocker 3 days before surgery.	to 15 min in 0.1- to 0.2-mg increments. Drug is compatible with D_5W and 0.45% and 0.9% NaCl and lactated Ringer's solutions. ▪ Give drug with meals. ▪ If severe hypotension occurs, notify doctor. ▪ Drug masks common signs of shock and hypoglycemia. ▪ For IV use, may be diluted and infused slowly.
propylthiouracil (PTU) Propyl-Thyracil† *Thyroid hormone antagonist* *Antihyperthyroid agent* Preg. Risk Category: D	*Hyperthyroidism* — **Adults:** 100 to 150 mg PO tid; up to 1,200 mg qd. Maint.: 100 to 150 mg qd in divided doses tid. **Children > 10 yr:** 150 to 300 mg PO qd in divided doses tid. **Children 6 to 10 yr:** 50 to 150 mg PO qd in divided doses tid. *Thyrotoxic crisis* — **Adults and children:** 200 mg PO q 4 to 6 hr on first day; once symptoms controlled, reduce dosage gradually to usual maintenance level.	▪ Monitor thyroid function studies in pregnant patients. Thyroid may be added to regimen. Drug may be stopped during last few weeks of pregnancy. ▪ Watch for hypothyroidism (depression; cold intolerance; hard, nonpitting edema); adjust dosage as ordered.

protamine sulfate

Antidote
Heparin antagonist
Preg. Risk Category: C

Heparin overdose — **Adults:** dosage based on blood coagulation studies, usually 1 mg for each 90 to 115 units heparin. Give by slow IV inj over 10 min, max 50 mg.

- **IV use:** Have emergency equipment available.
- Hypersensitivity reaction increased in hypersensitivity to fish, vasectomized or infertile males, and patients taking protamine-insulin.
- May act as anticoagulant in high doses.

---

pseudoephedrine hydrochloride

Children's Sudafed, Drixoral, Efidac/24, PediaCare Infant's Decongestant, Pseudofrint, Sudafed

pseudoephedrine sulfate

Afrin, Drixoral
Adrenergic
Decongestant
Preg. Risk Category: C

Nasal and eustachian tube decongestion — **Adults:** 60 mg PO q 4 hr. Max 240 mg daily. Or, 120 mg ext-release tab PO q 12 hr or 240 mg ext-release tab PO q 12 hr. **Children > 12 yr:** 120 mg PO q 12 hr, or 240 mg PO q.d. **Children 6 to 12 yr:** 30 mg PO reg-release form q 4 to 6 hr. Max 120 mg daily. **Children 2 to 6 yr:** 15 mg PO reg-release form q 4 to 6 hr. Max 60 mg/day. **Children 1 to 2 yr:** 7 drops (0.2 ml)/kg q 4 to 6 hr, up to 4 doses/day. **Children 3 to 12 mo:** 3 drops/kg q 4 to 6 hr, up to 4 doses/day.

- Elderly patients more sensitive to drug effects.
- Warn against using OTC products containing other sympathomimetics.
- Tell not to take within 2 hr of bedtime.
- Don't use with MAO inhibitors.
- Tell not to crush or break forms.
- Instruct to stop drug and notify doctor if unusual restlessness occurs.

---

psyllium

Fiberall, Maalox Daily Fiber Therapy, Metamucil, Mylanta Natural Fiber Supplement, Pro-Lax
Absorbent
Bulk laxative
Preg. Risk Category: NR

Constipation; bowel management — **Adults:** 1 to 2 tsp (rounded) PO in full glass of liquid q.d, b.i.d, or t.i.d, followed by second glass of liquid; or 1 packet dissolved in water q.d, b.i.d, or t.i.d. **Children > 6 yr:** 1 tsp (level) PO in half glass of liquid hs.

- Mix with at least 8 oz (240 ml) of cold, pleasant-tasting liquid, such as orange juice, to mask grittiness; stir only few seconds. Have patient drink immediately. Follow with additional glass of liquid.

†Canadian ‡Australian

DRUG / CLASS / CATEGORY	INDICATIONS / DOSAGES	KEY NURSING CONSIDERATIONS
pyrazinamide Pyrazinamide†, Tebrazid† *Synthetic pyrazine analogue* Antituberculosis agent Preg. Risk Category: C	*Adjunctive treatment of TB* — **Adults:** 15 to 30 mg/kg PO qd. Max 2 g daily. Or, if patient noncompliant, 50 to 70 mg/kg PO twice weekly.	• Given for initial 2 mo of ≥ 6-mo regimen. Patients with HIV infection may require longer course. • Reduce dosage in renal impairment. • Watch for signs of gout and liver impairment. Notify doctor if present.
pyridostigmine bromide Mestinon, Mestinon Timespans, Mestinon Timespans, Regonol *Cholinesterase inhibitor* Muscle stimulant Preg. Risk Category: NR	*Antidote for nondepolarizing neuromuscular blockers* — **Adults:** 10 to 20 mg IV preceded by atropine sulfate 0.6 to 1.2 mg IV. *Myasthenia gravis* — **Adults:** 60 to 120 mg PO q 3 or 4 hr. Usual dosage. 600 mg qd but higher dosage may be needed (up to 1,500 mg qd). For IM or IV use, give 1⁄30 of oral dosage. Adjust dosage for each patient, based on response and tolerance. Or, 180 to 540 mg ext-rel tab (1 to 3 tab) PO bid, with at least 6 hr between doses. **Children:** 7 mg/kg or 200 mg/m² qd in 5 or 6 divided doses. *Supportive treatment of neonates born to myasthenic mothers* — **Neonates:** 0.05 to 0.15 mg/kg IM q 4 to 6 hr. Decrease dosage qd until drug can be stopped.	• Stop other cholinergics before giving drug. • **I.V. use:** Give IV injection no faster than 1 mg/min or bradycardia and seizures may occur. Monitor vital signs. Position patient to ease breathing. Be ready to give atropine injection; provide respiratory support prn. • Don't crush ext-rel (Timespans) tablets. • Monitor and document patient's response. • If muscle weakness is severe, be aware that doctor determines if caused by drug-induced toxicity or exacerbation of disease. Test dose of edrophonium IV aggravates drug-induced weakness but temporarily relieves weakness caused by disease. • Know that Regonol (only US) contains benzyl ethanol that may cause toxicity in neonates if given in high doses.

pyridoxine hydrochloride (vitamin B₆)

Beesix, Hexa-Betalin, Nestrex, Rodex

Water-soluble vitamin

Nutritional supplement

Preg. Risk Category: A

Dietary vitamin B₆ deficiency — **Adults:** 10 to 20 mg PO, IM, or IV daily for 3 wk, then 2 to 5 mg daily as supplement to proper diet.

Seizures related to vitamin B₆ deficiency or dependency — **Adults and children:** 100 mg IM or IV in single dose.

- Protect from light. Don't use solution if it contains precipitate, although slight darkening acceptable.
- High doses (2 to 6 g/day) may cause difficulty walking.
- Monitor diet. Excessive protein intake increases daily pyridoxine requirements.

---

pyrimethamine

Daraprim

pyrimethamine with sulfadoxine

Fansidar

Aminopyrimidine derivative (folic acid antagonist)

Antimalarial

Preg. Risk Category: C

Malaria prophylaxis and transmission control (pyrimethamine) — **Adults and children ≥ 10 yr:** 25 mg PO/wk; **4 to 10 yr:** 12.5 mg PO/wk; **< 4 yr:** 6.25 mg PO/wk. Continue 6 to 10 wk after leaving endemic areas.

Acute attacks of malaria (Fansidar) — **Adults and children ≥ 14 yr:** 2 to 3 tab as single dose; **9 to 14 yr:** 2 tab/wk; **4 to 8 yr:** 1 tab/wk; **< 4 yr:** ¾ tab/wk.

Malaria prophylaxis (Fansidar) — **Adults and children ≥ 14 yr:** 1 tab/wk; **9 to 14 yr:** ¾ tab/wk; **4 to 8 yr:** ½ tab/wk; **< 4 yr:** ¼ tab/wk.

Acute attacks of malaria (pyrimethamine) — **Adults and children ≥ 15 yr:** 25 mg PO qd for 2 days. **Children < 15 yr:** 12.5 mg PO qd for 2 days.

Toxoplasmosis (pyrimethamine) — **Adults:** 100 mg PO, then 25 mg PO qd for 4 to 5 wk; **Children:** 1 mg/kg PO (< 100 mg) in 2 equally divided doses for 2 to 4 days, then 0.5 mg/kg qd for 4 wk.

- Obtain twice-weekly blood counts, including platelets, for toxoplasmosis patient.
- Fansidar should be used in areas where chloroquine-resistant malaria prevalent and if traveler plans to stay > 3 wk.
- Tell to take with meals.
- Instruct to stop drug and notify doctor at first sign of rash.
- Not recommended alone in nonimmune patients; should be used with faster-acting antimalarials for 2 days to initiate transmission control and suppressive cure.
- Sulfadiazine given with pyrimethamine to treat toxoplasmosis.

DRUG/CLASS/ CATEGORY	INDICATIONS/ DOSAGES	KEY NURSING CONSIDERATIONS
quazepam Doral *Benzodiazepine* *Hypnotic* Preg. Risk Category: X Controlled Sub. Sched.: IV	*Insomnia* — **Adults:** 15 mg PO hs. Some patients may respond to lower dosages. Lower dosage in elderly after 2 days.	• Prevent hoarding or self-overdosing if patient depressed, suicidal, or drug-dependent or has history of drug abuse. • Withdrawal symptoms may occur if suddenly stopped after 6 wk continuous use.
quinapril hydrochloride Accupril, Asig† *ACE inhibitor* *Antihypertensive* Preg. Risk Category: C (1st trimester), D (2nd and 3rd)	*Hypertension* — **Adults:** initially, 10 mg PO daily or 5 mg daily if patient takes diuretic. Adjust based on response at 2-wk intervals. *Heart failure* — **Adults:** 5 to 10 mg PO bid. Increase at weekly intervals.	• Advise to report angioedema (including laryngeal edema). • Monitor BP for effectiveness. • Observe for lightheadedness and syncope. • Monitor serum potassium.
quinidine gluconate Quinaglute, Dura-Tabs, Quinalan, Quinatet† **quinidine sulfate** Apo-Quinidine†, Cin-Quin, Quinidex Extentabs *Cinchona alkaloid* *Antiarrhythmic* Preg. Risk Category: C	*Atrial flutter or fib* — **Adults:** 200 mg PO q 2 to 3 hr for 5 to 8 doses, then increase qd. Max 3–4 g qd. *PSVT* — **Adults:** 400 to 600 mg IM or PO q 2 to 3 hr. *PACs, PVCs, PAT, PVT, maint. after cardioversion of atrial fib* — **Adults:** test dose 200 mg PO or IM. Then 200 to 400 mg (sulf. or equiv. base) PO q 4 to 6 hr; or 600 mg (gluc.) IM, then 400 mg q 2 hr prn; or 800 mg (gluc.) in 40 ml D₅W IV infusion at 16 mg/min. **Children:** test dose 2 mg/kg PO, then 30 mg/kg/24 hr PO or 900 mg/m²/24 hr PO in 5 divided doses.	• Use cautiously in impaired renal or hepatic function, asthma, muscle weakness, or infection with fever. • Check apical pulse and BP before therapy. • Monitor patient response. Adverse GI reactions signal toxicity. Check blood drug levels: > 8 mcg/ml toxic. • Give with meals to prevent GI symptoms. • Give sulfate or equivalent base for atrial flutter or fib only if AV node has been blocked by another agent to prevent in- creased AV conduction.

ramipril

Altace, Ramace‡, Tritace‡

ACE inhibitor

Antihypertensive

Preg. Risk Category: C (1st trimester); D (2nd and 3rd trimesters)

Hypertension — **Adults:** initially, 2.5 mg PO qd for patient not taking diuretic; 1.25 mg PO qd for patient taking diuretic. Increase prn based on response. Maint. 2.5 to 20 mg qd as single or divided doses.

Heart failure — **Adults:** 2.5 mg PO bid. If hypotension, decrease to 1.25 mg PO bid. May increase slowly to max 5 mg PO bid prn.

- Advise to report angioedema (including laryngeal edema).
- Monitor BP regularly.
- Watch for light-headedness and syncope.
- Monitor serum potassium.

ranitidine hydrochloride

Apo-Ranitidine†, Zantac, Zantac-C†, Zantac 75

Histamine₂-receptor antagonist

Antiulcer agent

Preg. Risk Category: B

Duodenal and gastric ulcer (short-term treatment); pathologic hypersecretory conditions, such as Zollinger-Ellison syndrome — **Adults:** 150 mg PO bid or 300 mg qd hs. Or, 50 mg IV or IM q 6 to 8 hr. Patients with Zollinger-Ellison syndrome may need up to 6 g PO qd.

Maintenance therapy for duodenal or gastric ulcer — **Adults:** 150 mg PO hs.

GERD — **Adults:** 150 mg PO bid.

- *IV use:* When giving IV push, dilute to total volume of 20 ml and inject over 5 min.
- For intermittent IV infusion, dilute 50 mg on 100 ml compatible solution, and infuse over 15 to 20 min.
- For continuous IV infusion: 150 mg in 250 ml compatible solution. Administer at 6.25 mg/hr using infusion pump.
- Incompatible with aluminum.

respiratory syncytial virus immune globulin intravenous, human (RSV-IGIV)

RespiGam

Immunoglobulin G

Immune serum

Preg. Risk Category: C

Prevention of serious lower respiratory tract infections caused by RSV in children with bronchopulmonary dysplasia (BPD) or premature birth — **Premature infants and children < 2 yr:** single infusion monthly. Give 1.5 ml/kg/hr IV for 15 min; then may increase to 3 ml/kg/hr for 15 min to max 6 ml/kg/hr until infusion ends. Max total per monthly infusion 750 mg/kg.

- Assess cardiopulmonary status and vital signs before infusion, each rate increase, and q 30 min until 30 min after infusion.
- May use slower rate in critically ill children with BPD.
- Monitor for fluid overload.
- *IV use:* Enter single-use vial only once; don't shake, avoid foaming. Begin infusion within 6 hr and complete by 12 hr.

RSV-IGIV   261

†Canadian ‡Australian

DRUG / CLASS / CATEGORY	INDICATIONS / DOSAGES	KEY NURSING CONSIDERATIONS
reteplase, recombinant Retavase *Tissue plasminogen activator* *Thrombolytic* Preg. Risk Category: C	*Management of acute MI* — **Adults:** double-bolus of 10 + 10 U. Give each bolus IV over 2 min. If no complications after 1st bolus, give 2nd bolus 30 min after start of 1st.	• Carefully monitor ECG during treatment. Be prepared to treat bradycardia or ventricular irritability. • Monitor for bleeding. Avoid IM injections, invasive procedures, and nonessential patient handling. If local measures don't control serious bleeding, stop concomitant anticoagulant and notify doctor. • *IV use:* Administer as double-bolus injection. If bleeding or anaphylactoid reactions occur after 1st bolus, notify doctor. • Don't give with other IV medications through same IV line.
ribavirin Virazole *Synthetic nucleoside* *Antiviral agent* Preg. Risk Category: X	*Hospitalized infants and young children infected by respiratory syncytial virus (RSV)* — **Infants and young children:** sol in conc of 20 mg/ml delivered via Viratek Small Particle Aerosol Generator (SPAG-2) and mechanical ventilation or via O_2 mask, hood, or tent at flow rate of 12.5 L/min mist. Treat for 12 to 18 hr/day for 3 to 7 days, with flow rate of 12.5 L/min of mist.	• Administer aerosol form by SPAG-2 only. • Use sterile USP water for injection, *not* bacteriostatic water. • Discard solutions placed in SPAG-2 unit ≥ q 24 hr before adding newly reconstituted solution. • Eye irritation and headache reported in health care personnel exposed to aerosolized drug. • Monitor ventilator function frequently.

riboflavin (vitamin B₂)

Vitamin B complex vitamin

Preg. Risk Category: NR

Riboflavin deficiency or adjunct to thiamine treatment for polyneuritis or cheilosis secondary to pellagra — **Adults and children ≥ 12 yr:** 5 to 30 mg PO daily, depending on severity. **Children < 12 yr:** 3 to 10 mg PO daily, depending on severity.

- Deficiency often accompanies other vitamin B complex deficiencies; may require multivitamin therapy.
- Tell to take with meals; food increases absorption.
- Stress proper nutritional habits.
- Urine may appear bright yellow.

---

rifabutin

Mycobutin

Semisynthetic ansamycin

Antibiotic

Preg. Risk Category: B

Prevention of disseminated Mycobacterium avium complex in advanced HIV infection — **Adults:** 300 mg PO daily as single dose or divided bid, with food.

- Use cautiously in preexisting neutropenia and thrombocytopenia.
- Perform baseline hematologic studies; repeat periodically.

---

rifampin (rifampicin)

Rifadin, Rifadin IV, Rimactane, Rimycin‡, Rofact†

Semisynthetic rifampin B derivative (macrocyclic antibiotic)

Antituberculosis agent

Preg. Risk Category: C

Pulmonary TB — **Adults:** 600 mg PO or IV in single dose 1 hr before or 2 hr after meals. **Children > 5 yr:** 10 to 20 mg/kg PO or IV daily in single dose 1 hr before or 2 hr after meals. Max 600 mg/day. Give with other antituberculars.

Meningococcal carriers — **Adults:** 600 mg PO or IV bid for 2 days, or 600 mg/day PO or IV for 4 days. **Children 1 mo to 12 yr:** 10 mg/kg PO or IV bid for 2 days, ≤ 600 mg/day, or 10 to 20 mg/kg/day PO for 4 days. **Neonates:** 5 mg/kg PO or IV bid for 4 days.

Prophylaxis of H. influenzae type b — **Adults and children:** 20 mg/kg/day PO for 4 days; max 600 mg/day.

- Give 1 hr before or 2 hr after meals.
- *IV use:* Reconstitute with 10 ml sterile water for injection to make solution containing 60 mg/ml. Add to 100 ml D₅W and infuse over 30 min, or add to 500 ml D₅W and infuse over 3 hr.
- Give with at least one other antitubercular.
- May discolor urine, feces, saliva, sweat, sputum, and tears red-orange.

DRUG / CLASS / CATEGORY	INDICATIONS / DOSAGES	KEY NURSING CONSIDERATIONS
riluzole Rilutek *Benzothiazole* *Neuroprotector* Preg. Risk Category: C	*Amyotrophic lateral sclerosis —* **Adults:** 50 mg PO q 12 hr, on empty stomach.	▪ Give ≥ 1 hr before or 2 hr after meal. ▪ Tell to take at same time daily. ▪ Instruct to report fever. ▪ Caution to avoid hazardous activities. ▪ Perform liver function tests periodically; elevations in baseline test preclude use.
rimantadine hydrochloride Flumadine *Adamantine* *Antiviral* Preg. Risk Category: C	*Influenza A (preventative) —* **Adults and children ≥ 10 yr:** 100 mg PO bid. **Children < 10 yr:** 5 mg/kg (max 150 mg) PO daily. **Elderly, severe hepatic or renal dysfunction, or adverse effects at normal dosage:** 100 mg PO daily. *Influenza A —* **Adults:** 100 mg PO bid, within 24 to 48 hr of symptom onset and for 48 hr after symptoms disappear.	▪ Use cautiously in renal or hepatic impairment and in history of seizures. Pregnant patients should compare risks vs benefits before starting. ▪ Should take several hr before bedtime. ▪ Tell patient to take infection-control precautions. ▪ Resistant strains may emerge during therapy.
rimexolone Vexol 1% Ophthalmic Suspension *Ophthalmic steroid* *Ophthalmic anti-inflammatory agent* Preg. Risk Category: C	*Postop inflammation after ocular surgery —* **Adults:** 1 to 2 drops in conjunctival sac qid 24 hr after surgery and for 2 wk. *Anterior uveitis —* **Adults:** 1 to 2 drops in conjunctival sac q hr during waking hours for wk 1, 1 drop q 2 hr during waking hours of wk 2; then taper until uveitis resolved.	▪ Apply light finger pressure on lacrimal sac for 1 min after instillation. ▪ Don't use leftover for new eye inflammation. ▪ Monitor BP during therapy. ▪ Advise to have IOP checked frequently.

risperidone
Risperdal
Benzisoxazole derivative
Antipsychotic
Preg. Risk Category: C

Psychosis — **Adults:** initially, 1 mg bid, increased in 1-mg increments bid on days 2 and 3 to 3 mg bid. Wait ≥ 1 wk before adjusting dosage. Safety of > 16 mg/day not known. **Elderly or debilitated, hypotension, or severe renal or hepatic impairment:** 0.5 mg PO bid. Increase by 0.5-mg increments bid on days 2 and 3 to 1.5 mg PO bid. Wait ≥ 1 wk before increasing.

- Obtain baseline BP; monitor often.
- Look for orthostatic hypotension and tardive dyskinesia.
- Assess for neuroleptic malignant syndrome.

ritonavir
Norvir
Human immunodeficiency virus (HIV) protease inhibitor
Antiviral agent
Preg. Risk Category: B

Treatment of HIV infection with nucleoside analogues or as monotherapy when antiretroviral therapy needed — **Adults:** 600 mg PO bid before meals. If nausea occurs, adjust dosage: 300 mg bid for 1 day, 400 mg bid for 2 days, 500 mg bid for 1 day, and 600 mg bid thereafter.

- Give before meals to decrease nausea.
- May be given alone or with nucleoside analogues.
- With combination regimen, patient may benefit by taking ritonavir alone and then adding nucleosides before completing 2 wk of ritonavir.

rubella and mumps virus vaccine, live
Biavax II
Vaccine
Viral vaccine
Preg. Risk Category: C

Rubella and mumps immunization — **Adults and children ≥ 1 yr:** 0.5 ml SC.

- Obtain history of allergies and reaction to antibiotics or immunization.
- Keep epinephrine 1:1,000 available.
- Use only diluent supplied. Discard 8 hr after reconstituting.
- Inject SC into outer upper arm.
- Refrigerate and protect from light. Reconstituted solution clear yellow; discard if discolored.
- Allow ≥ 3-wk interval between BCG and rubella vaccines.

RUBELLA AND MUMPS VIRUS VACCINE, LIVE   265

DRUG/CLASS/ CATEGORY	INDICATIONS/ DOSAGES	KEY NURSING CONSIDERATIONS
rubella virus vaccine, live attenuated (RA 27/3) Meruvax II *Vaccine* *Viral vaccine* Preg. Risk Category: C	*Rubella immunization* — **Adults and children ≥ 1 yr:** 0.5 ml (1,000 U) SC.	- Obtain history of allergies and reaction to immunization. - Keep epinephrine 1:1,000 available. - Use only diluent supplied. Discard 8 hr after reconstituting. - Inject SC into outer upper arm.
S		
salmeterol xinafoate Serevent *Selective beta$_2$-adrenergic stimulating agonist* *Bronchodilator* Preg. Risk Category: C	*Long-term maintenance of asthma; prevention of bronchospasm for nocturnal asthma or reversible obstructive airway disease* — **Adults and children >12 yr:** 2 inhalations bid. *Prevention of exercise-induced bronchospasm* — **Adults and children ≥12 yr:** 2 inhalations 30 to 60 min before exercise.	- Use cautiously in coronary insufficiency, arrhythmias, hypertension, other CV disorders, thyrotoxicosis, or seizure disorders and in patients unusually responsive to sympathomimetics. - Take at 12-hr intervals. - Instruct to use 30 to 60 min before exercise. - Don't use for acute bronchospasm.
saquinavir mesylate Invirase *Protease inhibitor* *Antiviral agent* Preg. Risk Category: B	*Adjunct treatment of advanced HIV infection in selected patients* — **Adults:** 600 mg PO tid given 2 hr after full meal and with nucleoside analogue.	- Monitor hydration if adverse GI reactions occur. - Adverse reactions include headache, nausea, and diarrhea.

		• Don't add other medications to infusion sol. • Don't give within 24 hr of last chemotherapy dose or within 12 hr of last radiotherapy dose. • Monitor CBC with differential. • Transient rash and local reactions at injection site may occur.
sargramostim (granulocyte-macrophage colony-stimulating factor, GM-CSF) Leukine *Biologic response modifier* *Colony-stimulating factor* Preg. Risk Category: C	*Acceleration of hematopoietic reconstitution after autologous bone marrow transplantation (BMT)* — **Adults:** 250 mcg/m²/day for 21 days given as 2-hr IV infusion starting 2 to 4 hr after BMT. *BMT failure or engraftment delay* — **Adults:** 250 mcg/m²/day for 14 days as 2-hr IV infusion. May repeat dose after 7 days of no therapy.	
scopolamine (hyoscine) Isopto Hyoscine, Scop‡, Transderm-Scop, Transderm-V† **scopolamine butylbromide (hyoscine butylbromide** Buscopan‡ **scopolamine hydrobromide (hyoscine hydrobromide)** *Anticholinergic* *Antimuscarinic/cycloplegic mydriatic* Preg. Risk Category: C	*Spastic states* — **Adults:** 10 to 20 mg PO tid or qid. Adjust dosage prn. Or 10 to 20 mg (butylbromide) SC, IM, or IV tid or qid. *Delirium, preanesthetic sedation and obstetric amnesia with analgesics* — **Adults:** 0.3 to 0.65 mg IM, SC, or IV. **Children:** 0.006 mg/kg IM, SC, IV; max 0.3 mg. *Prevention of motion sickness* — **Adults:** 1 Transderm-Scop or Transderm-V patch applied to skin behind ear several hr before antiemetic required. Or 300 to 600 mcg (hydrobromide) SC, IM, or IV. **Children:** 6 mcg/kg or 200 mcg/m² (hydrobromide) SC, IM, or IV.	• Use cautiously in autonomic neuropathy, hyperthyroidism, CAD, arrhythmias, heart failure, hypertension, hiatal hernia associated with reflux esophagitis, hepatic or renal disease, or ulcerative colitis; in children < 6 yr; or in hot or humid environments. • **IV use:** Avoid intermittent and continuous infusions. For direct IV use, dilute with sterile water. • Protect IV solutions from freezing and light; store at room temperature. • Tolerance may develop with long-term use.

†Canadian ‡Australian

DRUG / CLASS / CATEGORY	INDICATIONS / DOSAGES	KEY NURSING CONSIDERATIONS
scopolamine hydrobromide Isopto Hyoscine *Anticholinergic* *Antimuscarinic/cycloplegic mydriatic* Preg. Risk Category: NR	*Cycloplegic refraction* — **Adults:** 1 to 2 drops 0.25% sol 1 hr before refraction. **Children:** 1 drop 0.25% sol bid for 2 days before refraction. *Iritis, uveitis* — **Adults:** 1 to 2 drops 0.25% sol daily to qid. **Children:** 1 drop qd to qid.	▪ Warn to avoid hazardous activities until temporary blurring subsides. ▪ Observe for adverse CNS effects. ▪ Advise to wear dark glasses. ▪ May use in patients sensitive to atropine.
secobarbital sodium Novosecobarb†, Seconal Sodium *Barbiturate* *Sedative-hypnotic/anticonvulsant* Preg. Risk Category: D Controlled Sub. Sched.: II	*Preop sedation* — **Adults:** 200 to 300 mg PO 1 to 2 hr before surgery or 1 mg/kg IM 15 min before procedure. **Children:** 2 to 6 mg/kg PO. Max single dose 100 mg. *Insomnia* — **Adults:** 100 to 200 mg PO or IM. *Status epilepticus* — **Adults:** 250 to 350 mg IM or IV. **Children:** 15 to 20 mg IV over 15 min.	▪ *IV use:* IV injection for emergency use; give by direct injection. Administer at rate not > 50 mg/15 sec. ▪ IV use may cause respiratory depression, laryngospasm, or hypotension; keep emergency resuscitation equipment available. ▪ Assess mental status before initiating.
selegiline hydrochloride Eldepryl *MAO Inhibitor* *Antiparkinsonian agent* Preg. Risk Category: C	*Adjunctive treatment with carbidopa-levodopa in managing Parkinson's disease* — **Adults:** 10 mg/day PO (5 mg at breakfast and 5 mg at lunch). After 2 or 3 days, slowly decrease carbidopa-levodopa dosage.	▪ Some patients may experience more adverse reactions with levodopa and need 10% to 30% reduction of carbidopa-levodopa dosage. ▪ May cause dizziness at start of therapy.

senna
Fletcher's Castoria, Senexon, Senokot
Anthraquinone derivative
Stimulant laxative
Preg. Risk Category: C

Acute constipation; preparation for bowel or rectal exam — **Adults:** dosage for Senokot 1 to 8 tab PO; ½ to 4 tsp of granules added to liquid PO; 1 to 2 supp PR hs; or 1 to 4 tsp syrup PO hs.

- Don't expose drug to excessive heat or light.

sertraline hydrochloride
Zoloft
Serotonin uptake inhibitor
Antidepressant
Preg. Risk Category: B

Depression — **Adults:** 50 mg/day PO; adjust dosage as tolerated and needed (clinical trials used 50 to 200 mg/day). Adjust dosage at ≥1-wk intervals.
Obsessive-compulsive disorder — **Adults:** 50 mg/day PO. If no response, may increase to max 200 mg/day. Adjust dosage at ≥1-wk intervals.

- Use cautiously in patients at risk for suicide and in seizure disorders, major affective disorder, or conditions that affect metabolism or hemodynamic responses.
- Give without regard to food.
- Monitor for suicidal tendencies, and allow minimum drug supply.

silver sulfadiazine
Flamazine†, Flint SSD, Silvadene, Thermazene
Synthetic anti-infective
Topical antibacterial
Preg. Risk Category: B

Prevention and treatment of wound infection in 2nd- and 3rd-degree burns — **Adults:** apply ¹⁄₁₆″ thickness to clean, debrided burn daily or bid.

- Use sterile application technique.
- Use only on affected areas; keep medicated at all times.
- Inspect skin daily, and note changes. Notify doctor of burning or excessive pain.
- Discard darkened cream.

simethicone
Gas-X, Mylanta, Mylicon
Dispersant
Antiflatulent
Preg. Risk Category: NR

Flatulence, functional gastric bloating — **Adults and children > 12 yr:** 40 to 160 mg before meals and hs; **Children 2 to 12 yr:** 40 mg (drops) PO qid; **Children < 2 yr:** 20 mg (drops) PO qid, up to 240 mg/day.

- Don't use for infant colic.
- Doesn't prevent gas formation.

†Canadian ‡Australian

DRUG/CLASS/CATEGORY	INDICATIONS/DOSAGES	KEY NURSING CONSIDERATIONS
simvastatin (synvinolin) Lipext, Zocor *HMG-CoA reductase inhibitor* *Antilipemic* Preg. Risk Category: X	*Reduction of LDL and total cholesterol levels in primary hypercholesterolemia (types IIa and IIb) —* **Adults:** initially, 5 to 10 mg/day PO in pm. Adjust dosage q 4 wk based on tolerance and response; max 40 mg/day.	▪ Use cautiously in patients who use excessive alcohol or in history of liver disease. ▪ Assess liver function before therapy and periodically thereafter; if liver enzyme elevations persist, liver biopsy may be done.
sodium phosphates Fleet Enema *Acid salt* *Saline laxative* Preg. Risk Category: C	*Constipation —* **Adults:** 20 ml sol mixed with 120 ml cold water PO, or as enema; 120 ml PR. **Children:** 5 to 10 ml sol mixed with 120 ml cold water PO; or as enema, 60 ml PR.	▪ Use cautiously in patients with large hemorrhoids or anal excoriations. ▪ Before giving for constipation, assess for adequate fluid intake, exercise, and diet. ▪ Up to 10% of sodium content may be absorbed.
sodium bicarbonate Bell/ans, Citrocarbonate, Soda Mint *Alkalinizing agent* *Systemic and urinary alkalinizer* Preg. Risk Category: C	*Cardiac arrest —* **Adults and children:** 1 mEq/kg IV of 7.5% or 8.4% sol, followed by 0.5 mEq/kg IV q 10 min, based on ABGs. If ABG results unavailable, use 0.5 mEq/kg IV q 10 min until spontaneous circulation returns. **Infants < 2 yr:** ≤ 8 mEq/kg/day IV of 4.2% sol. *Metabolic acidosis —* **Adults and children:** usually, 2 to 5 mEq/kg IV over 4 to 8 hr. *Systemic or urinary alkalinization —* **Adults:** initially, 4 g PO, then 1 to 2 g q 4 hr. **Children:** 84 to 840 mg/kg/day PO.	▪ **IV use:** May add to other IV fluids. Don't mix with IV norepinephrine, dopamine, or calcium. ▪ Obtain blood pH, Pao$_2$, Paco$_2$, and serum electrolytes; report results to doctor. ▪ Not routinely used in cardiac arrest or during early resuscitation stages unless pre-existing acidosis exists. ▪ Monitor vital signs often; when used as urinary alkalinizer, monitor urine pH. ▪ Dosage based on blood CO_2 content, pH, and clinical condition.

sodium chloride

Electrolyte
Sodium and chloride replacement
Preg. Risk Category: C

Hyponatremia caused by electrolyte loss or in severe salt depletion — **Adults:** dosage individualized. Use 3% or 5% sol only with frequent electrolyte determination and give only slow IV. With 0.45% sol: 3% to 8% of body weight, according to deficiencies, over 18 to 24 hr; with 0.9% sol: 2% to 6% of body weight, according to deficiencies, over 18 to 24 hr.

Heat cramp caused by excessive perspiration — **Adults:** 1 g PO with water.

- Never give without diluting. Read labels carefully.
- **IV use:** Infuse 3% and 5% solutions slowly and cautiously. Use only for critical situations. Observe patient continually.
- Monitor serum electrolytes, acid-base balance, and changes in fluid balance.
- Never use bacteriostatic NaCl injection with newborns.
- Tell to report adverse reactions promptly.

sodium poly-styrene sulfonate

Kayexalate, Resonium A, SPS
Cation-exchange resin
Potassium-removing resin
Preg. Risk Category: C

Hyperkalemia — **Adults:** 15 g PO daily to qid in water or sorbitol (3 to 4 ml/g of resin). Or, mix powder with appropriate medium (aqueous suspension or diet appropriate for renal failure) and instill through NG tube. Or, 30 to 50 g/100 ml of sorbitol q 6 hr as warm emulsion deep into sigmoid colon (20 cm). **Children:** 1 g/kg of body weight/dose PO or PR prn. PO route preferred (drug should be in intestine ≥ 30 min).

- Monitor serum potassium at least daily. Stop drug when level falls to 4 or 5 mEq/L.
- Watch for signs of hypokalemia and digitalis toxicity in digitalized patients.
- Monitor for other electrolyte deficiencies. Monitor serum calcium in patients receiving drug for > 3 days.
- Watch for sodium overload.
- Prevent fecal impaction in elderly patients by giving resin PR. Give cleansing enema first. Have patient retain enema for 6 to 10 hr if possible, but 30 to 60 min acceptable.

SODIUM POLYSTYRENE SULFONATE 271

DRUG / CLASS / CATEGORY	INDICATIONS / DOSAGES	KEY NURSING CONSIDERATIONS
sotalol Betapace, Sotacor‡ *Beta-adrenergic blocker* *Antiarrhythmic* Preg. Risk Category: B	*Documented, life-threatening ventricular arrhythmias* — **Adults:** initially, 80 mg PO bid. Increase q 2 to 3 days as needed and tolerated; most respond to 160 to 320 mg/day.	• Proarrhythmic events may occur at start of therapy and at dosage adjustments. Use cardiac rhythm monitoring. • Withdraw other antiarrhythmics first. • Monitor serum electrolytes regularly.
sparfloxacin Zagam *Fluoroquinolone* *Anti-infective* Preg. Risk Category: C	*Community-acquired pneumonia and acute bacterial exacerbation of chronic bronchitis caused by susceptible organisms* — **Adults > 18 yr:** 400 mg PO on day 1 as loading dose, then 200 mg/day for total 10 days.	• Use cautiously in renal impairment. • If patient experiences excessive CNS stimulation, discontinue and notify doctor. Institute seizure precautions.
spectinomycin hydrochloride Trobicin *Aminocyclitol* *Antibiotic* Preg. Risk Category: B	*Acute gonococcal urethritis and proctitis (men) and cervicitis and proctitis (women); alternative for patients allergic to beta-lactam antibiotics* — **Adults:** 2 to 4 g IM as single dose injected deeply into upper outer quadrant of buttock.	• Shake vial vigorously after reconstitution and before withdrawing dose. Store at room temp after reconstitution; use within 24 hr. • Use 20G needle to administer. Divide 4-g dose (10 ml) into two 5-ml injections; give one in each buttock.
spironolactone Aldactone, Novospiroton‡ *Potassium-sparing diuretic* *Management of edema/anti-hypertensive/treatment of diuretic-induced hypokalemia* Preg. Risk Category: NR	*Edema* — **Adults:** 25 to 200 mg PO daily or in divided doses. **Children:** 3.3 mg/kg PO daily or in divided doses. *Hypertension* — **Adults:** 50 to 100 mg PO daily or in divided doses. *Diuretic-induced hypokalemia* — **Adults:** 25 to 100 mg PO daily.	• Instruct to take in am; if 2nd dose needed, tell to take in early pm. Take with food. • Warn to avoid excessive ingestion of potassium-rich foods, salt substitutes, and potassium supplements.

stanozolol
Winstrol
Anabolic steroid
Angioedema prophylactic
Preg. Risk Category: X
Controlled Sub. Sched.: III

Prevention of hereditary angioedema —
Adults: initially, 2 mg PO tid. After response, slowly reduce dosage at 1- to 3-mo intervals to 2 mg/day PO. **Children < 6 yr:** 1 mg/day PO during attack only. **Children 6 to 12 yr:** up to 2 mg/day PO during attack only.

- Don't use in women until pregnancy ruled out.
- Administer before or with meals.
- Periodically evaluate hepatic function.
- Monitor weight routinely. Edema generally controllable.

stavudine
Zerit
Synthetic thymidine nucleoside analogue
Antiviral
Preg. Risk Category: C

Treatment of HIV-infected patients who have received prolonged zidovudine therapy —
Adults ≥ 60 kg: 40 mg PO q 12 hr. **Adults < 60 kg:** 30 mg PO q 12 hr.

- Monitor CBC, serum creatinine, AST, ALT, and alkaline phosphatase levels.
- Instruct not to take with other drugs for HIV or AIDS unless doctor approves.

streptokinase
Kabikinase, Streptase
Plasminogen activator
Thrombolytic enzyme
Preg. Risk Category: C

Arteriovenous cannula occlusion — **Adults:** 250,000 IU in 2 ml IV sol by IV pump infusion into each occluded limb of cannula over 25 to 35 min. Clamp off cannula for 2 hr. Then aspirate, flush, and reconnect.
Venous thrombosis, PE, arterial thrombosis and embolism — **Adults:** loading dose 250,000 IU IV over 30 min. Sustaining dose 100,000 IU/hr IV for 72 hr for DVT and 100,000 IU/hr over 24 to 72 hr for PE and arterial thrombosis or embolism.
Lysis of coronary artery thrombi — **Adults:** loading dose 20,000 IU bolus via coronary catheter; then 2,000 IU/min infusion over 60 min. Or, give as IV infusion. Usual adult dose 1.5 million IU IV over 60 min.

- Before initiating, draw blood for coagulation studies, Hct, platelet count, and type and crossmatching. Keep aminocaproic acid and corticosteroids available.
- Avoid IM injections and other invasive procedures during therapy.
- Check for hypersensitivity reactions. Monitor vital signs and neurologic status often.
- Monitor closely for excessive bleeding. If bleeding occurs, stop therapy and notify doctor.
- Monitor pulses, color, and sensation of extremities q hr.
- Avoid unnecessary patient handling; pad side rails.

DRUG / CLASS / CATEGORY	INDICATIONS / DOSAGES	KEY NURSING CONSIDERATIONS
streptozocin Zanosar *Antibiotic antineoplastic nitrosurea (cell cycle–phase nonspecific)* *Antineoplastic* Preg. Risk Category: C	*Metastatic islet cell carcinoma of pancreas* — **Adults and children:** 500 mg/m² IV for 5 consecutive days q 6 wk until max benefit or toxicity observed. Or, 1,000 mg/m² at weekly intervals for 1st 2 wk. Max single dose 1,500 mg/m². Infuse diluted sol over 15 min.	• Obtain renal function tests before therapy. • Monitor CBC and liver function ≥ weekly. • Make sure patient receiving antiemetic. • Test urine for protein and glucose each shift; notify doctor of even mild proteinuria. • If extravasation occurs, stop infusion and notify doctor. • Obtain urinalysis, BUN, creatinine, serum electrolyte levels, and creatinine clearance ≥ weekly and for 4 wk after each course.
sucralfate Carafate, SCF‡, Sulcrate† Pepsin *Antiulcer agent* Preg. Risk Category: B	*Short-term (≤ 8 wk) treatment of duodenal ulcer* — **Adults:** 1 g PO qid 1 hr after meals and hs. *Maintenance therapy for duodenal ulcer* — **Adults:** 1 g PO bid.	• Low incidence of adverse reactions. • Monitor for severe, persistent constipation. • May be as effective as cimetidine in healing duodenal ulcers.
sulconazole nitrate Exelderm *Imidazole derivative* *Antifungal agent* Preg. Risk Category: C	*Tinea cruris, tinea corporis, tinea pedis, or tinea versicolor* — **Adults:** massage small amount into affected area daily to bid for 3 wk. Treat tinea pedis with cream bid for 4 wk.	• Tell to avoid touching eyes with drug and to wash hands thoroughly after applying. • Explain need to complete full course of therapy to prevent recurrence. • If irritation develops during treatment, tell to discontinue and contact doctor.
sulfamethoxazole Apo-Sulfamethoxazole†, Gantanol	*UTIs and systemic infections* — **Adults:** initially, 2 g PO, then 1 g PO bid or tid for severe infections.	• Monitor urine cultures, CBC, and urinalysis before and during therapy.

Sulfonamide *Antibiotic* Preg. Risk Category: C (contraindicated at term)	C. trachomatis — **Adults:** 1 g PO bid for 21 days. **Children and infants > 2 mo:** initially, 50 to 60 mg/kg PO, then 25 to 30 mg/kg bid. Max dosage 75 mg/kg/day.	• Monitor fluid I&O. Intake should be sufficient to produce output of 1,500 ml/day. If fluid intake not adequate, may give sodium bicarbonate. Monitor urine pH daily.
sulfasalazine (sala- **zosulfapyridine,** **sulphasalazine)** Azulfidine *Sulfonamide* *Antibiotic* Preg. Risk Category: B	*Mild to moderate ulcerative colitis, adjunctive therapy in severe ulcerative colitis,* *Crohn's disease —* **Adults:** 3 to 4 g/day PO in evenly divided doses; usual maint: 2 g/day PO in divided doses q 6 hr. **Children > 2 yr:** 40 to 60 mg/kg/day PO, divided into 3 to 6 doses; then 30 mg/kg/day in 4 doses.	• Administer after food; space doses evenly. • May start at lower dose if GI intolerance occurs. • Advise to maintain adequate fluid intake. • Discontinue immediately and notify doctor if hypersensitivity occurs. • Warn to avoid ultraviolet light.
sulfinpyrazone Anturan, Anturane *Uricosuric agent* *Renal tubular-blocking* *agent/platelet aggregation* *inhibitor* Preg. Risk Category: NR	*Intermittent or chronic gouty arthritis —* **Adults:** 200 to 400 mg PO bid 1st wk, then 400 mg PO bid. Max 800 mg/day.	• Give with milk, food, or antacids. • Monitor I&O closely. Force fluids to maintain minimum output of 2 to 3 L/day. • May increase severity of acute gout attacks during 1st 6 to 12 mo. • Instruct to take drug regularly.
sulfisoxazole ~~zolet~~	*UTI and systemic infections —* **Adults:** initially, 2 to 4 g PO, then 4 to 8 g/day divided in 4 to 6 doses. **Children > 2 mo:** initially, 75 mg/kg/day PO or 2 g/m² PO, then 150 mg/kg or 4 g/m² PO daily in divided doses q 6 hr. Max total dose 6 g/day. C. trachomatis — **Adults:** 500 mg PO for 10 to 21 days.	• Obtain specimen for culture and sensitivity tests before first dose. • Monitor urine cultures, CBC, PT, and urinalyses before and during therapy. • Watch for superinfection. • Monitor fluid I&O. Intake should be sufficient to produce output of 1,500 ml/day. If fluid intake not adequate, may give sodium bicarbonate. Monitor urine pH daily.

DRUG / C
CATEG

SULFISOXAZOLE ACETYL 275

CLASS / CATEGORY	INDICATIONS / DOSAGES	KEY NURSING CONSIDERATIONS
sulindac Aclin†, Apo-Sulin†, Clinoril, Novo-Sundac† *Nonsteroidal anti-inflammatory* *Nonnarcotic analgesic/anti-inflammatory* Preg. Risk Category: NR	*Osteoarthritis, rheumatoid arthritis, ankylosing spondylitis* — **Adults:** initially, 150 mg PO bid; increase to 200 mg bid, prn. *Acute subacromial bursitis or supraspinatus tendinitis; acute gouty arthritis* — **Adults:** 200 mg PO bid for 7 to 14 days. Reduce dosage as symptoms subside.	▪ Give with food, milk, or antacids. ▪ May mask signs and symptoms of infection. ▪ May cause peptic ulceration and bleeding. ▪ Periodically monitor hepatic and renal function and CBC with long-term therapy.
sumatriptan succinate Imitrex *Selective 5-hydroxytryptamine receptor agonist* *Antimigraine agent* Preg. Risk Category: C	*Acute migraine attacks (with or without aura)* — **Adults:** 6 mg SC. Max recommended dosage two 6-mg injections daily, with at least 1 hr between. Or, initial dose of 25 to 100 mg PO and 2nd dose of up to 100 mg in 2 hr, prn. Further doses may be given q 2 hr, prn, to max oral dosage 300 mg/day.	▪ After SC injection, most experience relief within 1 to 2 hr. ▪ Instruct to immediately report persistent or severe chest pain. ▪ Tell to stop taking and report if pain, tightness in throat, wheezing, heart throbbing, rash, lumps, hives, or swelling of eyelids, face, or lips develops.
t		
tacrine hydrochloride Cognex *Cholinesterase inhibitor* *Psychotherapeutic agent* Preg. Risk Category: C	*Mild to moderate dementia of Alzheimer's type* — **Adults:** initially, 10 mg PO qid. After 6 wk and if tolerated with no transaminase elevations, increase to 20 mg qid. After 6 wk, titrate to 30 mg qid. If still tolerated, increase to 40 mg qid after another 6 wk.	▪ Doesn't alter underlying disease but can alleviate symptoms. ▪ Abrupt discontinuation or large reduction in daily dosage (≥ 80 mg/day) may cause behavioral disturbances and loss of cognitive function.

tacrolimus
Prograf
Bacteria-derived macrolide
Immunosuppressant
Preg. Risk Category: C

Prophylaxis of organ rejection in allogenic liver transplantation — **Adults:** 0.05 to 0.1 mg/kg/day IV as cont inf ≥ 6 hr after transplantation. Initial PO dosage 0.15 to 0.3 mg/kg/day in 2 divided doses q 12 hr. Start 8 to 12 hr after stopping IV. Titrate per response. **Children:** 0.1 mg/kg/day IV, then 0.3 mg/kg/day PO on schedule similar to adults; adjusted prn.

- Monitor for anaphylaxis continuously during 1st 30 min and frequently thereafter. Keep epinephrine 1:1,000 available.
- Observe for hyperkalemia.
- Monitor for neurotoxicity and nephrotoxicity.
- Check blood glucose regularly.
- Increases risk for infections, lymphomas, and other malignant diseases.

tamoxifen citrate
Nolvadex, Nolvadex-D†‡,
Nonsteroidal antiestrogen
Antineoplastic
Preg. Risk Category: D

Advanced premenopausal and postmenopausal breast cancers — **Adults:** 10 to 20 mg PO bid.

- Monitor serum calcium. May compound hypercalcemia at start of therapy.
- Monitor CBC.
- Exacerbation of bone pain during therapy often indicates good response.

temazepam
Restoril
Benzodiazepine
Sedative-hypnotic
Preg. Risk Category: X
Controlled Sub. Sched.: IV

Insomnia — **Adults:** 7.5 to 30 mg hs. **Adults > 65 yr:** 7.5 mg PO hs.

- Assess mental status before initiating therapy. Elderly patients more sensitive to adverse CNS effects.
- Prevent hoarding or self-overdosing by depressed, suicidal, or drug-dependent patients or those with drug abuse history.

terazosin hydrochloride
α₁ blocker
Antihypertensive
Preg. Risk Category: C

Hypertension — **Adults:** initially, 1 mg PO hs. Adjust dosage gradually based on response. Usual range 1 to 5 mg/day; max. 20 mg/day.
Symptomatic BPH — **Adults:** initially, 1 mg PO hs. Increase in stepwise fashion to 2, 5, or 10 mg/day; most need 10 mg/day.

- Monitor BP frequently.
- If discontinued for several days, retitrate using initial dosing regimen.
- Advise not to discontinue suddenly and to call doctor if adverse reactions occur.
- Caution to avoid hazardous activities for 12 hr after 1st dose.

TERAZOSIN HYDROCHLORIDE 277

DRUG/CLASS/ CATEGORY	INDICATIONS/ DOSAGES	KEY NURSING CONSIDERATIONS
terbinafine hydrochloride Lamisil *Synthetic allylamine derivative* *Antifungal* Preg. Risk Category: B	*Interdigital tinea pedis, tinea cruris, and tinea corporis* — **Adults:** cover affected and immediate surrounding area bid for at least 1 wk.	▪ Use as directed for full course, even if symptoms disappear. ▪ Don't apply near eyes, mouth, or mucous membranes or use occlusive dressings. ▪ Tell to discontinue and contact doctor if irritation or sensitivity develops. ▪ Therapy shouldn't exceed 4 wk.
terbutaline sulfate Brethaire, Brethine, Bricanyl *Adrenergic (beta₂ agonist)* *Bronchodilator/premature labor inhibitor (tocolytic)* Preg. Risk Category: B	*Bronchospasm in patients with reversible obstructive airway disease* — **Adults and children ≥ 12 yr:** dosage varies with form. *Aerosol inhaler* — 2 inhalations separated by 60-sec interval, repeated q 4 to 6 hr. *Inj* — 0.25 mg SC. May repeat in 15 to 30 min, prn. Max 0.5 mg in 4 hr. *Tab in adults* — 2.5 to 5 mg PO q 6 hr tid. Max 15 mg/day. *Tab in children 12 to 15 yr* — 2.5 mg PO q 6 hr tid during waking hours. Max 7.5 mg/day.	▪ Use cautiously in CV disorders, hyperthyroidism, diabetes, or seizure disorders. ▪ Give SC injections in lateral deltoid area. ▪ Protect injection from light; discard if discolored. ▪ May use tablets and aerosol together. Monitor for toxicity. ▪ Teach to perform oral inhalation correctly. ▪ Advise to discontinue drug and call if paradoxical bronchospasm occurs.
terconazole Terazol 3 Vaginal Suppositories, Terazol 7 Vaginal Cream *Triazole derivative* *Antifungal* Preg. Risk Category: C	*Vulvovaginal candidiasis* — **Adults:** 1 applicatorful of cream or 1 supp inserted into vagina hs. 0.4% cream used for 7 days; 0.8% cream or 80-mg supp for 3 days. Course repeated, prn, after reconfirmation by smear or culture.	▪ Discontinue and notify doctor if fever, chills, flulike symptoms, or signs of sensitivity develop. ▪ Persistent infection may be caused by reinfection. Evaluate for possible sources. ▪ Continue treatment during menses. Avoid tampons.

- Monitor fluid and electrolyte levels.
- Force fluids and encourage exercise.
- Notify doctor if patient vomits shortly after dose given.
- Tell to report numbness or tingling in fingers, toes, or face.
- Inform that therapeutic response isn't immediate; 3 mo is adequate trial.

- Use cautiously in elderly patients and in renal, hepatic, or cardiac disease.
- Don't use in women of childbearing age until pregnancy ruled out.
- Give daily dosage requirement in divided doses for best results.
- Assess liver function tests, serum lipid profiles, Hgb and Hct, and PSA antigen levels.

testolactone
Teslac
Androgen
Antineoplastic
Preg. Risk Category: C
Controlled Sub. Sched.: III

Advanced postmenopausal breast cancer; advanced premenopausal breast cancer in women whose ovarian function has been terminated — **Women:** 250 mg PO qid.

testosterone
Andro 100, Andronaq-50, Histerone, Tesamone 100
testosterone cypionate
Depo-Testosterone, Testa-C
testosterone propionate
Malogent, Testex
testosterone transdermal system
Androderm, Testoderm
Androgen
Androgen replacement/antineoplastic
Preg. Risk Category: X
Controlled Sub. Sched.: III

Male hypogonadism — **Adults:** 10 to 25 mg (testosterone or propionate) IM 2 to 3 times/wk or 50 to 400 mg (cypionate) IM q 2 to 4 wk.
Metastatic breast cancer in women 1 to 5 yr postmenopausal — **Adults:** 100 mg IM 2 times weekly; 50 to 100 mg (propionate) IM 3 times weekly; or 200 to 400 mg (cypionate) IM q 2 to 4 wk.
Postpartum breast pain and engorgement — **Adults:** 25 to 50 mg/day IM for 3 to 4 days.
Primary or hypogonadotropic hypogonadism in men — **Adults:** (Testoderm) One 4-6-mg/day patch on scrotal area daily. Patch worn for 22 to 24 hr/day.
Adults: (Androderm) 2 systems applied nightly. Apply to clean, dry skin on back, abdomen, upper arms, or thigh.

†Canadian ‡Australian

DRUG / CLASS / CATEGORY	INDICATIONS / DOSAGES	KEY NURSING CONSIDERATIONS
tetracycline hydrochloride Achromycin V, Panmycin P↓, Robitet, Sumycin, Tetralant *Tetracycline* *Antibiotic* Preg. Risk Category: D	*Infections caused by susceptible organisms* — **Adults:** 250 to 500 mg PO q 6 hr. **Children > 8 yr:** 25 to 50 mg/kg/day PO, in divided doses q 6 hr. *C. trachomatis infections* — **Adults:** 500 mg PO qid for 7 to 21 days. *Brucellosis* — **Adults:** 500 mg PO q 6 hr for 3 wk with 1 g of streptomycin IM q 12 hr for 1st wk; once daily for 2nd wk.	• Use with extreme caution in impaired renal or hepatic function. Use with extreme caution (if at all) during last half of pregnancy and in children < 9 yr. • Check tongue for candidal infection. Stress good oral hygiene.
tetracycline hydrochloride Achromycin, Topicycline *Tetracycline* *Antibiotic* Preg. Risk Category: B	*Acne vulgaris* — **Adults and children > 11 yr:** use bid; rub sol into affected areas until skin thoroughly covered. *Superficial skin infections caused by susceptible bacteria* — **Adults:** apply to affected area bid in am and pm or tid.	• Wash area before applying. • Tell not to share drug, towels, or washcloths. • Explain how to adjust applicator pressure against skin to control flow rate.
tetrahydrozoline hydrochloride Tyzine Drops, Tyzine Pediatric Drops *Sympathomimetic agent* *Vasoconstrictor/decongestant* Preg. Risk Category: C	*Nasal congestion* — **Adults and children > 6 yr:** 2 to 4 drops 0.1% sol into each nostril q 4 to 6 hr, prn. **Children 2 to 6 yr:** 2 to 3 drops 0.05% sol into each nostril q 4 to 6 hr, prn.	• Tell to hold head upright to minimize swallowing of drug, and then to sniff solution briskly. • Advise that product should be used by only 1 person. • Tell not to exceed recommended dosage and to use prn for 3 to 5 days.

theophylline

Immed-release liquids: Accurbron; immed-release tab and cap: Bronkodyl, Slo-Phyllin; timed-release tab: Theo-Dur; timed-release cap: Aerolate

theophylline sodium glycinate

Acet-Amt

Xanthine derivative
Bronchodilator
Preg. Risk Category: C

Acute bronchospasm if not on drug — For IV, loading dose 4.7 mg/kg IV slowly; then maint. **Adult (nonsmoker):** 6 mg/kg PO, then 2-3 mg/kg q 6 hr for 2 doses. Maint: 3 mg/kg q 8 hr. Or, 0.55 mg/kg/hr IV for 12 hr, then 0.39 mg/kg/hr. **Healthy adult smoker:** 6 mg/kg PO, then 3 mg/kg q 4 hr for 3 doses. Maint.: 3 mg/kg q 6 hr. Or, 0.79 mg/kg/hr IV for 12 hr, then 0.63 mg/kg/hr. **Adult, heart failure or liver disease:** 6 mg/kg PO, then 2 mg/kg q 8 hr for 2 doses. Maint.: 1-2 mg/kg q 12 hr. Or, 0.39 mg/kg/hr IV for 12 hr, then 0.08-0.16 mg/kg/hr. **9-16 yr:** 6 mg/kg PO, then 3 mg/kg q 4 hr for 3 doses. Maint.: 3 mg/kg q 6 hr. Or, 0.79 mg/kg/hr IV for 12 hr; then 0.63 mg/kg/hr. **6 mo-9 yr:** 6 mg/kg PO, then 4 mg/kg q 4 hr for 3 doses. Maint.: 4 mg/kg q 6 hr. Or, 0.95 mg/kg/hr IV for 12 hr; then 0.79 mg/kg/hr.

Chronic bronchospasm — **Adult, child:** 16 mg/kg or 400 mg PO qd in 3-4 divided doses q 6-8 hr, or 12 mg/kg or 400 mg PO qd in ext-release prep in 2-3 divided doses q 8 or 12 hr. Increase as tol q 2-3 day to max: **Over 16 yr:** 13 mg/kg or 900 mg PO qd. **12-16 yr:** 18 mg/kg PO qd. **9-12 yr:** 20 mg/kg PO qd. **Under 9 yr:** 24 mg/kg/day PO.

- For acute bronchospasm in patient already receiving drug, dosage adjusted per current level. Note that each 0.5 mg/kg IV or PO (load) increases levels by 1 mcg/ml.
- Ext-release preparations not for use in treatment of acute bronchospasm.
- Monitor vital signs; measure and record fluid I&O. Clinical effects include improved pulse quality and respirations.
- Don't confuse ext-release and reg form.
- **IV use:** Use commercially available infusion sol, or mix in D_5W. Use infusion pump for continuous infusion.
- Give around-the-clock, using ext-release product hs.
- Xanthine metabolism varies; dosage based on response, tolerance, pulmonary function, and theophylline levels (10 to 20 mcg/ml); toxicity reported with levels > 20 mcg/ml.
- Teach to swallow ext-release preparations whole. For children who can't swallow, sprinkle contents over soft food.
- Dosage in chronic bronchospasm adjusted to minimum necessary for response. Also adjust dosage for older adult with cor pulmonale.

DRUG / CLASS / CATEGORY	INDICATIONS / DOSAGES	KEY NURSING CONSIDERATIONS
thiabendazole Mintezol *Benzimidazole* *Anthelmintic* Preg. Risk Category: C	*Cutaneous infestations with larva migrans* — **Adults and children:** 25 mg/kg PO bid for 2 to 5 days. Max 3 g/day. If lesions persist, repeat. *Roundworm, threadworm, whipworm* — **Adults and children 13.6 to 70 kg:** 25 mg/kg PO bid daily for 2 days. **Adults and children >70 kg:** 1.5 g q 12 hr for 2 days. Max 3 g/day. *Trichinosis* — **Adults and children:** 25 mg/kg PO in 2 doses daily for 2 to 4 days.	▪ Give to family members to prevent spreading infection. ▪ No dietary restrictions, laxatives, or enemas as needed. ▪ Administer before meals. ▪ Shake oral suspension before dosing. ▪ Advise to chew tablets before swallowing.
thiamine hydrochloride (vitamin B₁) Betamint, Beta-Solt, Biamine, Thiamilate *Water-soluble vitamin* *Nutritional supplement* Preg. Risk Category: A	*Beriberi* — **Adults:** 10 to 20 mg IM tid for 2 wk, then diet correction and multivitamin supplement containing 5 to 10 mg/day thiamine for 1 mo. **Children:** depending on severity, 10 to 50 mg/day IM for several wk with adequate diet. *Wernicke's encephalopathy* — **Adults:** initially, 100 mg IV, followed by 50 to 100 mg/day IV or IM until patient eats balanced diet.	▪ **IV use:** Dilute before giving. Administer large doses cautiously; give skin test before therapy in history of hypersensitivity reactions. Have epinephrine available. ▪ Accurate dietary history important. Stress proper nutrition. ▪ Significant deficiency can occur in 3 wk of thiamine-free diet. Thiamine deficiency usually requires concurrent treatment for multiple deficiencies. ▪ Doses > 30 mg tid may not be fully used by the body. ▪ Don't use with materials that yield alkaline solutions.

thioguanine (6-thioguanine, 6-TG)
Lanvis†
Antimetabolite (cell cycle-phase specific, S phase)
Antineoplastic
Preg. Risk Category: D

Acute nonlymphocytic leukemia, chronic myelogenous leukemia — **Adults and children:** initially, 2 mg/kg/day PO (calculated to nearest 20 mg). If necessary, increase slowly to 3 mg/kg/day as tolerated.

- Monitor CBC and serum uric acid.
- Watch for jaundice.
- Avoid IM injections when platelet count < 100,000/mm³.
- Tell to watch for signs of infection and bleeding and take temp daily.

thioridazine hydrochloride
Aldazine†, Apo-Thioridazine†, Mellaril, Mellaril Concentrate, Novo-Ridazine†, PMS Thioridazine†
Phenothiazine (piperidine derivative)
Antipsychotic
Preg. Risk Category: NR

Psychosis — **Adults:** 50 to 100 mg PO tid, with gradual increases to 800 mg/day in divided doses, prn. Dosage varies.
Short-term treatment of moderate to marked depression with variable degrees of anxiety, treatment of multiple symptoms in geriatric patients — **Adults:** 25 mg PO tid. Maintenance 20 to 200 mg/day. Max 200 mg/day. **Children 2 to 12 yr:** 0.5 to 3 mg/kg PO qd in divided doses.

- Different liquid formulations have different concentrations. Check dosage carefully.
- Keep drug away from skin and clothes; wear gloves when preparing liquid forms.
- Monitor for tardive dyskinesia.
- Shake suspension well before use.
- Dilute liquid concentrate with water or fruit juice before use.

thiotepa (TESPA, triethylenethiophosphoramide, TSPA)
Thioplex
Alkylating agent (cell cycle-phase nonspecific)
Antineoplastic
Preg. Risk Category: D

Breast and ovarian cancers, lymphoma, Hodgkin's disease — **Adults and children > 12 yr:** 0.3 to 0.4 mg/kg IV q 1 to 4 wk or 0.2 mg/kg for 4 to 5 days at 2- to 4-wk intervals.

- If pain occurs at insertion site, dilute further or use local anesthetic. Make sure drug doesn't infiltrate.
- Monitor CBC weekly for 3 wk after last dose. Notify doctor if WBC count < 3,000/mm³ or if platelet count < 150,000/mm³.
- Monitor serum uric acid.
- Tell to watch for signs of infection and bleeding and take temp daily.

DRUG/CLASS/ CATEGORY	INDICATIONS/ DOSAGES	KEY NURSING CONSIDERATIONS
thiothixene Navane **thiothixene hydrochloride** Navane *Thioxanthene Antipsychotic* Preg. Risk Category: NR	*Mild to moderate psychosis* — **Adults:** 2 mg PO tid. Increase gradually to 15 mg/day. *Severe psychosis* — **Adults:** initially, 5 mg PO bid. Increase slowly to 20 to 30 mg/day. Max recommended 60 mg/day. Or, 4 mg IM bid or qid. Max 30 mg/day IM. PO should replace IM promptly.	• Watch for orthostatic hypotension. Keep patient supine for 1 hr afterward. • Keep drug off skin and clothes. Wear gloves when preparing liquid forms. • Dilute liquid concentrate with fruit juice, milk, or semisolid food before use. • Monitor for tardive dyskinesia.
ticarcillin disodium Ticar, Ticillin† *Extended-spectrum penicillin/alpha-carboxypenicillin Antibiotic* Preg. Risk Category: B	*Severe systemic infections caused by susceptible organisms* — **Adults:** 18 g/day IV or IM, in divided doses q 4 to 6 hr. **Children:** 50 to 300 mg/kg/day IV or IM, in divided doses q 4 to 6 hr.	• Before giving, ask about previous allergic reactions to penicillin. • Avoid continuous infusion. Change site q 48 hr. • For IM, use 2 ml diluent per gram of drug. Inject deep IM into large muscle. Don't exceed 2 g/injection.
ticarcillin disodium/clavulanate potassium Timentin *Beta-lactamase inhibitor Antibiotic* Preg. Risk Category: B	*Lower respiratory tract, urinary tract, bone and joint, and skin and skin-structure infections and septicemia when caused by beta-lactamase-producing strains of bacteria or by ticarcillin-susceptible organisms* — **Adults:** 3.1 g (3 g ticarcillin and 100 mg clavulanic acid) by IV infusion q 4 to 6 hr.	• Before giving, ask about previous allergic reactions to penicillin. • Check CBC and platelet counts frequently. May cause thrombocytopenia. • With large doses and prolonged therapy, bacterial or fungal superinfection may occur.

ticlopidine hydrochloride
Ticlid
Platelet aggregation inhibitor
Antithrombotic agent
Preg. Risk Category: B

To reduce risk of thrombotic stroke in patients with history of stroke or with stroke precursors — **Adults:** 250 mg PO bid with meals.

- Instruct to avoid aspirin and aspirin-containing products and to check with doctor or pharmacist before taking OTC products.
- Report unusual or prolonged bleeding. Advise to tell doctor of therapy.
- Report signs of infection immediately.

timolol maleate
Apo-Timol†, Blocadren
Beta-adrenergic blocker
Antihypertensive agent/adjunct in MI
Preg. Risk Category: C

Hypertension — **Adults:** 10 mg PO bid. Max 60 mg/day. Allow at least 7 days between dosage increases.
MI (long-term prophylaxis in patients who have survived acute phase) — **Adults:** 10 mg PO bid.
Migraine headache prophylaxis — **Adults:** 20 mg PO qd in 1 or divided doses bid. Increase prn to max 30 mg/day. Stop if no response after 6 to 8 wk at max dosage.

- Use cautiously in compensated heart failure, diabetes, hyperthyroidism, and hepatic, renal, or respiratory disease.
- Check apical pulse before giving. If extreme, withhold dose and call doctor immediately.
- Monitor BP frequently.
- May mask signs and symptoms of hypoglycemia. Monitor blood glucose in diabetics.

timolol maleate
Timoptic Solution, Timoptic-XE
Beta-adrenergic blocker
Antiglaucoma agent
Preg. Risk Category: C

Chronic open-angle, secondary, and aphakic glaucomas; ocular hypertension — **Adults:** initially, 1 drop 0.25% sol in each affected eye bid; maint. 1 drop/day. If no response, 1 drop 0.5% sol bid. If IOP controlled, reduce to 1 drop/day. Or, 1 drop gel daily.

- Administer other ophthalmic agents ≥ 10 min before gel drop.
- Can mask hypoglycemia signs.
- Some patients may need few wk of treatment to stabilize pressure-lowering response. Determine IOP after 4 wk.

DRUG / CLASS / CATEGORY	INDICATIONS / DOSAGES	KEY NURSING CONSIDERATIONS
tioconazole Vagistat *Imidazole derivative* *Antifungal* Preg. Risk Category: C	*Vulvovaginal candidiasis* — **Adults:** 1 applicatorful (about 4.6 g) inserted intravag hs once.	▪ Review proper use of drug. Written instructions available with product. Tell to insert drug high into vagina. ▪ Report irritation or sensitivity. ▪ Tell to open applicator just before use.
tobramycin Aktob, Tobrex *Aminoglycoside* *Antibiotic* Preg. Risk Category: B	*External ocular infections caused by susceptible bacteria* — **Adults and children:** in mild to moderate infections, 1 or 2 drops into affected eye q 4 hr, or thin strip (1 cm long) of oint q 8 to 12 hr. In severe infections, instill 2 drops into infected eye q 30 to 60 min until improvement; then reduce frequency. Or, thin strip of oint q 3 to 4 hr until improvement; then reduce frequency.	▪ Clean eye area before application. ▪ Advise to watch for itching lids, swelling, or constant burning. Tell to discontinue and notify doctor if these occur. ▪ Instruct not to share drug, washcloths, or towels and to notify doctor if family member develops same symptoms. ▪ Discontinue if keratitis, erythema, lacrimation, edema, or lid itching occurs.
tobramycin sulfate Nebcin *Aminoglycoside* *Antibiotic* Preg. Risk Category: D	*Serious infections caused by susceptible organisms* — **Adults:** 3 mg/kg IM or IV daily divided q 8 hr. Up to 5 mg/kg daily divided q 6 to 8 hr for life-threatening infections; reduce to 3 mg/kg daily as soon as indicated. **Children:** 6 to 7.5 mg/kg IM or IV daily in 3 or 4 equally divided doses. **Neonates < 1 wk or premature infants:** up to 4 mg/kg/day IV or IM in 2 equal doses q 12 hr.	▪ *IV use:* Infuse over 20 to 60 min. ▪ Notify doctor if tinnitus, vertigo, or hearing loss occurs. ▪ Obtain blood for peak level 1 hr after IM injection and ½ to 1 hr after infusion ends; trough level just before next dose. Don't collect blood in heparinized tube. ▪ Monitor renal function.

tocainide hydrochloride

Tonocard
Anesthetic
Ventricular antiarrhythmic
Preg. Risk Category: C

Suppression of symptomatic life-threatening ventricular arrhythmias — **Adults:** initially, 400 mg PO q 8 hr. Usual dosage 1,200 to 1,800 mg daily in 3 divided doses. May treat patients with renal or hepatic impairment with <1,200 mg/day.

- May ease transition from IV lidocaine to oral antiarrhythmic. Monitor carefully.
- Correct potassium deficit.
- Observe for tremor.
- Monitor blood levels. Therapeutic range 4 to 10 mcg/ml.

topotecan hydrochloride

Hycamtin
Semi-synthetic camptothecin derivative
Antineoplastic agent
Preg. Risk Category: D

Metastatic carcinoma of ovary after failure of initial or subsequent chemotherapy — **Adults:** 1.5 mg/m² IV infusion over 30 min daily for 5 days, starting on day 1 of 21-day cycle. Give minimum 4 cycles.

- Before 1st course, patient must have baseline neutrophil count > 1,500 cells/mm³ and platelet count > 100,000 cells/mm³. Frequently monitor peripheral blood cell counts.
- Prepare under vertical laminar flow hood while wearing protective clothing.
- Use reconstituted product immediately.

torsemide

Demadex
Loop diuretic
Diuretic/antihypertensive
Preg. Risk Category: B

Diuresis in patients with heart failure — **Adults:** 10 to 20 mg/day PO or IV. If response inadequate, double dose until response obtained. Max 200 mg/day.
Diuresis in patients with chronic renal failure — **Adults:** initially, 20 mg/day PO or IV. If response inadequate, double dose until response obtained. Max 200 mg/day.
Hypertension — **Adults:** 5 mg/day PO. Increase to 10 mg prn. If response inadequate, add another antihypertensive.

- *IV use:* May give by direct injection over at least 2 min. Rapid injection may cause ototoxicity. Don't give > 200 mg at a time. Immediately report ringing in ears.
- Monitor I&O, serum electrolytes, BP, weight, and HR.
- Watch for hypokalemia.
- Tell to take in am to prevent nocturia.

DRUG/CLASS/ CATEGORY	INDICATIONS/ DOSAGES	KEY NURSING CONSIDERATIONS
tramadol hydrochloride Ultram *Synthetic derivative* *Analgesic* Preg. Risk Category: C	*Moderate to moderately severe pain* — **Adults:** 50 to 100 mg PO q 4 to 6 hr, prn. Max 400 mg/day. In patients > 75 yr, max 300 mg/day in divided doses.	▪ Monitor CV and respiratory status. Withhold dose and notify doctor if respirations fall or resp rate < 12. ▪ Monitor bowel and bladder function. ▪ Give before onset of intense pain. ▪ Monitor patients at risk for seizures.
trandolapril Mavik *ACE inhibitor* *Antihypertensive* Preg. Risk Category: C (D in 2nd and 3rd trimesters)	*Hypertension* — **Adults:** for patients not receiving diuretics, initially 1 mg for nonblack patient and 2 mg for black patient PO daily. If control not adequate, can increase dosage at ≥ 1-wk intervals. Maintenance dosages generally 2 to 4 mg/day. Some patients receiving 4 mg/day may need bid doses. For patient receiving diuretic, give initial dose of 0.5 mg/day PO. Dosage per BP response.	▪ Angioedema associated with involvement of tongue, glottis, or larynx may be fatal. ▪ Monitor serum potassium closely. ▪ Monitor for hypotension. If possible, discontinue diuretics 2 to 3 days before starting trandolapril. If drug doesn't control BP, diuretics may be reinstituted cautiously. ▪ Assess renal function before and during therapy.
trazodone hydrochloride Desyrel, Trazon, Trialodine *Triazolopyridine derivative* *Antidepressant* Preg. Risk Category: C	*Depression* — **Adults:** initially, 150 mg PO daily in divided doses; increased by 50 mg/day q 3 to 4 days, prn. Average dosage 150 to 400 mg/day. Max daily dosage for inpatients 600 mg; for outpatients, 400 mg.	▪ Administer before meals or with light snack. ▪ Monitor for suicidal tendencies, and allow only minimum drug supply. ▪ Report presence of priapism immediately. ▪ Warn to avoid hazardous activities until CNS effects known.

tretinoin (vitamin A retinoic acid)

Renova, Retin-A, StieVAA†

Vitamin A derivative
Antiacne agent
Preg. Risk Category: C

Acne vulgaris — **Adults and children:** clean affected area and lightly apply daily hs.

Adjunct therapy to skin care and sun avoidance program — **Adults:** apply to affected area daily hs.

- Clean area thoroughly before application. Avoid getting in eyes, mouth, or mucous membranes. Instruct to wash face with mild soap no more than bid or tid. Warn against using products with alcohol, astringents, spices, or lime.
- Instruct to minimize exposure to sunlight, ultraviolet rays, wind, cold temperatures.

tretinoin

Vesanoid
Retinoid
Antineoplastic
Preg. Risk Category: D

Induction of remission in patients with acute promyelocytic leukemia (APL), French-American-British (FAB) classification M3 (including M3 variant), when anthracycline chemotherapy contraindicated or unsuccessful — **Adults and children ≥ 1 yr:** 45 mg/m²/day PO in 2 even doses. Discontinue 30 days after complete remission or after 90 days of treatment, whichever is first.

- Notify doctor if fever, dyspnea, or weight gain occurs.
- Monitor CBC and platelet counts regularly.
- Maintain infection control and bleeding precautions.
- Watch for infection or bleeding.

triamcinolone acetonide

Azmacort, Kenalog-10, Triamonide 40, Trilog

Glucocorticoid
Anti-inflammatory/antiasthmatic
Preg. Risk Category: C

Severe inflammation or immunosuppression — **Adults:** 4 to 48 mg PO daily in divided doses; 40 mg IM weekly; 1 mg IM into lesions; 2.5 to 40 mg into joints or soft tissue.

Persistent asthma — **Adults:** Azmacort 2 inh tid or qid. Max 16 inh daily. Total daily dosage may be given bid for maint. **6 to 12 yr:** Azmacort 1 to 2 inh tid or qid. Max 12 inh daily.

- For better results and less toxicity, give daily dose in am with food.
- Don't use diluents with preservatives.
- Monitor weight, BP, and serum electrolytes.

TRIAMCINOLONE ACETONIDE 289

†Canadian ‡Australian

DRUG / CLASS / CATEGORY	INDICATIONS / DOSAGES	KEY NURSING CONSIDERATIONS
triamcinolone acetonide Aristocort, Flutex, Kenalog, Kenalone‡, Triacet *Topical adrenocorticoid* *Anti-inflammatory* Preg. Risk Category: C	*Inflammation associated with corticosteroid-responsive dermatoses* — **Adults and children:** clean area; apply aerosol, cream, lotion, or oint sparingly bid to qid. *Inflammation associated with oral lesions* — **Adults and children:** apply paste hs and, if needed, bid or tid, preferably after meals. Apply small amount without rubbing, and press to lesion in mouth until thin film develops.	• Gently wash skin before applying. Rub in gently, leaving thin coat. Don't apply near eyes or in ear canal. • Change dressing. Discontinue and tell doctor for if infection, striae, or atrophy occurs. • Don't use occlusive dressing in place > 16 hr each day. Don't use occlusive dressings on infected or exudative lesions. • Stop drug and report signs of systemic absorption, skin irritation or ulceration, hypersensitivity, or infection.
triamcinolone acetonide Nasacort *Glucocorticoid* *Anti-inflammatory* Preg. Risk Category: C	*Relief of symptoms of seasonal or perennial allergic rhinitis* — **Adults and children ≥ 12 yr:** 2 sprays (110 mcg) in each nostril daily. Increase prn to 440 mcg/day as daily dosage or divided doses ≤ qid. Then decrease, if possible, to as little as 1 spray in each nostril daily.	• Instruct to instill properly. • Stress importance of using regularly. • Warn not to exceed dosage prescribed. • Instruct to report nasal infection. • Tell to notify doctor if symptoms worsen or don't diminish within 2 to 3 wk. • Discard canister after 100 actuations.
triamterene Dyrenium, Dytac‡ *Potassium-sparing diuretic* *Diuretic* Preg. Risk Category: B	*Edema* — **Adults:** initially, 100 mg PO bid after meals. Max total dosage 300 mg/day.	• Monitor BP, blood uric acid, CBC, blood glucose, BUN, and serum electrolytes. • Warn to avoid excessive ingestion of potassium-rich foods and supplements. • Inform that urine may turn blue.

triazolam
Apo-Triazo†, Halcion
Benzodiazepine
Sedative-hypnotic
Preg. Risk Category: X
Controlled Sub. Sched.: IV

Insomnia — **Adults:** 0.125 to 0.5 mg PO hs. **Adults > age 65:** 0.125 mg PO hs; increased, prn, to 0.25 mg PO hs.

- Assess mental status before initiating therapy. Elderly patients more sensitive to CNS effects.
- Prevent hoarding or self-overdosing if patient depressed, suicidal, or drug-dependent or has drug abuse history.

trifluoperazine hydrochloride
Apo-Trifluoperazine†, Calmazine†, Solazine†, Stelazine, Terfluzine†
Phenothiazine (piperazine derivative)
Antipsychotic/antiemetic
Preg. Risk Category: NR

Anxiety states — **Adults:** 1 to 2 mg PO bid. Max 6 mg/day. Don't give > 12 wk.
Schizophrenia and other psychotic disorders — **Adults:** 2 to 5 mg PO bid, gradually increased until response. Or 1 to 2 mg deep IM q 4 to 6 hr, prn. More than 6 mg IM in 24 hr rarely required. **6 to 12 yr (hospitalized or under close supervision):** 1 mg PO qd or bid; may increase gradually to 15 mg daily.

- Wear gloves when preparing liquid forms.
- Watch for orthostatic hypotension. Keep patient supine for 1 hr after administration.
- Dilute liquid conc with 60 ml tomato or fruit juice, carbonated beverages, coffee, tea, milk, water, or semisolid food.
- Protect from light. Slight yellowing of injection or conc common. Discard markedly discolored solutions.

trifluridine
Viroptic Ophthalmic Solution 1%
Flourinated pyrimidine nucleoside
Antiviral agent
Preg. Risk Category: C

Primary keratoconjunctivitis and recurrent epithelial keratitis caused by herpes simplex virus, types I and II — **Adults:** 1 drop of sol into affected eye q 2 hr while patient awake to max 9 drops/day until corneal ulcer reepithelialization occurs; then 1 drop q 4 hr (min 5 drops/day) for another 7 days.

- Watch for signs of increased IOP.
- Clean eye area before application. Wash hands before and after administering. Don't touch dropper tip to area.
- Apply light finger pressure on lacrimal sac for 1 min after drops instilled.
- Reassure that mild local irritation on instillation is usually temporary.

DRUG / CLASS / CATEGORY	INDICATIONS / DOSAGES	KEY NURSING CONSIDERATIONS
trihexyphenidyl hydrochloride Aparkane†, Apo-Trihex†, Artane†, Novohexidyl†, Trihexane *Anticholinergic* *Antiparkinsonian agent* Preg. Risk Category: NR	*All forms of parkinsonism, drug-induced parkinsonism, and adjunctive treatment to levodopa in parkinsonism management —* **Adults:** 1 mg PO 1st day, 2 mg 2nd day; then increased in 2-mg increments q 3 to 5 days until total of 6 to 10 mg/day. Usually given tid with meals, sometimes given qid (last dose hs) or switched to ext-release form bid. Postencephalitic parkinsonism may require 12 to 15 mg total daily dosage.	• Dosage may need to be increased if tolerance develops. • Adverse reactions dose-related and transient. Monitor patient. • May cause nausea if given after meals. • Gonioscopic evaluation and intraocular pressure monitoring required, especially in patients > 40 yr.
trimethoprim Proloprim, Trimpex, Triprim† *Synthetic folate antagonist* *Antibiotic* Preg. Risk Category: C	*Uncomplicated UTIs caused by susceptible organisms —* **Adults:** 200 mg PO daily as single dose or in divided doses q 12 hr for 10 days. Not recommended in children < age 12.	• Obtain urine specimen for culture and sensitivity tests before first dose. • Monitor CBC routinely. Sore throat, fever, pallor, and purpura may be early signs of serious blood disorders. • Prolonged use at high doses may cause bone marrow suppression.
trimetrexate glucuronate Neutrexin *Dihydrofolate reductase inhibitor* *Antimicrobial/antineoplastic* Preg. Risk Category: D	*Alternative treatment of moderate to severe P. carinii pneumonia in immunocompromised patients —* **Adults:** 45 mg/m² IV infusion over 60 to 90 min daily for 21 days, given with 20 mg/m² of leucovorin IV or PO q 6 hr for 24 days.	• Follow institutional policy when administering parenteral form. • **IV use:** After reconstitution, drug stable at room temp or refrigerated for 24 hr. • Use D₅W only for IV infusion. • Leucovorin therapy must accompany and extend for 3 days after drug therapy.

trimipramine maleate

Apo-Trimip†, Surmontil

Tricyclic antidepressant

Antidepressant/antianxiety agent

Preg. Risk Category: C

Depression — **Adults:** 75 to 100 mg PO daily in divided doses, increased to 200 to 300 mg/day. Dosages > 300 mg/day not recommended in hospitalized patients; ≤ 200 mg in outpatients. Total dosage requirement may be given hs. **Elderly and adolescent patients:** initially, 50 mg/day, gradually increased to 100 mg/day.

- Don't withdraw abruptly.
- Dosage should be gradually discontinued several days before surgery.
- If signs of psychosis occur or increase, expect to reduce dosage. Monitor for suicidal tendencies, and allow only minimum drug supply.
- Relieve dry mouth with sugarless hard candy or gum.

triprolidine hydrochloride

Actidil, Alleract, Myidyl

Alkylamine antihistamine derivative

Antihistamine (H₁-receptor antagonist)

Preg. Risk Category: C

Colds and allergy symptoms — **Adults and children ≥ 12 yr:** 2.5 mg PO q 4 to 6 hr. Max 10 mg/day. **6 to 12 yr:** 1.25 mg PO q 4 to 6 hr. Max 5 mg/day. **4 to 6 yr:** 0.938 mg PO q 4 to 6 hr. Max 3.744 mg/day. **2 to 4 yr:** 0.625 mg PO q 4 to 6 hr. Max 2.5 mg/day. **4 mo to 2 yr:** 0.313 mg PO q 4 to 6 hr. Max 1.252 mg/day.

- Use with extreme caution in increased IOP, angle-closure glaucoma, hyperthyroidism, CV disease, hypertension, bronchial asthma, prostatic hyperplasia, bladder-neck obstruction, and stenosing peptic ulcerations and in children < 12 yr.
- Give with food or milk to reduce GI distress.

troglitazone

Rezulin

PPAR gamma activator

Antidiabetic

Preg. Risk Category: B

Adjunct to diet and insulin therapy in type 2 diabetes if hyperglycemia inadequately controlled with insulin > 30 U/day as multiple injections — **Adults:** for patients on insulin, continue with current insulin dose and begin therapy with 200 mg/day PO, with meal. May increase after 2 to 4 wk. Usual daily dose 400 mg; max 600 mg/day. Insulin dose may be decreased 10% to 25% when fasting glucose < 120 mg/dl in patients on troglitazone and insulin.

- Should be used by pregnant patient only if benefit justifies risk to fetus.
- Shouldn't be used to treat type 1 diabetes or ketoacidosis.
- Monitor for hypoglycemia. Insulin dose may need to be reduced.

DRUG/CLASS/CATEGORY	INDICATIONS/DOSAGES	KEY NURSING CONSIDERATIONS
U		
urokinase Abbokinase, Abbokinase Open-Cath, Ukidant‡ *Thrombolytic enzyme* *Thrombolytic enzyme* Preg. Risk Category: B	*Lysis of acute massive PE or PE accompanied by unstable hemodynamics* — **Adults:** for IV infusion *only* by constant infusion pump. Priming dose: 4,400 IU/kg in 0.9% NaCl or D₅W sol admixture over 10 min. Then 4,400 IU/kg/hr for 12 hr. *Coronary artery thrombosis* — **Adults:** after bolus dose of heparin from 2,500 to 10,000 units, infuse 6,000 IU/min of urokinase into occluded artery for up to 2 hr. Avg total dosage 500,000 IU. Initiate within 6 hr of symptoms. Follow with IV infusion of heparin, then oral anticoagulants. *Venous catheter occlusion* — **Adults:** 5,000 IU/ml sol into occluded line, then after 5 min, aspirate. Repeat aspiration attempts q 5 min for 30 min. If not patent, cap line and leave for 30 to 60 minutes before aspirating again. May require 2nd instillation.	▪ Be prepared with RBCs, whole blood, plasma expanders other than dextran, and aminocaproic acid to treat bleeding, and corticosteroids, epinephrine, and antihistamines to treat allergic reactions. ▪ IM injections and other invasive procedures contraindicated during therapy. ▪ Monitor for excessive bleeding q 15 min for 1st hr, q 30 min for 2nd through 8th hr; then q 4 hr. Pretreatment with drugs affecting platelets increases risk of bleeding. ▪ Monitor pulses, color, and sensation of extremities q hr. Monitor vital signs and neurologic status as ordered. ▪ *IV use:* Reconstitute according to manufacturer's directions. Don't mix with other drugs. Administer through separate line.
V		
valacyclovir hydrochloride Valtrex	*Herpes zoster infection (shingles)* — **Adults:** 1 g PO tid for 7 days. Adjust for impaired renal function based on creatinine clearance.	▪ Use cautiously in renal impairment, elderly patients, and those receiving other nephrotoxic drugs. ▪ Alert doctor if patient breast-feeding.

Synthetic purine nucleoside
Antiviral
Preg. Risk Category: B

For first episode of genital herpes —
Adults: 1 g PO bid for 10 days. If creatinine clearance ≥ 30 ml/min, 1 g PO q 12 hr; for 10 to 29 ml/min, 1 g PO q 24 hr; for < 10 ml/min, 500 mg PO q 24 hr.
Recurrent genital herpes — **Adults:** 500 mg PO bid for 5 days, given at first sign.

- Inform that drug may be taken without regard to meals.
- Teach about signs and symptoms of herpes infection and to notify doctor if they occur. Treatment should begin within 48 hr.

---

valproate sodium
Depakene Syrup, Epilim†, Myproic Acid Syrup
valproic acid
Depakene, Myproic Acid
divalproex sodium
Depakote, Depakote Sprinkle, Epival†, Valcote‡
Carboxylic acid derivative
Anticonvulsant
Preg. Risk Category: D

Simple and complex absence seizures, mixed seizure types — **Adults and children:** 15 mg/kg PO daily, divided bid or tid; increase by 5 to 10 mg/kg daily q wk to max 60 mg/kg qd.
Mania (delayed-release capsules) — **Adults and children:** 750 mg qd in divided doses. Adjust per response: max 60 mg/kg/day.
Prophylaxis for migraine (Depakote only) — **Adults:** initially, 250 mg PO bid. Some patients may need up to 1,000 mg/day.

- Serious or fatal hepatotoxicity may follow nonspecific symptoms. Notify doctor; drug must be discontinued if hepatic dysfunction suspected.
- Administer with food or milk.
- Don't give syrup to patients on sodium restriction.
- Never withdraw suddenly. Call doctor if adverse reactions develop.

---

valsartan
Diovan
Angiotensin II antagonist
Antihypertensive
Preg. Risk Category: C (1st trimester), D (2nd, 3rd)

Hypertension — **Adults:** initially, 80 mg PO qd. Expect BP reduction in 2 to 4 wk. For additional effect, increase to 160 or 320 mg daily, or add diuretic. (Adding diuretic has greater effect than increases beyond 80 mg.) Usual dosage range: 80 to 320 mg daily.

- Correct volume and salt depletions before starting.
- Monitor for hypotension.
- Advise to notify doctor if pregnancy occurs; drug should be discontinued.
- Inform that drug may be taken with or without food.

DRUG / CLASS / CATEGORY	INDICATIONS / DOSAGES	KEY NURSING CONSIDERATIONS
vancomycin hydrochloride Lyphocin, Vancocin, Vancoled *Glycopeptide Antibiotic* Preg. Risk Category: C	*Serious infections when other antibiotics ineffective or contraindicated —* **Adults:** 1 to 1.5 g IV q 12 hr. **Children:** 10 mg/kg IV q 6 hr. **Neonates and young infants:** 15 mg/kg IV loading dose, then 10 mg/kg IV q 12 hr if < 1 wk old, and 10 mg/kg IV q 8 hr if > 1 wk but < 1 mo. *Antibiotic-associated pseudomembranous and staphylococcal enterocolitis —* **Adults:** 125 to 500 mg PO q 6 hr for 7 to 10 days. **Children:** 40 mg/kg PO qid, in divided doses q 6 hr for 7 to 10 days. Max 2 g/day. *Endocarditis prophylaxis for dental procedures —* **Adults:** 1 g IV slowly over 1 hr, starting 1 hr before procedure. **Children:** > 27 kg, adult dose; < 27 kg, 20 mg/kg.	• Check daily for phlebitis and irritation. Report pain at infusion site. Avoid extravasation. • Refrigerate IV solution after reconstitution; use within 96 hr. • Monitor for 'red-neck' syndrome. If present, stop infusion and report to doctor.
vasopressin (ADH) Pitressin *Posterior pituitary hormone Antidiuretic hormone / hemostatic agent* Preg. Risk Category: C	*Nonnephrogenic, nonpsychogenic diabetes insipidus —* **Adults:** 5 to 10 units IM or SC bid to qid, prn; or intranasally in individualized dosages, based on response. **Children:** 2.5 to 10 units IM or SC bid to qid, prn; or intranasally in individualized doses.	• Never inject during first stage of labor. • Monitor for signs of water intoxication. • Monitor BP if patient taking bid. Watch for elevated BP or lack of response. • Monitor daily weight, urine specific gravity, and fluid I&O.

venlafaxine hydrochloride

Effexor

Serotonin, norepinephrine, dopamine reuptake inhibitor

Antidepressant

Preg. Risk Category: C

Depression — **Adults:** initially, 75 mg PO daily, in 2 or 3 divided doses with food. Increase as needed by 75 mg/day at intervals of ≥ 4 days. For moderate depression, usual max 225 mg/day; certain severely depressed patients may receive 375 mg/day.

- Closely monitor BP.
- If patient has received drug for 6 wk or more, taper over 2 wk as instructed by doctor.
- Warn to avoid hazardous activities until CNS effects known.

verapamil

Apo-Verap†, Calan, Isoptin, Novo-Veramil†, Nu-Verap†

verapamil hydrochloride

Calan, Calan SR, Isoptin, Isoptin SR, Verelan

Calcium channel blocker

Antianginal/antihypertensive/antiarrhythmic

Preg. Risk Category: C

Vasospastic angina and classic chronic, stable angina pectoris; chronic atrial fibrillation — **Adults:** 80 to 120 mg PO tid. Increase, q wk prn. Max 480 mg qd.

Supraventricular arrhythmias — **Adults:** 0.075 to 0.15 mg/kg by IVP over 2 min. 0.15 mg/kg in 30 min if no response. **1 to 15 yr:** 0.1 to 0.2 mg/kg IV over 2 min. **Under 1 yr:** 0.1 to 0.3 mg/kg IV over 2 min. For children, may repeat in 30 min.

Hypertension — **Adults:** 80 mg PO tid. Max 480 mg. Or, 120 to 240 mg ext-release tab PO qd in am. May add ½ tab daily.

- Monitor BP and ECG during and after I.V. administration.
- Assist with ambulation.
- **IV use:** Give by direct inj into vein or into tubing of free-flowing, compatible IV solution. Administer over ≥ 3 min to minimize adverse reactions.
- Monitor R-R interval for IV use. All patients should be on a cardiac monitor.

vidarabine

Vira-A

Purine nucleoside

Antiviral agent

Preg. Risk Category: C

Acute keratoconjunctivitis, superficial keratitis, and recurrent epithelial keratitis caused by herpes simplex — **Adults and children:** 1 cm oint into lower conjunctival sac 5 times daily at 3-hr intervals.

- Explain that ointment may produce temporary visual haze.
- Advise to watch for signs of sensitivity. Instruct to discontinue and notify doctor if present.

DRUG/CLASS/ CATEGORY	INDICATIONS/ DOSAGES	KEY NURSING CONSIDERATIONS
vinblastine sulfate (VLB) Alkaban-AQ, Velban, Velbe‡‡, Velsar *Vinca alkaloid* *Antineoplastic* Preg. Risk Category: D	*Breast or testicular cancer, Hodgkin's disease and malignant lymphoma* — **Adults:** 3.7 mg/m² IV q 1 to 2 wk. Max 18.5 mg/m² IV q wk per response. Don't repeat if WBC < 4,000/mm³. **Children:** 2.5 mg/m² IV q wk. Increase by 1.25 mg/m² until WBC < 3,000/ mm³ or tumor response seen. Max 12.5 mg/ m² IV q wk.	• Give antiemetic first. • **IV use:** Inject directly into vein or tubing of running IV line over 1 min. If extravasation occurs, stop infusion and notify doctor. • Don't administer limb with compromised circulation. • Monitor for acute bronchospasm. • Assess hands and feet for numbness and tingling. Assess gait for footdrop.
vincristine sulfate (VCR) Oncovin, Vincasar PFS *Vinca alkaloid* *Antineoplastic* Preg. Risk Category: D	*Acute lymphoblastic and other leukemias, Hodgkin's disease* — **Adults:** 1.4 mg/m² IV weekly. Max weekly dosage 2 mg. **Children >10 kg:** 2 mg/m² IV weekly. **Children 10 kg and under or with BSA < 1 m²:** initially 0.05 mg/kg IV weekly.	• **IV use:** Inject into vein or tubing of running IV line slowly over 1 min. If extravasation occurs, stop and notify doctor. • Monitor for acute bronchospasm and hyperuricemia. Maintain adequate hydration.
vinorelbine tartrate Navelbine *Vinca alkaloid* *Antineoplastic agent* Preg. Risk Category: D	*Alone or with cisplatin for 1st-line treatment of ambulatory patients with nonresectable advanced nonsmall-cell lung cancer (NSCLC); alone or with cisplatin in stage IV of NSCLC; with cisplatin in stage III of NSCLC* — **Adults:** 30 mg/m² IV weekly. In combination treatment, same dosage used with 120 mg/m² cisplatin, given on days 1 and 29, then q 6 wk.	• Check granulocyte count giving. If < 1,000 cells/mm³, withhold and notify doctor. • Dilute before administering. • If extravasation occurs, stop and inject remaining dose into different vein. • Monitor deep tendon reflexes.

warfarin sodium

Coumadin, Panwarfin, Sofarin, Warfilone Sodium†

Coumarin derivative

Anticoagulant

Preg. Risk Category: X

Pulmonary embolism with DVT, MI, rheumatic heart disease with heart valve damage, prosthetic heart valves, chronic atrial fibrillation — **Adults:** 2 to 5 mg PO daily for 2 to 4 days, then dosage based on daily PT and INR. Usual maintenance dosage 2 to 10 mg PO daily.

- PT determinations essential for proper control. INR values based on specific indication; refer to package insert.
- Inspect for bleeding gums, bruises on arms or legs, petechiae, nosebleeds, melena, tarry stools, hematuria, and hematemesis.
- Withhold and call doctor if fever or rash occurs.
- Anticoagulant can be neutralized by vitamin K injections.

x-y

xylometazoline hydrochloride

4-Way Long Acting, Neo-Synephrine II, Otrivin, Sinex Off Nasal Spray, Sinex-L.A.

Sympathomimetic

Decongestant/vasoconstrictor

Preg. Risk Category: NR

Nasal congestion — **Adults and children ≥ 12 yr:** 2 to 3 drops or sprays 0.1% sol in each nostril q 8 to 10 hr. **Children 2 to 12 yr:** 2 to 3 drops 0.05% sol in each nostril q 8 to 10 hr. **Children 6 mo to 2 yr:** 1 drop 0.05% sol in each nostril q 6 hr, p.r.n.

- Have patient hold head upright to minimize swallowing of drug, then sniff spray briskly.
- Product should be used by only 1 person.
- Instruct to report insomnia, dizziness, weakness, tremor, or irregular heartbeat.
- Use only as needed ≤ 5 days.

N

DRUG/CLASS/CATEGORY	INDICATIONS/DOSAGES	KEY NURSING CONSIDERATIONS
zafirlukast Accolate Antileukotriene Anti-inflammatory Preg. Risk Category: B	*Prophylaxis and chronic treatment of asthma* — **Adults and children ≥ 12 yr:** 20 mg PO bid 1 hr before or 2 hr after meals.	• Not for reversing bronchospasm in acute asthma attacks. • Advise to keep taking even if symptoms disappear. • Instruct to take 1 hr before or 2 hr after meals.
zalcitabine (dideoxycytidine, ddC) Hivid Nucleoside analogue Antiviral agent Preg. Risk Category: C	*Monotherapy for advanced HIV disease in patients who can't tolerate zidovudine or with disease progression while on zidovudine* — **Adults and children ≥ 13 yr:** 0.75 mg PO q 8 hr. *Combination therapy for advanced HIV disease* — **Adults and children ≥ 13 yr:** 0.75 mg PO q 8 hr given with zidovudine 200 mg PO q 8 hr.	• Don't give with food. • Assess for peripheral neuropathy; can progress to sharp shooting pain or severe continuous burning pain. May not be reversible.
zidovudine (azidothymidine, AZT) Apo-Zidovudine†, Novo-AZT†, Retrovir Thymidine analogue Antiviral agent Preg. Risk Category: C	*Symptomatic HIV infection, including AIDS* — **Adults and children ≥ 12 yr:** 100 mg PO q 4 hr or 300 mg PO q 12 hr; IV inf 1 mg/kg (over 1 hr) q 4 hr to 6 mg/kg/day. **3 mo to 12 yr:** 180 mg/m² PO q 6 hr (720 mg/m²/day), ≤ 200 mg q 6 hr. *Asymptomatic HIV infection* — **Adults and children ≥ 12 yr:** 100 mg PO q 4 hr while awake; IV inf 1 mg/kg (over 1 hr) q 4 hr while awake to 5 mg/kg/day. **3 mo to 12 yr:**	• **IV use:** Dilute first. Infuse at constant rate over 1 hr. Avoid rapid infusion or bolus injection. Don't add to biological or colloidal fluids. After dilution, stable for 24 hr at room temp and 48 hr if refrigerated at 35.6° to 46.4° F (2° to 8° C). Store undiluted vials at 59° to 77° F (15° to 25° C); protect from light.

180 mg/m² PO q 6 hr (720 mg/m²/day), max 200 mg q 6 hr.
To reduce risk of HIV transmission from mother with CD4+ lymphocyte count > 200 cells/mm³ to newborn — **Adults:** 100 mg PO 5 times daily between 14 and 34 wks' gestation and continued through pregnancy. During labor, loading dose of 2 mg/kg IV over 1 hr, followed by continuous IV infusion of 1 mg/kg/hr until umbilical cord clamped. **Neonates:** 2 mg/kg PO (syrup) q 6 hr for 6 wk, starting within 12 hr of birth. Or, 1.5 mg/kg IV (infuse over 30 min) q 6 hr.

- Monitor blood studies every 2 wk.
- Administer on empty stomach. Have patient sit up and drink adequate fluids.

---

zileuton
Zyflo
Antileukotriene
Anti-inflammatory
Preg. Risk Category: C

Prophylaxis and chronic treatment of asthma — **Adults and children ≥ 12 yr:** 600 mg PO qid.

- Caution that drug not bronchodilator and shouldn't be used to treat acute asthma attack.

---

zolpidem tartrate
Ambien
Imidazopyridine
Hypnotic
Preg. Risk Category: B
Controlled Sub. Sched.: IV

Short-term management of insomnia — **Adults:** 10 mg PO immed before bedtime. In elderly or debilitated patients and in hepatic insufficiency, 5 mg PO immed before bedtime. Max 10 mg daily.

- Give only for short-term management of insomnia, usually 7 to 10 days.
- Prevent hoarding or self-overdosing in depressed, suicidal, or drug-dependent patient or one with drug abuse history.
- Give with or immed after meals.

Appendix 1
Table of equivalents
Metric system equivalents

Metric weight

1 kilogram (kg or Kg)	=	1,000 grams (g or gm)
1 gram	=	1,000 milligrams (mg)
1 milligram	=	1,000 micrograms (µg or mcg)
0.6 g	=	600 mg
0.3 g	=	300 mg
0.1 g	=	100 mg
0.06 g	=	60 mg
0.03 g	=	30 mg
0.015 g	=	15 mg
0.001 g	=	1 mg

Metric volume

1 liter (l or L)	=	1,000 milliliters (ml)*
1 milliliter	=	1,000 microliters (µl)

Household		Metric
1 teaspoon (tsp)	=	5 ml
1 tablespoon (T or tbs)	=	15 ml
2 tablespoons	=	30 ml
1 measuring cupful	=	240 ml
1 pint (pt)	=	473 ml
1 quart (qt)	=	946 ml
1 gallon (gal)	=	3,785 ml

*1 ml = 1 cubic centimeter (cc); however, ml is the preferred measurement term today.

Weight conversions

1 oz = 30 g	1 lb = 453.6 g	2.2 lb = 1 kg

Temperature conversions

FAHRENHEIT DEGREES	CELSIUS DEGREES	FAHRENHEIT DEGREES	CELSIUS DEGREES	FAHRENHEIT DEGREES	CELSIUS DEGREES
106.0	41.1	100.6	38.1	95.2	35.1
105.8	41.0	100.4	38.0	95.0	35.0
105.6	40.9	100.2	37.9	94.8	34.9
105.4	40.8	100.0	37.8	94.6	34.8
105.2	40.7	99.8	37.7	94.4	34.7
105.0	40.6	99.6	37.6	94.2	34.6
104.8	40.4	99.4	37.4	94.0	34.4
104.6	40.3	99.2	37.3	93.8	34.3
104.4	40.2	99.0	37.2	93.6	34.2
104.2	40.1	98.8	37.1	93.4	34.1
104.0	40.0	98.6	37.0	93.2	34.0
103.8	39.9	98.4	36.9	93.0	33.9
103.6	39.8	98.2	36.8	92.8	33.8
103.4	39.7	98.0	36.7	92.6	33.7
103.2	39.6	97.8	36.5	92.4	33.6
103.0	39.4	97.6	36.4	92.2	33.4
102.8	39.3	97.4	36.3	92.0	33.3
102.6	39.2	97.2	36.2	91.8	33.2
102.4	39.1	97.0	36.1	91.6	33.1
102.2	39.0	96.8	36.0	91.4	33.0
102.0	38.9	96.6	35.9	91.2	32.9
101.8	38.8	96.4	35.8	91.0	32.8
101.6	38.7	96.2	35.7	90.8	32.7
101.4	38.6	96.0	35.6	90.6	32.6
101.2	38.4	95.8	35.4	90.4	32.4
101.0	38.3	95.6	35.3	90.2	32.3
100.8	38.2	95.4	35.2	90.0	32.2

Appendix 2
Common pharmacologic abbreviations

To transcribe medication orders and document drug administration accurately, review the following commonly used abbreviations for drug measurements, dosage forms, routes and times of administration, and related terms. Remember that abbreviations are often subject to misinterpretation, especially if written carelessly or quickly. If an abbreviation seems unusual or doesn't make sense, given your knowledge of the patient or the drug, always question the order, clarify the terms, and clearly write out the correct term in your revision and transcription.

Drug and solution measurements

cc	cubic centimeter
g or GM	gram
gal	gallon
gr	grain
gtt	drop
IU	International Units
kg	kilogram
L	liter
mcg	microgram
mEq	milliequivalent
mg	milligram
ml	milliliter
M_x	minim
ss	one half
oz	ounce
pt	pint
qt	quart
Tbs	tablespoon
tsp	teaspoon
U	unit

Drug dosage forms

amp	ampule
cap	capsule
CD	controlled dose
DS	double-strength
elix	elixir
ER	extended release
LA	long-acting
liq	liquid
loz	lozenge
S.A.	sustained action
S.R.	sustained release
sol	solution
sp	spirits
supp	suppository
susp	suspension
syr	syrup
tab	tablet
tinct	tincture
trans	transdermal
troc	troche
ung or oint	ointment

Routes of drug administration

AD	right ear
AS	left ear
AU	each ear
ID	intradermal
IM	intramuscular
IT	intrathecal
IV	intravenous
INH	inhaler
inj	injection
IVB/IVP	intravenous bolus/push
IVPB	intravenous piggy back
Ⓛ	left
Neb	nebulizer
NGT	nasogastric tube
OD	right eye
OS	left eye
OU	each eye
ophth	ophthalmic
PO or po	by mouth

Rect. or PR	by rectum
®	right
S&S	swish and swallow
SC or SQ	subcutaneous
SL or sl	sublingual
V or PV	vaginally

Times of drug administration

ac	before meals
ad lib	as desired
bid	twice a day
hs	at bedtime
pc	after meals
prn	as needed
PCA	patient-controlled analgesia
qam or QM	every morning
qd or QD	every day
qh	every hour
qid	four times a day
qn	every night
qod	every other day
q2h, q3h	every 2 hours, every 3 hours, and so on
STAT	immediately
tid	three times a day

Miscellaneous

AMA	against medical advice
$\approx$	approximately equal to
ASAP	as soon as possible
D/C or dc	discontinue
$\rightarrow$	decrease
$>$	greater than
$\geq$	greater than or equal to
HO	house officer
$\leftarrow$	increase
KVO	keep vein open
$<$	less than
$\leq$	less than or equal to
MR	may repeat
NPO	nothing by mouth
NKA	no known allergies
OTC	over the counter
Rx	prescription, treatment
TO	telephone order
VO	verbal order
$\bar{c}$	with
$\bar{s}$	without

Appendix 3

Pharmacologic abbreviations to avoid

The Joint Commission on Accreditation of Healthcare Organizations mandates that every health care facility develop a list of approved abbreviations for staff use. Certain abbreviations should be avoided whenever possible, however, because they can be misunderstood easily, especially when handwritten. Here's a list of abbreviations to avoid.

Abbreviation	Intended meaning	Misinterpretation	Correction
Apothecaries' symbols			
℥	fluidounce	Frequently misinterpreted	Use metric equivalents.
ʒ	fluidram	Frequently misinterpreted	Use metric equivalents.
♏	minim	Frequently misinterpreted	Use metric equivalents.
Drug names			
MTX	methotrexate	mustargen	Use complete spelling.
CPZ	Compazine (prochlorperazine)	chlorpromazine	Use complete spelling.
HCl	hydrochloric acid	potassium chloride (H may be misinterpreted as K)	Use complete spelling.
MgSO4	morphine sulfate	magnesium sulfate (MgSO$_4$)	Use complete spelling.
DIG	digoxin	digitoxin	Use complete spelling.
MVI	Multivitamins without fat-soluble vitamins	Multivitamins with fat-soluble vitamins	Use complete spelling.
HCTZ	hydrochlorothiazide	hydrocortisone (HCT)	Use complete spelling.
ara-a	vidarabine	cytarabine (ara-C)	Use complete spelling.

Dosage directions			
AU	auris uterque (each ear)	Frequently misinterpreted as *OU* (*oculus uterque*, each eye)	Write it out.
μg	microgram	Frequently misinterpreted as mg	Use *mcg*.
OD	once daily	Frequently misinterpreted as *OD* (*oculus dexter*, right eye)	Don't abbreviate *daily*. Write it out.
OJ	orange juice	Frequently misinterpreted as *OD* (*oculus dexter*, right eye) or *OS* (*oculus sinister*, left eye)	Write it out.
OS	once daily	Misinterpreted as tid (three times daily)	Write it out.
per os	orally	os frequently misinterpreted as OS (*oculus sinister*, left eye)	Use P.O., by mouth, or orally.
q.d.	every day	Period after the *q* misinterpreted as *i*, incorrectly indicating qid (4 times a day)	Write it out.
qn	nightly or at bedtime	Misinterpreted as qh (every hour)	Use *h.s.* or *nightly*.
qod	every other day	Misinterpreted as qd (daily) or qid (4 times a day)	Use *q other day or every other day.*
Subq	subcutaneous	*q* misinterpreted as *every*, may lead to misinterpretations in abbreviations to follow (Ex: A S.Q. heparin dose meant to be given 2 hours before surgery may be given every 2 hours instead.)	Use *subcut*, or write out *subcutaneous.*
u	unit	Misinterpreted as a *0* or *4*	Write it out.

Appendix 4
Estimating surface area in children

Pediatric drug dosages should be calculated on the basis of body surface area or body weight. If your pediatric patient is of average size, find his weight and corresponding surface area in the box. Otherwise, to use the nomogram, lay a straightedge at the correct height and weight points for your patient. Observe the point where the straightedge intersects on the surface area scale in the center.

Note: Do not calculate drug dosages based on body surface area in a premature or full-term newborn. Use body weight instead.

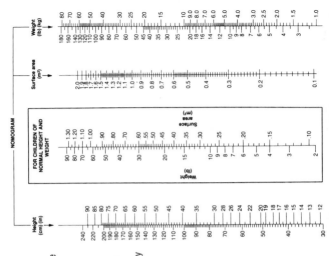

Nelson Textbook of Pediatrics, 15th edition. Courtesy W.B. Saunders Co., Philadelphia, 1996.

Appendix 5
Estimating surface area in adults

Lay a straightedge from the patient's height in the left-hand column to his weight in the right-hand column. The intersection of this line with the center scale reveals the body surface area. The adult nomogram is especially useful in calculating dosages for chemotherapy.

Height

cm 200 — 79 in
195 — 78
— 77
190 — 76
— 75
185 — 74
— 73
180 — 72
— 71
175 — 70
— 69
170 — 68
— 67
165 — 66
— 65
160 — 64
— 63
155 — 62
— 61
150 — 60
— 59
145 — 58
— 57
140 — 56
— 55
135 — 54
— 53
130 — 52
— 51
125 — 50
— 49
120 — 48
— 47
115 — 46
— 45
110 — 44
— 43
105 — 42
— 41
cm 100 — 40
39 in

Body surface

2.80 m²
2.70
2.60
2.50
2.40
2.30
2.20
2.10
2.00
1.95
1.90
1.85
1.80
1.75
1.70
1.65
1.60
1.55
1.50
1.45
1.40
1.35
1.30
1.25
1.20
1.15
1.10
1.05
1.00
0.95
0.90
0.86 m²

Mass

kg 150 — 330 lb
145 — 320
140 — 310
135 — 300
— 290
130 — 280
125 — 270
120 — 260
115 — 250
110 — 240
105 — 230
— 220
100 — 210
95 — 200
90 — 190
85 — 180
80 — 170
75 — 160
70 — 150
65 — 140
60 — 130
55 — 120
50 — 110
— 105
45 — 100
— 95
40 — 90
— 85
35 — 80
— 75
kg 30 — 66 lb

Geigy Scientific Tables, 1990, 8th edition, Vol. 5, p. 105. © Novartis.

Appendix 6

Dangerous drug interactions

Many drugs can cause severe adverse reactions when they interact with other drugs. The following chart lists drug interactions for selected drugs. Especially dangerous interactions are shown in *italic* type.

Drug	Interacting drug	Possible effect
allopurinol	mercaptopurine	*Increased potential for bone marrow suppression*
amikacin	bumetanide, ethacrynic acid, furosemide	Possible enhanced ototoxicity
	ceftazidime, ceftizoxime, cephalothin	Possible enhanced nephrotoxicity
atenolol	verapamil	Enhanced pharmacologic effects of beta[1] and beta[2] adrenergic blockers and verapamil
captopril	amiloride, spironolactone, triamterene	Possible hyperkalemia
	indomethacin	Decreased antihypertensive effect of ACE inhibitors
carbamazepine	erythromycin, isoniazid, propoxyphene	Increased risk of carbamazepine toxicity
ciprofloxacin	aluminum hydroxide, magnesium oxide antacids	Decreased plasma levels and effectiveness of ciprofloxacin
clonidine	sotalol	Enhanced rebound hypertension following clonidine withdrawal
cyclosporine	erythromycin	Possible elevated cyclosporine concentrations and nephrotoxicity
	phenytoin	Reduced plasma levels of cyclosporine
digoxin	amiodarone, verapamil	Elevated serum digoxin levels
	bendroflumethiazide, chlorothiazide, hydrochlorothiazide, methyclothiazide, metolazone, quinethazone, trichloromethiazide	Increased risk of cardiac arrhythmias due to hypokalemia
	quinidine	*Elevated serum digoxin levels*

enalapril	indomethacin	Decreased antihypertensive effect of ACE inhibitors
epinephrine	nadolol, pindolol, propranolol	*Increased systolic and diastolic pressures; marked decrease in heart rate*
erythromycin	astemizole	Increased risk of arrhythmias
esmolol	verapamil	Enhanced pharmacologic effects of beta₁ and beta adrenergic blockers and verapamil
ethanol	acetohexamide, chlorpropamide, disulfiram, metronidazole, tolbutamide	*Acute alcohol intolerance reaction*
gentamicin	bumetanide, ethacrynic acid, furosemide	Possible enhanced ototoxicity
	ceftazidime, ceftizoxime, cephalothin	Possible enhanced nephrotoxicity
heparin	aspirin	Enhanced risk of bleeding
lisinopril	indomethacin	Decreased antihypertensive effect of ACE inhibitors
lithium	bendroflumethiazide, chlorothiazide, hydrochlorothiazide, methyclothiazide, polythiazide, trichlormethiazide	*Decreased lithium excretion, which increases risk of lithium toxicity*
methotrexate	aspirin	*Increased risk of methotrexate toxicity*
	probenecid	*Decreased methotrexate elimination, increasing risk of methotrexate toxicity*
metoprolol	verapamil	Enhanced pharmacologic effects of beta₁ and beta₂ adrenergic blockers and verapamil
nadolol	verapamil	Enhanced pharmacologic effects of beta₁ and beta₂ adrenergic blockers and verapamil
neomycin	bumetanide, ethacrynic acid, furosemide	Possible enhanced ototoxicity
	ceftazidime, ceftizoxime, cephalothin	Possible enhanced nephrotoxicity
penicillin	tetracycline	Reduced effectiveness of penicillins
potassium	amiloride, spironolactone, triamterene	*Increased risk of hyperkalemia*

Drug	Interacting drug	Possible effect
propranolol	verapamil	Enhanced pharmacologic effects of beta$_1$ and beta$_2$ adrenergic blockers and verapamil
quinidine	amiodarone	Increased risk of quinidine toxicity
tetracyclines	aluminum carbonate, aluminum hydroxide, aluminum phosphate, calcium carbonate, dihydroxyaluminum sodium carbonate, magaldrate, magnesium oxide antacids	*Decreased plasma levels and effectiveness of tetracyclines*
timolol	verapamil	Enhanced pharmacologic effects of beta$_1$ and beta$_2$ adrenergic blockers and verapamil
tobramycin	bumetanide, furosemide	Possible enhanced ototoxicity
	ceftazidime, ceftizoxime, cephalothin	Possible enhanced nephrotoxicity
	ethacrynic acid	*Possible enhanced ototoxicity*
warfarin sodium	amiodarone, aspirin, cefamandole, cefoperazone, cefotetan, chloral hydrate, cimetidine, clofibrate, desipramine, erythromycin, glucagon, imipramine, nortriptyline, protriptyline, trimipramine	Increased risk of bleeding
	carbamazepine	Reduced effectiveness of warfarin
	cholestyramine	May bind with oral anticoagulants, resulting in impaired absorption
	cotrimoxazole, disulfiram, methimazole, metronidazole, propylthiouracil, sulfinpyrazone	*Increased risk of bleeding*
	griseofulvin	Decreased pharmacologic effect of oral anticoagulants
	rifampin	*Decreased pharmacologic effect of oral anticoagulants*

Index